Tetraplegia and Paraplegia

Within the book, the author makes references to and comments upon a variety of lifts. Whether the lifts are appropriate in any particular situation will depend upon all the circumstances and, in particular, the training of those involved in the lift. The author and publisher do not accept any responsibility for any injury which may result from reliance on the material contained in this publication.

For Churchill Livingstone

Editorial director: Mary Law
Project manager: Valerie Burgess
Project development editor: Dinah Thom
Design direction: Judith Wright
Project controller: Pat Miller
Copy editor: Adam Campbell
Sales promotion manager: Hilary Brown

Tetraplegia and Paraplegia

A Guide for Physiotherapists

Ida Bromley MBE FCSP

Illustrated by

Janet Plested AIIP AMPA
Jane Upton DipAD(Hons) ATD

FIFTH EDITION

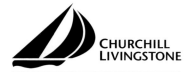

EDINBURGH LONDON NEW YORK MADRID PHILADELPHIA SAN FRANCISCO SYDNEY TORONTO 1998

CHURCHILL LIVINGSTONE
An imprint of Harcourt Publishers Limited

First published 1998
Reprinted 2002

ISBN 0 443 05872 5

British Library Cataloguing in Publication Data
A catalogue record for this book is available from the British
Library.

Library of Congress Cataloging in Publication Data
A catalog record for this book is available from the Library
of Congress.

Note
Medical knowledge is constantly changing. As new
information becomes available, changes in treatment,
procedures, equipment and the use of drugs become
necessary. The author, contributors and publishers have, as
far as it is possible, taken care to ensure that the information
given in this text is accurate and up to date. However,
readers are strongly advised to confirm that the information,
especially with regard to drug usage, complies with the
latest legislation and standards of practice.

The
publisher's
policy is to use
**paper manufactured
from sustainable forests**

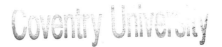

Contents

Contributors

Ebba M. K. Bergström
Research Physiotherapist, National Spinal
Injuries Centre, Stoke Mandeville Hospital,
Aylesbury, UK

Sarah Brownlee
Formerly Senior Staff Member, Stoke
Mandeville Hospital, Aylesbury, UK

Susan Edwards
Lead Professional Adviser, Physiotherapy, The
National Hospital for Neurology and
Neurosurgery, London, UK

Lone Rose
Responsible for Posture and Seating Clinics
and postgraduate physiotherapy education,
National Spinal Injuries Centre, Stoke
Mandeville Hospital, Aylesbury, UK

Preface to the Fifth Edition

Spinal cord injury can occur in any country in the world. Sometimes there is access to well developed, sophisticated and specialized medical services but this is often not the case. The advantages for patients receiving knowledgeable phyiotherapy with a well-motivated and collaborative team is self-evident. The emphasis in text and layout in this book is for student and post-graduate physiotherapists who have little experience in this field. Therefore, I hope it will particularly assist those physiotherapists who do not work in spinal injury centres to treat and encourage people who sustain such a shattering injury.

The text is not exhaustive but suggests methods of treatment which have been tried and found valuable for a large number of patients. The principles of treatment were originally laid down by Sir Ludwig Guttmann at the National Spinal Injuries Centre in England, and his interest in and enthusiasm for physiotherapy are well known. Unlike many other textbooks on the subject, this book outlines the rehabilitation programme from the day of admission with an acute lesion to the achievement of maximum independence. Treatment for children and those with incomplete lesions is also included. In this edition, as well as updating existing material, new sections have been added on a variety of developments including functional electrical stimulation for the upper limb, posture and seating, the treatment of patients with lesions above C2, and the problems which appear as patients with spinal cord injury grow older.

I am deeply indebted to many people for their contribution to this and previous volumes:

To Ebba Bergstrom for agreeing to revise her chapter; to Lone Rose for updating her previous contribution and providing additional material to chapter 6; to both these colleagues for their outstanding patience with my many requests for assistance from the National Spinal Injuries Centre, Stoke Mandeville Hospital; to Susan Edwards for the vast task she gave herself in re-writing the majority of her chapter on The Incomplete Lesion; to Mr El Masry for his warm welcome on my visit to the unit at Oswestry and for assisting me to revise the medical chapter; to the superintendents and staff of the 7 spinal injury centres I visited in the UK, for their friendly hospitality and eagerness to discuss new approaches and other issues; to the many colleagues who have read and re-read sections of the text over the years and who have unstintingly given me their expert advice; to Janet Plested in the early volumes, and more recently, to Jane Upton for their excellent diagrams without which it would be difficult for this book to fulfil its function; and to my personal friends for their understanding and practical help and support without which *none* of the editions would have been completed. The assistance of the members of staff of Churchill Livingstone has been unfailing for over 20 years and I am most grateful to them all.

I. B.

1

Spinal cord injury

Spinal cord injury is not a notifiable disease and so figures for the annual incidence are inaccurate and may vary according to the source. In the UK, approximately 1000 new injuries are estimated to occur per year, excluding non-traumatic cases (De Vivo et al 1992). These numbers are augmented by the group of people with spinal cord damage caused by disease or other forms of injury, e.g. stab wounds. Until Sir Ludwig Guttmann pioneered a positive approach to the treatment of spinal cord lesions at Stoke Mandeville Hospital in the mid-1940s, most people died of the resultant complications (Guttmann 1946a). Regrettably this can still happen today where appropriate skills, knowledge and facilities are not readily available. Spinal injury units now exist worldwide and international symposia on the treatment of those with spinal cord lesions take place regularly.

The life expectancy of this group of people has steadily increased over the last five decades, and with constantly improving methods of treatment this trend should continue.

Patients with spinal cord injury are initially totally dependent on those around them and need expert care if they are once again to become independent members of the community. It is an exciting challenge to be involved in and contribute to the metamorphosis which occurs when a tetraplegic or paraplegic patient evolves into a spinal man (Fig. 1.1).

In this book, maximum detail has been given in the sections dealing with the tetraplegic patient. Solutions to the majority of problems

REHABILITATION

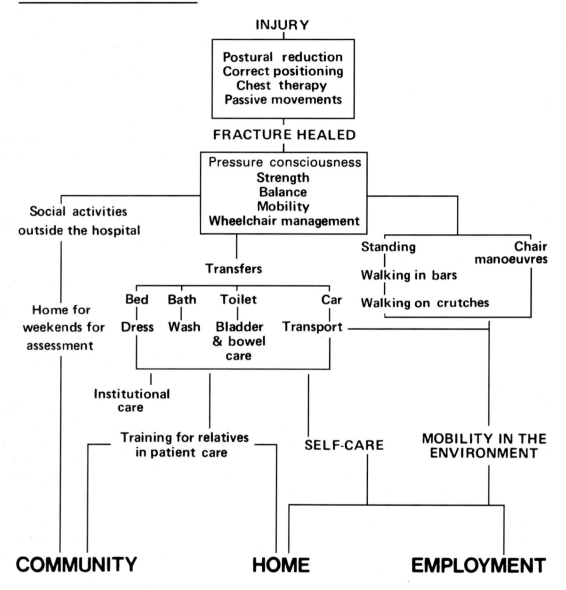

Figure 1.1 Dependence to independence.

facing those with paraplegia have now been found, whereas many of the social, professional and industrial rehabilitation problems of those with tetraplegia have still to be solved. The tetraplegic patient needs a longer period of rehabilitation to achieve maximum independence and overcome the sometimes apparently insurmountable obstacles. With the increased expertise of paramedical personnel in the ambulance service, the lives of patients who have fractures as high as C2 are saved at the scene of the accident and they now reach hospital alive.

Of the cases admitted to spinal units, the majority are traumatic, and about half of these involve the cervical spine.

The major causes of spinal cord injury in the UK are road traffic accidents, industrial accidents, sporting injuries and accidents in the home. Causes differ according to the prevailing circumstances in the country in which they occur – for example, industrial accidents are more prevalent in countries where there is little legislation regarding safety at work. The majority of the traumatic cases are found to have fractures/dislocations, less than a quarter have fractures only, and a very small number are found to have involvement of the spinal cord with no obvious bony damage to the vertebral column, e.g. those with whiplash injuries. The most vulnerable areas of the vertebral column would appear to be:

- lower cervical, C5–7
- mid-thoracic, T4–7
- thoracolumbar, T10–L2.

The non-traumatic cases are mainly the result of transverse myelitis, tumours and vascular accidents. Thrombosis or haemorrhage of the anterior vertebral artery causes ischaemia of the cord with resulting paralysis.

Spinal cord damage resulting from either injury or disease may produce tetraplegia or paraplegia depending upon the level at which the damage has occurred, and the lesion may be complete or incomplete.

'**Tetraplegia.** This term refers to impairment or loss of motor and/or sensory function in the cervical segments of the spinal cord due to damage of neural elements within the spinal canal. Tetraplegia results in impairment of function in the arms as well as in the trunk, legs and pelvic organs. It does not include brachial plexus lesions or injury to peripheral nerves outside the neural canal.

Paraplegia. This term refers to impairment or loss of motor and/or sensory function in the thoracic, lumbar or sacral (but not cervical) segments of the spinal cord, secondary to damage of neural elements within the spinal canal. With paraplegia, arm function is spared, but depending on the level of injury, the trunk, legs and pelvic organs may be involved. The term is used in referring to cauda equina and conus medullaris injuries, but not to lumbosacral plexus lesions or injury to peripheral nerves outside the neural canal' (Ditunno et al 1994)

Definition of the level of lesion

There are 30 segments in the spinal cord: 8 cervical, 12 thoracic, 5 lumbar and 5 sacral. As the spinal cord terminates opposite the first lumbar vertebra, there is a progressive discrepancy between spinal cord segments and vertebral body levels.

All cervical nerve roots pass through the intervertebral foramen adjacent to the vertebra of equivalent number. Roots C1 to C7 inclusive leave above the appropriate vertebral body, whereas root C8 and the remainder exit below the appropriate vertebral body. The higher the root, the more laterally it is situated within the spinal cord. Although there is little difference between spinal cord segments and vertebral body levels in the cervical area, the nerve roots below C8 travel increasing distances in the canal before exiting.

The 12 thoracic segments lie within the area covered by the upper 9 thoracic vertebrae; the 5 lumbar segments lie within that covered by vertebrae T10 and T11; and the 5 sacral segments lie within T12 and L1 vertebrae.

Several methods of classification of the level of lesion are in use throughout the world. The system most often used in the UK is to give the most distal uninvolved segment of the cord

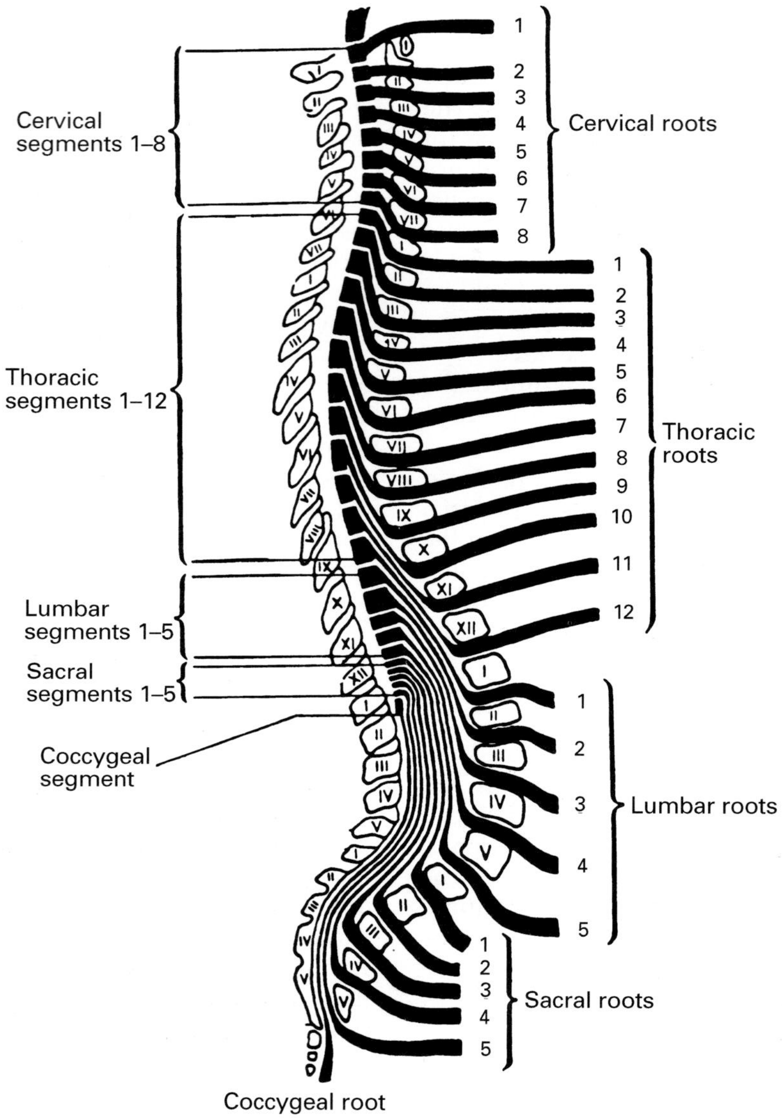

Figure 1.2 Topographical correlation between spinal cord segments and vertebral bodies, spinous processes and intervertebral foramina. (From Haymaker 1969.)

together with the skeletal level, e.g. paraplegia, complete or incomplete, below T11, due to fracture/dislocation of vertebrae T9–10 (Fig. 1.2). A lesion may not be the same on both sides, e.g. C5L/C7R. To give some idea of the neurological involvement in incomplete lesions, the most distal uninvolved segment is given together with the last segment transmitting any normal function, e.g. incomplete below C5, complete below C7. In this case, some motor power or sensation supplied by C6 and C7 is present.

The inadequacy of the neurological level to define function and disability has long been recognized. The degree of paralysis, loss of sensation and the inability to perform activities of daily living demonstrate the severity of an injury, and in order to identify that level of disability measurements are required in all these areas. Many researchers, including those interested in the regeneration of the central nervous system (Davies et al 1995), require an accredited system of monitoring changes in the neurological level and the abilities of patients with spinal cord lesions. Such measures are necessary not only for the comparison of research results but also to facilitate communication between clinicians.

International agreement on a classification has now been reached and the booklet *The international standards for neurological and functional classification of spinal cord injury* (Ditunno et al 1994) has been published. These standards provide a tool to determine neurological level and to calculate a motor, sensory and functional score for each patient. They represent a valid, precise and reliable minimum data set.

The neurological levels are determined by examination of the following:

- a key sensory point within 28 dermatomes on each side of the body
- a key muscle within each of 10 myotomes on each side of the body. The sensation and motor power present are quantified, giving a final numerical score.

This is achieved by using the American spinal cord injuries impairment (ASIA) scale to grade impairment of sensation and motor power (Appendix 1), and the functional independence measure (FIM) to measure disability and grade function (Appendix 2).

The ASIA scale (Table 1.1) is based on the Frankel scale (1969) (Table 1.2). The letters A–E are used to denote degrees of impairment. The Frankel scale has broader bands than the ASIA scale, so unless there is marked improvement or deterioration it is more difficult to show change.

The FIM, as its name states, is devised to measure function for any disability. Each area of function is evaluated in terms of independence using a seven point scale. A total score from all these measures is calculated each time an assessment is carried out and progress can be readily seen.

Table 1.1 The ASIA scale

Grade	Description
A	Complete: no motor or sensory function is preserved in the segments
B	Incomplete: sensory (but not motor) function is preserved below the neurological level and extends through the sacral segments S4–S5
C	Incomplete: motor function is preserved below the neurological level, and the majority of key muscles below the neurological level have a muscle grade less than 3
D	Incomplete: motor function is preserved below the neurological level, and the majority of key muscles below the neurological level have a muscle grade greater than or equal to 3
E	Normal: motor and sensory function are normal

Table 1.2 The Frankel scale

Grade	Description
A	Complete
B	Sensory only
C	Motor non-functional
D	Motor functional
E	Recovered

Clinicians are using the ASIA scale and reporting that its accuracy is greater than the Frankel scale in classifying injuries and monitoring progress (Capaul et al 1994, Tetsuo et al 1996). Others are suggesting amendments (El Masry et al 1996).

In addition to these measures, some therapists and other professionals are using the Ashworth scale of muscle spasticity (Table 1.3).

Therapists now have tools to measure the outcome of treatment and to identify landmarks in the recovery of patients with spinal cord lesions. Interesting data should be collected within units, both nationally and internationally, which will undoubtedly determine future therapy.

Table 1.3 The Ashworth scale

Grade	Description
0	Normal muscle tone
1	Slight increase in muscle tone, 'catch' when limb is moved
2	More marked increase in muscle tone, but limb easily flexed
3	Considerable increase in muscle tone
4	Limb rigid in flexion or extension

2

Physiological effects and their initial management

CLINICAL EFFECTS OF SPINAL CORD INJURY

Severe injury to the vertebral column can occur from any direction and result in dislocation, fracture or fracture/dislocation with or without resultant displacement. As a result, extensive trauma can occur to the spinal cord as it is compressed, crushed or stretched within the spinal canal (Hughes 1984). Yet there appears to be no absolute relationship between the severity of the damage to the vertebral column and that to the spinal cord and roots. A patient may sustain a severe fracture dislocation and yet the spinal cord may be undamaged or only partially damaged. Another may exhibit no obvious vertebral damage on X-ray and yet have sustained an irreversibly complete tetraplegia.

The spinal cord conveys impulses to and from the brain, and through its various afferent and efferent pathways provides a vital link in the control of involuntary muscle. Transection of the cord will result in loss of:

- motor power
- deep and superficial sensation
- vasomotor control
- bladder and bowel control
- sexual function.

Frequently, at the actual level of the lesion there is complete destruction of nerve cells, disruption of the reflex arc and flaccid paralysis of the muscles supplied from the destroyed segments of the spinal cord. This segmental reflex loss is of little importance when the lesion involves the mid-thoracic region, but when the cervical or lumbar enlargements are involved, some important muscles in the upper or lower limbs are inevitably affected with flaccid paralysis. In the same way, a lesion at the level of the lumbar enlargement or cauda equina may destroy the reflex activity of the bladder and rectum and thus deprive the paraplegic not only of voluntary, but also of involuntary (or automatic) control.

Lesions may be complete, where the damage is so extensive that no nerve impulses from the brain reach below the level of the lesion, or incomplete, where some or all of the nerves escape injury.

Immediately after injury the patient will be in a state of spinal areflexia. The nerve cells in the spinal cord below the level of the lesion (i.e. the isolated cord) do not function. No reflexes are present and the limbs are entirely flaccid. This depression of nerve cell activity can last for a few hours or days in young people, up to 6 weeks. Gradually the cells in the isolated cord recover independent function, although they are no longer controlled by the brain. The reflexes return and the stage of spasticity ensues. If complications exist, the return of reflex activity can be delayed (Guttmann 1970). As the spinal cord terminates at the level of the lower border of L1, vertebral lesions below this level do not cause spasticity. The damage in these cases occurs to nerve roots only or is due to direct injury of the conus terminalis.

Occasionally a cord lesion of higher level may also cause sustained flaccidity. This is due to injury in the longitudinal as well as the transverse plane, or to longitudinal vascular damage.

Oedema or bleeding within the spinal cord may cause the level of the lesion to ascend one or even two segments within the first few days after injury. This is nearly always temporary, and the final neurological lesion will probably be the same as or even lower than that found immediately after injury.

Other skeletal or internal injuries are often present in addition to the spinal injury. Diagnosis of these injuries is rendered more difficult by the lack of sensation. The most common associated injuries are those of the long bones, head and chest. Head injuries are frequently found in conjunction with cervical fractures. Crush injuries of the chest with fractured ribs, pneumothorax or haemopneumothorax are commonly associated with fractures of the thoracic spine (Frankel 1968). Abdominal injuries also occur in some cases.

Early complications

Chest complications

The paralysis of the muscles of respiration, including the abdominal muscles, can give rise to serious problems (see Ch. 5).

Deep venous thrombosis

Deep venous thrombosis is recognized clinically by characteristic swelling of the leg. Erythema and low grade temperature may also occur. Unless contraindicated, patients are given prophylactic anticoagulant therapy (Silver 1975).

The swelling is frequently discovered by the physiotherapist when examining the limbs before giving passive movements. If a deep venous thrombosis is diagnosed in either one or both legs, passive movements to both lower limbs are discontinued until the anticoagulation has been stabilized.

Pulmonary embolism

This usually occurs between the second and fourth week, occasionally later, but most commonly between the 10th and 15th days. If an undiagnosed deep venous thrombosis is present, it may give rise to an embolus when the physiotherapist begins to move the leg. Many patients have pulmonary embolism without prior evidence of deep venous thrombosis.

AIMS OF MANAGEMENT

In spinal cord injury centres, the aim of management is the simultaneous treatment of the spinal injury, the multisystems impairment and the non-medical effects of paralysis.

MANAGEMENT OF THE SPINE

The principles of management of the spine are to:

- enhance neurological recovery
- avoid neurological deterioration
- achieve biomechanical stability of the spine at the site of the fracture, preserving spared neural tissue until healing occurs.

Neurological recovery is expected in patients with incomplete spinal cord lesions, provided the physiological instability of the spinal cord and the biomechanical instability of the spinal column are well controlled. Any major complications from the paralysis, such as pressure sores, septicaemia or hypoxia, can further destabilize a physiologically unstable spinal cord which has lost its blood–brain barrier and its autoregulatory mechanisms. This can result in lack of neurological recovery or further neurological deterioration. (El Masry 1993).

In order to prevent further mechanical damage of the neural tissues due to displacement at the fracture site, it is important that the biomechanical stability of the spinal column is contained by either conservative or surgical means. If, however, biomechanical stability is to be obtained through surgery, it is important that the physiologically unstable spinal cord is not further destabilized by hypoxia hypotension during or after the surgical procedure.

Reduction of the spine can be achieved by conservative as well as surgical means, with or without anaesthesia and with or without traction depending on the type of injury. Oedema within the spinal cord is probably at a maximum 48 hours after injury. In view of this, some clinicians believe that it is dangerous to actively reduce the fracture dislocation after this time, especially in elderly people or in patients with degenerative changes in the spine. As some reduction of the size of the spinal canal is inevitable during the process of spinal reduction, the oedematous and swollen cord may be further damaged during the procedure. Early reduction

is therefore particularly important. To date there is no evidence that realignment results in improvement of neurological recovery.

The development of computerized tomography and, in particular, magnetic resonance imaging now enables clinicians to assess impingement on the cord within the spinal canal and the longitudinal extent of cord pathology. It is a useful tool in determining and re-evaluating different management procedures for different patterns of injury (El Masry 1993).

Postural reduction

Various surgical procedures are used to stabilize the fracture in spinal injury centres throughout the world. In other centres, including the Stoke Mandeville Centre, the initial treatment of the fracture/dislocation is usually conservative, i.e. by postural reduction (Guttmann 1945, Frankel et al 1969, Ersmarke et al 1990).

Postural reduction, with or without traction, is aimed at aligning the fractured vertebra and restoring and maintaining the normal curvature of the spine.

After the initial X-rays are taken, pillows and/or a roll are used to place the spine in the optimum position, to reduce the dislocation and allow healing of the fracture. The majority of injuries are the result of acute flexion, flexion/ rotation or extension of the spine, and the position has to be adjusted accordingly.

Control X-rays are taken over the next few days and weeks to check that the position is achieving the desired results. Plaster jackets or beds are *never* used because of the grave risk of pressure sores.

Fractured cervical spine. A firm small roll made of wool and covered with linen or tube gauze is used to support the fracture. This roll is placed on top of a single pillow which extends under the shoulders as well as under the head. If further extension is needed, the pillow is placed under the shoulders and the head is allowed to rest on a sheepskin pad on the bed. Two pillows are used to support the thorax and a single one is placed under the glutei and thighs, with a gap of approximately 8 cm in between the pillows to prevent pressure on the sacrum. A pillow is placed underneath the lower legs to avoid pressure on the heels by keeping them off the bed. A double pillow or several pillows bound together are set against the footboard to support the feet and toes in dorsiflexion.

If skull traction is necessary, as is the case in the majority of cervical injuries, Cones or Gardner Wells calipers are preferred and the weights are moderate, i.e. 2.7–6.8 kg for 6 weeks on average.

Fractured thoracic or lumbar spine. Two pillows are usually sufficient to extend and support fractures of the dorsolumbar spine. Occasionally, a third pillow or a roll may be necessary to obtain the correct degree of hyperextension.

Pillows have to be adjusted in such a way that the bony prominences are always free of pressure. The patient must be handled very carefully at all times. He must be lifted by four people or rolled in one piece with the fracture site well supported and the spine in correct alignment. Flexion and rotation particularly must be avoided.

There appears to be no difference in the outcomes of conservative or surgical treatment, although the complications can be greater following surgical intervention (Bravo et al 1996). In particular, there is less interference with the blood supply of the spinal cord, which may lead to further neurological damage. Occasionally a late surgical stabilization procedure may be indicated where a spinal fracture remains unstable in both complete or incomplete lesions. Even when conservative management is preferred, there will be occasions when surgery is indicated, for example when there is delayed onset of neurological deficit or gross bony displacement which does not respond to conservative management in the first few days (Frankel et al 1987).

Correct positioning of the patient

Correct positioning of the patient in bed (see Ch. 5) is important in order to:

- obtain correct alignment of the fracture
- prevent contractures
- prevent pressure sores
- inhibit the onset of severe spasticity.

Turning the patient

Patients are turned every 3 hours, day and night. The supine and side lying positions are used for the acute lesion. In cervical and upper thoracic injuries, the prone position is unsuitable as it may cause further embarrassment to the respiratory system by inhibiting the excursion of the diaphragm. This can result in hypoxia. Immediately prior to discharge home, the turning interval may be increased to 4 and then to 6 hours.

MULTISYSTEMS IMPAIRMENT

The aims of treatment for the multisystems impairment are to:

- prevent death by resuscitation and maintenance of respiration (Ch. 5)
- prevent avoidable complications such as pressure sores
- institute a regimen of treatment for the care of the paralysed bladder and bowels.

Management of the bladder

Disturbance of bladder function can produce many complications which constitute a lifelong threat to the patient. Statistics show that renal disease was responsible for the majority of deaths among patients with spinal lesions. This is not now the case, but assiduous and continuing bladder care is essential if complications are to be prevented.

The acute lesion

The effect on the bladder depends upon the length of time after injury, as well as the level of cord injury and the degree of cord damage.

Paralysis of the bladder during the first few days after acute spinal damage is total and flaccid. During this period of spinal areflexia, all bladder reflexes and muscle action are abolished. The patient will develop acute retention, followed by passive incontinence due to overflow from the distended bladder. Treatment will be directed to:

- achieving a satisfactory method of emptying the bladder
- maintaining sterile urine
- enabling the patient to remain continent.

During the period of spinal areflexia, the bladder may be emptied in several ways, including:

- urethral catheterization
  — intermittent
  — indwelling
- suprapubic drainage.

For acute lesions from whatever cause – traumatic, vascular or viral – the treatment of choice at the Stoke Mandeville Centre is intermittent catheterization (Frankel 1984). This method allows some distension of the bladder, which represents the physiological stimulus for micturition and triggers the appropriate impulses to the spinal bladder centre. This promotes return of detrusor activity. A long-term indwelling catheter is likely to be the source of bladder infection, vesical calculi, urethral strictures, diverticula and fistula and periurethral abscesses. A fine-bore suprapubic catheter is often the most appropriate treatment for female patients during the first 2 months post-injury, and for tetraplegic patients they are sometimes left permanently.

Patients with total transection of the spinal cord no longer feel the specific sensations which indicate that the bladder needs emptying. Many patients, however, feel other sensations related to bladder filling and learn to interpret these as an indication that the bladder is full. The most common of the substitute sensations is a vague feeling of abdominal fullness which is the result of an increase in intravesical and/or intra-abdominal pressure.

Bladder training

As spinal areflexia wears off, which may take from a few days to several weeks, two main types of bladder condition develop:

- the automatic bladder
- the autonomous bladder.

The automatic (or reflex) bladder. This type of bladder develops in most patients with transverse spinal cord lesions above T10–11.

As reflex tone returns, the detrusor muscle contracts in response to a certain degree of filling pressure. The returning power of the sphincter is overcome and micturition occurs. This reflex detrusor action may be triggered by stroking, kneading or rhythmic tapping over the abdominal wall above the symphysis pubis, or by stimulating other trigger points, e.g. stroking the inner aspect of the thigh or pulling the pubic hair.

With training, this reflex action will occur on stimulation of the trigger points and not at other times, so that the patient can learn to empty his bladder every 2 or 3 hours and remain dry in between.

The autonomous (or non-reflex) bladder. This bladder is virtually atonic and occurs where the reflex action is interrupted, i.e. with a longitudinal lesion of the spinal cord or a lower motor neurone lesion. There is no reflex action of the detrusor muscle. The patient is taught to catheterize himself to empty the bladder.

If the abdominal muscles are innervated the patient can raise the intra-abdominal pressure by straining, when the pressure on the kidneys is the same as that on the bladder. The disadvantage is that high pressure is also put on the rectum.

Both the automatic and autonomous bladders may be emptied provided their function is understood, gradual training takes place and active infection of the bladder is avoided.

When out of bed, the general increase in muscular activity, especially of the abdominal muscles if innervated, may make it more difficult to keep dry. Consequently, it may be necessary to express the bladder every hour at first.

Bladder training takes up a great deal of time and the patient may get discouraged, but it is important to persevere, for gradually the bladder will become trained and the time between the visits to the toilet lengthened to 1, 2, 3 and in some cases even 4 hours.

The same training is carried out for both sexes,

but it is essential for the female patient as there is no satisfactory urinal at present on the market. Pads and incontinence pants are the only protection in case of leakage between expressions or catheterizations. With encouragement, patience and perseverance, this method is successful for many patients and it is well worth the effort involved. Where bladder training is ineffective, the patient is taught to catheterize himself on an intermittent though not necessarily regular basis. Self-catheterization is most commonly used with female patients and children (Hill & Davies 1988).

Male urinals

There are several types of male urinals available. The best for any individual is that which he finds most convenient to use, but the following conditions must be fulfilled:

- it must not cause pressure sores
- it must contain a non-return valve
- if not disposable, it must be easily cleaned and sterilized.

Urinary sheath. The sheath is rolled onto the penis and an integral band, or collar, of non-irritant adhesive at the top of the sheath ensures that it remains in place. A non-return valve prevents a backflow of urine along the penile shaft, keeping the penis dry. A plastic tube connects the sheath to the leg bag which can have expandable side pleats. These allow outward expansion, enabling a greater volume of urine to be contained in a shorter bag (Fig. 2.1).

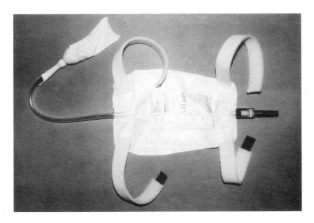

Figure 2.1 Urinary sheath.

Condom urinal. Where a proprietory brand of urinary sheath is not available, the condom urinal can be used. This consists of the condom, a nylon connector, a piece of rubber tubing and a bag for drainage (Fig. 2.2).

The nylon connector is first placed inside the end of the condom and the connection tube is pushed over from the outside. This clamps the condom, which is then pierced where it stretches across the lumen of the connector. An orange stick is useful for this purpose. The shaft of the penis is smeared with a suitable adhesive and the condom sheath is rolled on and held in place for at least 30 seconds to ensure that the glue becomes effective. The condom should extend at least 2.5 cm beyond the end of the penis. A finger stall may be more suitable than a condom for young boys. The connecting tube is then attached to the urine bag, which may be strapped to the

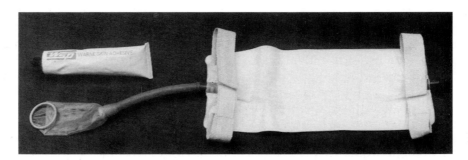

Figure 2.2 Condom urinal.

leg when the patient is up, and hung from the frame of the bed at night. Disposable bags can be used or the more durable suprapubic bag.

If the suprapubic bag is used, each patient must have two and use them alternately so that each can be thoroughly disinfected after use. The bag should be washed in warm soapy water, rinsed and soaked in, for example, Dakin's solution (16%) for 2 hours, rinsed well and hung up to dry for 12–14 hours.

Female pads

Incontinence garments with protective pads are available from many sources. When these are unavailable, pads can be made up by the patient. Size and thickness can be adjusted to suit individual needs, thin ones for use at home when the patient is in easy reach of the toilet, and thicker ones for travelling and visiting. The pads consist of 20 cm gauze tissue, white wool and cellulose tissue, and are approximately 12–15 cm wide and 30 cm long.

To make up the pad, use the following procedure:

1. Cut the wool and cellulose to the required size and the gauze tissue approximately 15 cm longer.
2. Open out the gauze tissue on a flat surface and ensure that it is free from creases.
3. Place the cellulose and the cotton wool, layered in that order, onto the gauze and fold the gauze over until the pad is completely enclosed.
4. Tuck the end of the gauze neatly into the layers of wool.

The pad is worn with the white wool side next to the skin.

Urinary hygiene

All patients must be taught urinary hygiene to avoid smell and must learn to watch for skin abrasions, redness and septic spots. If damage to the skin on the penis occurs, the urinal should not be worn until the lesion is fully healed. Severe pressure sores and fistulae can occur very rapidly if the urinal is applied over damaged skin. Difficult patches of adhesive may be removed with ether, but frequent use irritates the skin. Daily washing with soap and water and careful drying should be all that is required.

In order to have self-confidence, the incontinent patient must be prepared to cope either alone or with minimal help at all times, not only at home but also when a suitable toilet may not be available. For the female patient, receivers or bedpans can be useful and expression of the bladder can be successfully carried out on a suitable bedpan in a wheelchair. The incontinent female patient will find it essential to have a small travelling case containing:

- a plastic bedpan or receiver in a cover
- clean pads
- several plastic bags to receive soiled pads
- one plastic container of water for cleansing
- talcum powder.

Sacral anterior root stimulators

This is an alternative method of bladder stimulation for micturition. Radio-linked implants are successfully used to stimulate S2, S3 and S4. By activating these, the patient can empty the bladder at will. Resection of the posterior roots of S2, S3 and S4 has been found to improve the effectiveness of stimulation. This form of treatment is prescribed for female patients who are unsuccessful with simpler methods such as regular toileting and self-catheterization (Brindley 1984, Brindley & Rushton 1990) and is particularly useful for female patients with upper motor neurone lesions. In male patients, reflex micturition will be lost but stimulation will produce erectile function.

The Sacral Anterior Root Stimulation Implants (SARSIs) were still being used by 479 of the first 500 patients between 3 and 16 years after implantation (Brindley 1994, 1995)

Management of the bowels

Immediately after the onset of paralysis, fluids alone are given because of the danger of a paralytic ileus of neurogenic origin. The bowel training regime is instituted once the patient is on a full diet.

Bowel training

The aim is to deliver the bowel contents to the rectum at the same time either daily or every second day and remove them by reflex defaecation when the patient is prepared for it. This is achieved by:

- mild aperients in the evening, e.g. senna tablets (Senokot)
- two glycerine suppositories the following morning followed half an hour later by digital evacuation with a gloved finger
- correct diet and fluids.

Evacuation in bed. The previous evening senna tablets are given, 30 mg or as necessary depending on the results. Bulking agents may also be used.

The following morning, the patient is put on his left side and supported with sandbags and pillows. A plastic sheet and one or two disposable incontinence pads are placed under the buttocks. Two glycerine suppositories are inserted into the rectum as high as the gloved finger can reach. Care is taken to avoid overstretching the anus or damaging the rectal mucosa. The patient is kept warm and given a hot drink. Reflex defaecation usually occurs within 20–30 minutes but may take up to an hour. If the bowel has not emptied or not emptied completely, digital stimulation may be indicated. A gloved finger is inserted into the rectum. The anus contracts when the finger is inserted. It then relaxes and the bowel empties. It may be necessary to stimulate the anus in this way during bowel training but subsequently it becomes unnecessary for most patients.

Toilet training. When the patient is out of bed, he is taught to do his own evacuation on the toilet, once he has sufficient balance in sitting and is able to transfer with assistance. A bar is needed beside the toilet so that the patient can support himself whilst leaning forwards.

Aperients and/or suppositories are continued

as required. The development of a regular habit of bowel opening, usually every second day, is essential and with patience and perseverance it is possible to establish a satisfactory programme for all patients. Tetraplegic patients continue evacuations on the bed unless they can get onto a commode or toilet chair. Prior to the patient's discharge, the relatives or the district nurse are instructed in the procedure.

A patient with acute constipation may present with spurious diarrhoea, the impacted faeces allowing only liquids to pass through the gut. Although enemas as a routine are avoided, in this case they may be given before starting the bowel regime.

SEXUAL DYSFUNCTION
Male

Male patients with high lesions often have priapism for hours or several days after injury. Subsequently all sexual function is abolished during the stage of spinal areflexia. Later return of function will depend upon the level and completeness of the lesion. For patients with complete lesions above the reflex centre in the conus, automatic erections occur in response to local stimuli but there will be no sensation during sexual intercourse. Patients with low cord lesions above the sacral reflex centre may have not only reflex erections but also psychogenic erections if the sympathetic pathways are intact. Occasionally these may be accompanied by ejaculation. The seminal fluid will pass through the urethra only if there is an associated contraction of the internal bladder sphincter. Otherwise it refluxes into the bladder.

Mechanical assistive devices are now available, as well as various pharmacological agents which enhance erections.

Sexual function varies widely in patients with incomplete lesions, according to the degree of cord damage sustained. Any form of sensation on the penis may indicate some preservation of genital sex. Problems may remain in relation to locomotor and voluntary muscle activity.

Tests can be carried out to assess potency

and fertility. Patients can now undergo semen procurement predictably and safely. However, most couples will need assisted pregnancy techniques such as intrauterine insemination (Brindley 1984, Hirsch et al 1990).

Female

Menstruation

Interruption of the menstrual cycle occurs in the majority of women with complete or incomplete lesions who are not taking a contraceptive pill. This can last from a few months to more than a year. Eventually the menstrual cycle returns to normal.

Pregnancy

Apart from lacking genital sensation, sexual function is unimpaired for female patients with complete lesions.

Both paraplegic and tetraplegic women can become pregnant and have normal babies. These can be delivered vaginally or by caesarian section if indicated. Uterine contractions occur normally. Each uterine contraction in patients with complete lesions above T6 causes autonomic dysreflexia. Patients with complete lesions at T9 and below have uterine pain, but patients with complete lesions at T6, 7 or 8 may not be aware that labour has commenced, especially if it occurs during sleep. Therefore these patients should be kept under careful observation and are usually admitted to hospital before the expected delivery date.

AUTONOMIC DYSREFLEXIA

Autonomic dysreflexia is a vascular reflex which occurs in response to a stimulus from the bladder, bowel or other internal organ below the level of the lesion in a patient with a high lesion, i.e. above T6. The physiotherapist must be alert to recognize the symptoms of autonomic dysreflexia which are an outburst of sweating on the head, neck and shoulders, raised blood pressure, slow pulse and throbbing headache. Overdistension of the bladder caused by a blocked catheter can give rise to this reflex activity which presents quickly and which, if not dealt with immediately, can rapidly precipitate cerebrovascular accident, epileptic fits and even death (Calachis 1992). It can also be caused by strong spasms and by sudden changes of position, as, for example, with the tilt table. Tilting the body with the head up will reduce the blood pressure until further treatment can be given. The treatment is to remove the cause; antihypertensive drugs may be given as a temporary measure. Three cases of autonomic hyperreflexia were reported in the USA in 1980 which were precipitated by passive hip flexion. This occurred in young men with lesions at C5, C6 and T1. It was suggested that this response was evoked by stretching the hip joint capsule or proximal leg muscles innervated by L4, L5 and S1 (McGarry et al 1982).

Caution. All those involved in the care of patients with spinal cord lesions should be able to recognize the symptoms of autonomic dysreflexia and know what to do in an emergency.

3

Patient-centred practice

Spinal cord injury suddenly reduces an individual enjoying normal health and activity to a state of complete immobility and dependence upon others. He is precipitated into an unknown and unreal world full of fears and problems. He has to deal with pain and incapacity, cope with the stresses of hospital treatment, sustain relations with family and friends and prepare for an uncertain future. Understanding something about the psychological response of the patient to his condition is essential in planning care and treatment. This is a vast subject and only some brief comments are given here, with references for further reading.

Initially the patient is usually too dazed to appreciate his condition. This phase may pass in a dream-like state in which adaptation to the disability cannot begin (Horn 1989). This may be due to a variety of causes, e.g. medication, severe pain or total immobilization, and may be prolonged where there is anoxia due to respiratory dysfunction or an associated head injury. Within a day or two, in most cases, the patient becomes superficially aware of his disability. This knowledge gradually deepens and the patient begins to realize the enormity of what the loss of movement, bladder, bowel and sexual function will mean in daily life.

The emotional reaction to disability will vary from patient to patient (Shadish et al 1981) and there is no 'right' way to adapt to it (Woodbury & Radd 1987). Some people find it hard to believe and resist hearing the news that they will be paralysed: 'I just did not believe it. It took a month of total disbelief.' Others just face up to it: 'This has happened. Let's get on with it.' (Oliver et al 1991). Whilst there is no universal response to stress in general and to spinal cord injury in particular, it is quite normal for a person to grieve after becoming paralysed (Judd & Burrows 1986). Not all patients with spinal cord injury go through the same grief process, but Jacob et al (1995) suggests that mourning is essential for healthy adaptation.

Adjustment to such an injury is a lifelong process in which constant changes occur both in the patient and in his circumstances. It may be that a minimum of 2 years is needed to achieve some stability in life following spinal cord injury, although this will vary from person to person (Craig et al 1994).

Within the wide range of different personalities and individual responses to the immense disablement caused by the spinal injury, there are those patients who have a long psychiatric history prior to admission and others who sustain their injury while attempting to take their own lives. These patients present particular problems and are in need of special care.

The extent of the disability is brought home to the patient even more forcefully when he begins his rehabilitation in the wheelchair. During the acute phase in bed, others cared for his bodily needs, but once up, the patient is confronted by his dependent, heavy, useless limbs. Some patients cannot face the enormity of their problem and constantly affirm that they will walk again. In view of this, they refuse to learn the activities of daily living from a wheelchair or to consider any necessary alterations to the home. The therapist should not try to force the patient to face up to all his problems until he is ready.

Patients usually find it helpful to be in a spinal injuries unit, where they live with others with the same disability. Besides gaining confidence from the expertise of the staff, the patient is provided with visible evidence of what can be achieved through his contact with others who are similarly affected but who are in the later stages of rehabilitation, or already living at home. These positive characteristics seen in others who are well adjusted can be beneficial to successful adjustment (Cushman & Dijkers 1991).

Rehabilitation team

It is important that all members of the rehabilitation team act in the same supportive manner, as people who are adapting to recent disability are attentive to and influenced by the attitudes of health professionals (Nordholm & Westbrook 1986). No member of the team must contribute to a negative environment or reinforce a sense of powerlessness or hopelessness in the patient (Hammell 1995). Each member of the team is responsible for his or her own contribution to the atmosphere of hope and confidence in which the patient can most easily come to grips with his disability and regain his self-confidence. The expectations of the rehabilitation staff have an important influence on outcome (Bodenhammer et al 1983). The presence of a clinical psychologist in the rehabilitation team will be of particular importance, not only in the treatment of patients but also to assist colleagues.

Spinal cord injury is one of the most extreme examples of a situation where a person experiences severe loss of control of both body and environment. From the earliest days of treatment, the goal of all members of the rehabilitation team is to encourage independent thought, restore a sense of self-esteem and enable the patient to regain control over his life.

Perceived personal control

Perceptions of control have been shown to be important in terms of management of health care and disability: 'Perceived control is defined as the *belief* that one can determine one's own internal states and behaviours, influence one's environment and/or bring about desired outcomes' (Wallston et al 1987). Rotter (1966) described people who believe that they have a high degree of personal control over events in their lives as having an *internal* locus of control. These are people who want more information and are hopeful of, and persevere in, attaining goals. He described those who believe they have little or no control over what happens to them as having an *external* locus of control. Outcomes are seen as random occurrences controlled by fate, chance or powerful others. This may lead to the belief that their own efforts in rehabilitation will not be successful. It is not the actual reality of the extent of control that has been shown to be important, but rather the person's belief about his control over events (Hammell 1995). Even though a person may have a high lesion and little physical control over his immediate circumstances, this does not necessarily change his perception of the extent of control he has over his life (Trieschmann 1988). This belief is associated with the ability to influence others in order to achieve one's own ends (Johnson et al 1970).

The background to the concept of perceived personal control initially came from social learning theory research and has received a significant amount of attention in behavioural research (Wallston et al 1987) and more recently in the health care field. It is a complex subject and is mentioned briefly here because the patient's perceptions and beliefs are an integral part of his learning in rehabilitation, and health professionals need to take account of them in planning rehabilitation programmes. Patient compliance with externally imposed routines is highly rated by professionals, but it does not facilitate independence and problem-solving skills (Tucker 1984). Independence encompasses thinking and acting for oneself as well as the performance of physical skills. Those patients who believe that they are as physically independent as possible have more positive self-concepts than those who perceive themselves as less independent than they are capable of being (Green et al 1984).

Those who believe that they are primarily responsible for their health show less depression and more adaptive behaviour than those who have more externalized beliefs (Frank & Elliott 1989). A Recovery Locus of Control scale (RLOC) was developed by Partridge & Johnston (1989) on which patients with stroke were assessed at the start of rehabilitation and on recovery from physical disability. Their study showed that greater perceived control was associated with faster recovery from disability and greater

achievements in terms of function. They suggest that 'It may be useful to encourage patients' belief in their own control which is in contrast to most hospital care, including physiotherapy, where the emphasis is on external control, with reliance on the skill and expertise of the professionals'.

In a further study, Johnston et al (1992) showed that information given to patients can influence their perceptions of control over events in their lives and it is possible to change perceived control over recovery from physical disability. Those patients who were given information designed to increase their personal control scored significantly higher on the RLOC scale at discharge some weeks later than those who received standard information.

A greater belief in perceived personal control has also been shown to be associated with better health outcomes in patients with spinal cord injuries (Shadish et al 1981). Rehabilitation is an intensive process with a great deal for the patient to learn, particularly in the early stages. If learning is to be effective, patients need to define their own problems, decide on the action to be taken and evaluate the consequences of their decisions (Hammell 1995). In describing the value of rehabilitation, Banja (1990) offers the idea of empowerment as a key concept. Patients will differ in their desire for personal control, and in the extent to which they believe they have it. However, it is as destructive to insist that a patient who has little belief in his control takes charge as it is to take control away from someone who has strong beliefs in personal control.

The rehabilitation programme should place strong emphasis on individual responsibility and be oriented to encourage the patient to make choices regarding treatment (Wallston & Wallston 1978). The technical side of the therapy given remains the prerogative of the therapist.

Patient/physiotherapist relationship

The relationship between patient and professional needs to be a partnership where the professional uses expert knowledge and skills and the patient contributes his expectations and perspective of what is important to him in his life (Stocking 1996). The therapist is sensitive to the patient's needs and provides time and space for him to discuss fears, worries and values. Their relationship should be characterized by trust, commitment and respect (Peloquin 1990).

Goal setting

For collaborative goal setting, the therapist needs to understand the patient's goals for living at home and the impact the spinal cord injury will have upon his lifestyle. It is also essential that the patient should be given intelligible explanations of the treatment methods offered. Some patients will want more information than others, or at different times, and some more choice than others. Ozer (1988) suggests that the professional starts by asking open-ended questions such as: 'What do you expect to gain from your physiotherapy programme?' If this elicits no response, the therapist should provide multiple choice lists of questions from which the patient selects an answer. If this fails, the therapist finally recommends an answer and requires agreement.

Both patient and therapist then agree long- and short-term goals for therapy and make a contract to work towards the final goal by taking a series of steps. An objective, which should be a specific, measurable activity, is set to attain the first step. Shared treatment goals enable the patient to develop more achievable expectations, more confidence in his abilities to implement appropriate courses of action and more faith in the health care team (Steele et al 1987). Goal planning is informative about the injury and gives a sense of control over rehabilitation (MacLeod & MacLeod 1996).

Living at home

When the patient goes home, whether for the first weekend or on discharge, he is transferred from a sheltered life amongst others in wheelchairs into the hurly-burly of the able-bodied world where he may be patronized, stared at, or ignored. In consequence, there may be an initial tendency to shun social contacts until this barrier is overcome. Strong encouragement is needed from family or friends to go out and take part in social activities. Social adjustment is a continuous process and patients need to be told that they are going to find difficulty in adjusting to life at home. 'You have to relearn to live with other people again' (Oliver et al 1991). Patients feel guilty or concerned about the strain imposed on parents or other family members caring for them. Initial health problems often coincide with periods of depression, lethargy, irritability and loss of self-confidence (Oliver et al 1991). Depression was found to correlate with the 'Reintegration To Normal Living Index' but not to be related to neurological impairment. Whether the depression was the cause of the difficulties in reintegrating to normal living conditions or a consequence of poor integration is not known (Daverat et al 1995). Perceived control, social support, social integration, occupation and mobility all contribute to life satisfaction (Furher et al 1992).

The patient will have many anxieties, giving rise to questions regarding prognosis, home and family life, sex, employment, rehabilitation and practical environmental and financial problems. Many spinal units provide an educational programme for those patients, relatives and friends who wish to take advantage of it (Houston 1984, McGowan & Roth 1987). The aim of the programme is to assist the patient and members of his family to understand what has happened (Pachalski & Pachalski 1984). Subjects covered may include relevant anatomy, bladder and bowel function, spasm, skin care, sex, sexuality and personal relationships, citizens' rights and benefits, aids and adaptations in the home, and employment. In addition to information given in groups, sexual counselling needs to be undertaken on an individual basis. It will be particularly important at certain stages in rehabilitation, for example before and after weekends at home. The Stoke Mandeville Hospital Centre gives a comprehensive manual about the issues discussed to each patient who attends the course.

In addition to instruction on patient care, the

relatives need constant individual counsel and support both to assist them in adjusting and to support their paralysed relative. Psychologists and sociologists suggest, and experience proves, that the family provides the most effective link in the reintegration of the paraplegic or tetra-plegic patient into his social environment (Ray 1984). Communication between the patient and his family needs to be encouraged, as patients and relatives will often talk freely about the deeper issues involved with everyone except each other.

Medical and social follow-up is essential if long-term resettlement is to be successful. Domiciliary visits provide the opportunity for the patient and family to discuss any difficulties, such as those relating to housing, employment or attitude to the disability, which are found after leaving hospital.

Peripatetic services are organized from some spinal centres where a specialist team is available to follow up the ongoing needs of patients with spinal cord injury (Judd & Burrows 1986, Judd et al 1988).

4

The acute lesion

EXAMINATION OF THE PATIENT

For the therapist to gain maximum information regarding the patient, she should be present at the initial neurological examination carried out by the doctor in charge of the case. In this way she will gain information regarding:

- the patient's injury
- general condition
- the site and condition of the fracture, if any
- the presence of associated fractures or injuries, including any skin lesions
- condition of the chest, including the results of lung function tests
- motor function
- sensory function
- presence or absence of reflexes
- previous medical history and current medical conditions, e.g. ankylosing spondylitis, rheumatoid arthritis, diabetes
- occupation
- family history
- diagnosis of the level of the lesion
- immediate medical treatment.

The therapist will subsequently wish to make her own examination, adding to the above information her assessment of:

- respiratory function (see Ch. 5)
- the range of motion of all joints involved and the presence of contractures
- the strength of innervated muscles with particular regard to

—completely paralysed muscles
—unopposed innervated muscle groups
—imbalance of muscle groups
• the degree of spasticity, if present
• the presence of oedema.

When the doctor and therapist discuss the treatment required, factors such as the following will be given special attention:

• respiratory therapy, especially in relation to the treatment of patients on ventilators
• the danger of muscle shortening due to unopposed muscle action and the required positioning of the joints involved
• severe spasticity and the positioning required to reduce tone
• the necessity for splinting.

After her own initial assessment, the physiotherapist will need to discuss treatment with the other members of the multidisciplinary team.

Physiotherapy programme

On the basis of the physiotherapist's examination and assessment, the patient and therapist together set short- and long-term goals and plan the treatment schedule to achieve the initial short-term goals (Ch. 3).

Detailed records are kept of the initial assessment, treatment and progress of the patient. Everyday incidents are also noted, such as the occurrence of bladder infections, slight injury or pressure marks, the first outing and the first weekend home.

TREATMENT OF THE PATIENT IN BED

From the outset, the combined efforts of everyone are concentrated on assisting the patient to achieve maximum independence. When the patient cannot do something for himself, he must learn how to teach others to do it for him. Gaining knowledge and accepting responsibility both start whilst the patient is in bed. He must know where others can find his belongings in the locker and when, for example, he needs more soap or toothpaste.

The patient with a spinal fracture will be in bed from 6 to 12 weeks. Those paralysed from other causes or who have had surgery will spend considerably less time in bed.

Correct positioning of the patient

Correct positioning in bed is vitally important not only to maintain the correct alignment of the fracture, but also to prevent pressure sores (Ch. 6) and contractures, and to inhibit the onset of extreme spasticity.

The supine position (Fig. 4.1a)

When supine, the patient is positioned in the following way.
Lower limbs

• Hips – extended and slightly abducted
• Knees – extended but not hyperextended
• Ankles – dorsiflexed
• Toes – extended.

One or two pillows are kept between the legs to maintain abduction and prevent pressure on the bony points, i.e. medial condyles and malleoli.
Upper limbs (for patients with tetraplegia)

• Shoulders – adducted and in mid-position or protracted, but not retracted
• Elbows – extended; this is particularly important when the biceps is innervated and the triceps paralysed. If the biceps is overactive, extension can be maintained by wrapping a pillow round the forearms, or by using a vacuum splint
• Wrists – dorsiflexed to approximately 45°
• Fingers – slightly flexed
• Thumb – opposed to prevent the development of a 'monkey' hand, which is functionally useless.

The arms are placed on pillows at the sides. The pillows should be high enough under the shoulders to ensure that the shoulders are not retracted when damage to the anterior capsule can occur. If the shoulders are painful and protraction is required, a small sorbo wedge can be placed behind the joint on either or both sides. If necessary, two pillows should be used under the forearms and hands, as it is important that the hands are kept higher than the shoulders to prevent gravitational swelling in the static limbs.

In some units the arms are placed in alternative positions for periods during the day (see Ch. 14).

The side-lying or lateral position (Fig. 4.1b)

When lying on the side, the patient is positioned in the following manner.

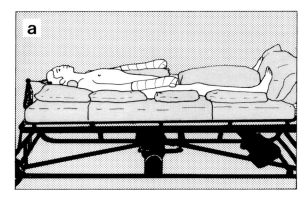

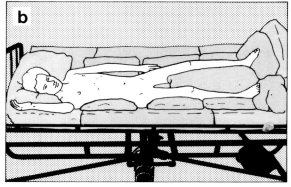

Figure 4.1 a: Supine position of a patient with a cervical fracture (right arm pillow was removed for clarity). The patient is lying on an Egerton–Stoke Mandeville 'electric turning bed'. b: Lateral position of a patient with a low thoracic fracture.

Lower limbs

- Hips and knees – flexed sufficiently to obtain stability with two pillows between the legs and with the upper leg lying slightly behind the lower one
- Ankles – dorsiflexed
- Toes – extended.

Upper limbs

- Lower arm – shoulder flexed and lying in the trough between the pillows supporting the head and thorax to relieve pressure on the shoulder
- Elbow – extended
- Forearm – supinated and supported either on the arm board attached to the more sophisticated beds or on a pillow on a table
- Upper arm – as in the supine position, but with a pillow between the arm and the chest wall.

The hand

If the hand is to be functional even when paralysed, the maintenance of a good position in the acute phase is essential. The hand must remain mobile as it will be used in different positions – flat for transfers and flexed for all gripping movements as described on page 29.

Gravitational swelling must be avoided. If it is allowed to occur unchecked, contractures easily develop.

Cheshire & Rowe (1971) maintained that swelling can be prevented if the collateral ligaments of the metacarpophalangeal joints are kept at their maximum tension, i.e. when the joint is kept in 90° flexion. In order to prevent swelling and maintain a good functional position, Cheshire developed the 'boxing glove' splint (Fig. 4.2). It consists of a light, well-padded, cock-up splint and a palmar roll. The wrist is maintained at 45° dorsiflexion, the metacarpophalangeal joints at 90° flexion, the interphalangeal joints at 30° flexion and the abductor web of the thumb in full stretch with opposition of the thumb. A layer of wool is placed over the dorsum of the hand and fingers and the whole is bandaged as for an amputation. The splint

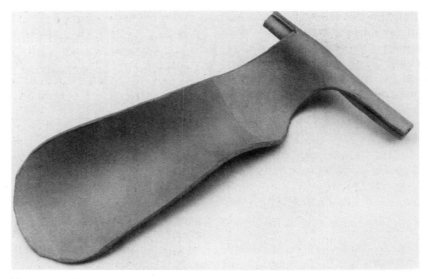

Figure 4.2 Unpadded cock-up support for the boxing glove splint.

is removed several times a day for washing, physiotherapy and occupational therapy, and the skin is checked for pressure marks. It is used constantly until the patient is using his hands and then is applied at night only.

If the boxing glove splint is not employed, the hand can be kept in a useful functional position with a small palmar roll. Light straps keep the fingers in flexion and the thumb in opposition around the roll. Cock-up or paddle splints may be used depending on the presenting problem and the level of the lesion. These splints are usually worn at night.

PHYSIOTHERAPY

During the period in bed, the following treatment is given:

- respiratory therapy – to maintain good ventilation (as the need for respiratory care may extend throughout life, this is dealt with separately in Ch. 5)
- passive movements – to assist the circulation and to ensure full mobility of all paralysed structures
- active movements – to maintain or regain muscle strength.

Passive movements

Passive movements of the paralysed limbs are essential to stimulate the circulation and preserve full range of movement in joints and soft tissues. Treatment is commenced the first day after injury or when anticoagulant therapy has started and the prothrombin times are within the therapeutic range (El Masry & Silver 1981). During the period of spinal areflexia, i.e. for approximately 6 weeks, treatment is given twice daily. Movements are continued once a day until the patient is mobile and capable of ensuring full mobility through his own activities. Approximately 10 minutes are spent on the movement of each limb. A high proportion of this time is given to slowly moving the limb as a whole to improve the circulation.

In addition, each joint – starting proximally and working distally and including the metatarsal and metacarpal joints – is moved several times through its full range, and appropriate movements are given to prevent muscle shortening. The patella should be mobilized before moving the knee. The movements are performed slowly, smoothly and rhythmically to avoid injury to the insensitive, unprotected joints and paralysed structures. Any limitations imposed by previous medical history and/or age must be taken into consideration.

When reflex activity returns, the limb must be handled with extreme care, so as not to elicit spasm and reinforce the spastic pattern. A pinch grip or any sudden brisk movement must be avoided. If a spasm occurs during a movement, the therapist holds the limb firmly and waits for the spasm to relax before completing the movement. Forced passive movements against spasticity may cause injury or even fracture of a limb. Sometimes, however, the only way to overcome ankle clonus is to completely dorsiflex the ankle, against the spasm, and hold it until the foot relaxes. The movement must be performed firmly but gently. Before moving any limb when tone is increased, the other limbs should be placed in positions which oppose their spastic pattern. For example, the lower limbs can be placed in the 'frog position' where the hips are abducted, laterally rotated and flexed to 40° before moving the upper limbs.

The importance of detail when giving passive movements cannot be overemphasized if the functional range in all structures is to be maintained.

If the patient has not had any passive movements for a week or more since being injured, the movements should be commenced extremely cautiously, avoiding full range for a few days. It is possible that minor contractures are present which, if torn, may give rise to heterotopic ossification (Silver 1996).

Cautions

1. *Extreme* range of movement must be avoided, particularly at the hip or knee, as the tearing of any structures may be a predisposing factor in the formation of para-articular ossification.
2. Only 45° abduction is given, to avoid tearing any structures on the medial side of the thigh. The medial side of the knee must always be supported to prevent stretching the medial ligament.
3. Flexion of the hip with the knee flexed is cautiously carried out where there is a fracture of the lower thoracic or lumbar spine to ensure that movement does not occur around the fracture site. If pain occurs on

movement, flexion is limited to the pain-free range. The range of movement is gradually increased as the pain at the fracture site diminishes. When the patient is supine, full flexion of the knee can only be obtained by combining knee flexion with lateral rotation of the hip.
4. Straight leg raising is taken only to 30° because of the danger of putting a stretch on the dura mater for the first 6 weeks post-injury. After that, with medical agreement, this can be increased to 60°. This angle is not increased further whilst the patient is on bed rest.
5. Combined flexion of the wrist and fingers is never given. This movement can cause trauma of the extensor tendons, resulting in loss of mobility and function.

Maintenance of muscle length

Gross contractures occur when a paralysed limb is not moved, but contractures can also occur in individual muscles or muscle groups in a limb which is receiving daily treatment. For example, contractures readily occur in the following situations:

- where the muscle on one side of a joint is innervated and the opposing muscle is paralysed
- where a paralysed muscle passes over more than one joint – in this case, individual joint movements are insufficient to maintain the muscle length
- when the patient lies with the spine in hyperextension to heal a fracture, the degree of hyperextension necessary to correct fracture dislocations of the lower thoracic and lumbar spine inevitably produces slight flexion of the hip joints. Where the cervical spine is fractured, the shoulders are held in elevation and retraction due to gravity and unopposed muscle pull.

For these reasons, the following movements must be given in addition to the full range of passive movements.

The shoulder girdle. Particular attention needs to be given to the shoulder girdle. It is so freely movable that its habitual position depends upon the relative tension in the following six muscles which act indirectly on the shoulder girdle through the arms:

- trapezius – cranial 11, C3, C4
- levator scapulae – C3, C4, C5
- rhomboids – C5
- serratus anterior – C5, C6, C7
- pectoralis minor – C8, T1
- subclavius – C5, C6

together with the tension produced by:

- pectoralis major – C5, C6
- latissimus dorsi – C6, C7, C8.

The mobility of the shoulder girdle is largely maintained through adequate unilateral and bilateral passive movements to the arms, which will prevent shortening of these muscles.

The scapula. Mobility of the scapula must be maintained. Movements are performed passively in lying or side-lying with the elbow well supported by the therapist.

Passive depression is particularly important where the muscles of elevation are innervated and unopposed.

In situations where passive movements of the limbs are impractical, accessory gliding techniques should be applied locally to the joints involved to maintain mobility.

To prevent shortening of the:

Rhomboids. With the arms in horizontal flexion, adduct both shoulders at the same time. Both elbows are flexed and each hand moves towards the opposite shoulder.

Long head of triceps. With the arm held in elevation, flex the elbow.

Pectoral muscles. With the opposite shoulder lying in abduction to 90° outward rotation and extension and supported on a padded board, abduct and extend the shoulder with the elbow and wrist extended and with the forearm supinated.

The arms can be placed in the cruciform position whilst giving passive movements to the lower limbs.

Biceps. Pronate and supinate the forearm with the elbow flexed and with the elbow extended. (Pronation is particularly important for patients with lesions at C5, since biceps pulls the forearm into supination, which is not a functional position.)

Flexor tendons of the fingers. Extend the wrist and fingers together.

Flexor muscles of the arm. Elevate and laterally rotate the arm with the forearm supinated and the elbow, wrist and fingers extended and with the arm held close to the side of the head.

Hip flexors, quadriceps and anterior fascia of the thigh. In side-lying, extend the hip through the last 15° of movement, keeping the knee flexed. The posterior aspect of the hip must be well supported to prevent movement occurring in the spine.

Tensor fascia lata. Adduct and medially rotate the leg beyond the midline.

Tendo Achillis. Dorsiflex the ankle with the knee extended.

Flexor muscles of the toes. Extend the toes, dorsiflex the ankle and extend the knee. Clawing of the toes occurs easily and not only hinders walking and increases spasticity but may lead to pressure sores on the dorsal and/or plantar aspect of the toes.

Careful attention must also be given to movements involving rotation and flexion of the limb. For example, flexion and lateral rotation of the hip with flexion of the knee are important for self-dressing.

Inspection of the lower limbs

Before commencing treatment, the therapist examines the legs for signs of swelling or pressure. Deep vein thrombosis is a common complication during the early weeks after injury, and the possibility of pressure sores is an ever present danger. If a deep vein thrombosis is diagnosed, passive movements to both lower limbs are discontinued because of the possibility of causing a pulmonary embolus. Movements are recommenced when the anticoagulation therapy is successful.

Active movements

Cervical cord lesions

Gentle, assisted, active movements are given to all innervated muscles from the first day after injury. Progression is made to unassisted active exercises and the patient is encouraged to move his arms independently and functionally as soon as possible.

Where possible, the following movements are taught.

Extension of the elbow without triceps. The patient laterally rotates and protracts his shoulder, relaxes biceps and allows gravity to extend the elbow. Independence in this movement should be achieved as soon as possible to prevent shortening of the biceps tendon.

Flexion of the shoulder without flexion of the elbow. The patient is encouraged to lift the arm off the bed, allowing gravity to keep the elbow extended. Lateral rotation of the shoulder may be necessary initially.

Grip without finger movements – wrist extension grip. The grip is obtained by first allowing gravity to flex the wrist when the fingers and thumb fall into extension. The hands or the first finger and thumb are placed over the object to be lifted. Extension of the wrist by extensor carpi radialis places passive tension on the flexors and enables a light object to be held in position. If the object is heavier, the pull of gravity can be partially overcome by supinating the forearm.

Although the efficacy of the wrist extension grip can be augmented by allowing some shortening of the finger flexors, not all therapists agree with this approach. Of those who do, some advocate that this shortening should be allowed to develop from the outset, while others believe that it should be allowed to occur only when there is no further hope of functional recovery.

Resisted movements. Gentle resisted movements can be gradually introduced as indicated. Strong unilateral exercise for the whole arm involves head movement and is therefore completely avoided until the fracture is healed. All movements must be given with carefully graded resistance, avoiding any neck movements.

Neck exercises. Gentle static neck exercises are given 6 weeks post-injury if there are no contraindications.

Thoracic cord lesions

Patients with thoracic cord lesions are given frequent resisted arm exercises, manually or by using a chest expander of suitable strength, hand weights or other equipment. All movements are given bilaterally and in a controlled manner when the patient is supine, so that resistance is constant and there is no unequal pull on the unstable spine.

5

Respiratory therapy

Ida Bromley   Sarah Brownlee
Lone Rose

When the spinal cord is damaged, the respiratory muscles innervated below the level of the lesion become paralysed. This interferes with the power and integration of the remaining muscles and reduces their ability to drive the chest wall efficiently. Patients with injuries to the cervical spine have serious problems, whilst those with lower thoracic and lumbar lesions have very little impairment of lung function. All acute lesions need prophylactic respiratory therapy as all are subject to hypostatic pneumonia. The patient with partial or complete paralysis of any of the muscles of respiration will need special care.

FUNCTION OF THE CHEST WALL AND RESPIRATORY MUSCLES

The current view of the action of the respiratory muscles on the chest wall is that an integrated activity of many muscles is probably required to expand the ribcage in the most efficient way.

The respiratory muscles comprise three main groups: the diaphragm, the intercostal/accessory muscles and the abdominal muscles. These muscles act upon the chest wall either as prime movers or to strengthen the ribcage and facilitate the action of the others.

Diaphragm – innervation C3, C4, C5

The diaphragm is the main muscle of inspiration. As the diaphragm contracts, the central tendon is pulled downwards and forwards, pushing before it the abdominal viscera. It expands the ribcage, using the abdominal viscera as a fulcrum. The efficiency of the diaphragm depends on this balance of both ribcage and abdominal compliance.

In patients with spinal cord lesions above C5, the diaphragm may be partially or completely paralysed. Its function can be assessed by inspecting or palpating the upper abdomen during inspiration. When the diaphragm's function is impaired, the negative intrathoracic pressure during inspiration sucks the diaphragm up into the chest and the upper abdomen will move inwards. The findings of Sinderby et al (1992), who investigated eight tetraplegic patients, imply that the diaphragm acts as a trunk extensor in addition to its respiratory function in these patients.

Intercostal muscles – innervation T1–T7

The internal and external intercostal muscles have both inspiratory and expiratory action. At lower lung volumes, their function is inspiratory and at higher volumes it is expiratory. When breathing is stressed, the intercostals may alternate with other inspiratory muscles; for example, when the diaphragm becomes fatigued, the intercostals may take over as the main inspiratory muscle until the diaphragm recovers. The ability to rotate the use of inspiratory muscles when fatigued is reduced if the intercostal muscles are paralysed. The reduction in respiratory muscle reserve makes fatigue and failure more likely. The intercostal muscles also stabilize the chest wall, in full inspiration they contract to prevent the intercostal spaces being sucked inwards by the negative intrathoracic pressure generated by contraction of the diaphragm. When the intercostal muscles are paralysed, paradoxical movement of the intercostal spaces on inspiration may occur.

Accessory muscles – innervation C1–C8

Scaleni

The scaleni muscles are now considered to be primary respiratory muscles. They lift, expand and stabilize the ribcage from their insertion on its upper part.

Sternomastoid and trapezius

The sternomastoid and trapezius are inspiratory muscles and contribute to inspiration only during exercise or stress. Usually they are incapable of providing long-term ventilation. In complete lesions above C3 where there is paralysis of the diaphragm, the accessory muscles become the main inspiratory muscles and can produce a vital capacity of 700 ml, particularly the sternomastoid and trapezius (Danon et al 1979). Diaphragmatic pacing may be considered if indicated in these situations (Glenn et al 1986). Clinical observation of the hypertrophy of the accessory muscles demonstrates their inspiratory role in tetraplegic patients (Short et al 1991).

De Troyer & Estenne (1991) attribute an expiratory function to the clavicular portion of pectoralis major in patients with lesions between C5 and C8. With the arms fixed, contraction of the clavicular portion on both sides of the chest pulls the clavicle and manubrium sterni downwards, taking with them the upper part of the ribcage. The anteroposterior diameter of the upper ribcage is thus reduced. This action was associated with a rise in intrathoracic pressure, which was transmitted through the diaphragm to the abdominal cavity. The anteroposterior diameter of the abdomen increased. It is suggested that latissimus dorsi and teres major (C5, 6, 7) fix the humerus and prevent pectoralis major from shortening excessively. Thereby, they facilitate the action of pectoralis major in pulling down the manubrium sterni. It is also suggested that cough is active and not passive in patients with lesions at this level.

Abdominal muscles – innervation T6–T12

The internal and external recti, oblique and transversus abdominal muscles are the most important muscles of expiration (De Troyer et al 1983). In quiet breathing, expiration is usually a passive process achieved by relaxation of inspiratory muscles. In forced expiration, e.g. coughing or sneezing, the abdominal muscles contract strongly. The action of the abdominal muscles is also important in maintaining the position of the diaphragm and hence its efficiency. In the erect posture, the abdominal muscles contract to maintain the diaphragm in the dome-shaped position above the lower ribs by pressing on the abdominal contents and raising intra-abdominal pressure (De Troyer et al 1983).

Paralysis of the abdominals, as in high thoracic or cervical cord injuries, results in severe impairment of forced expiration. Sputum retention may occur, causing microatelectasis, major segmental, lobar or lung collapse and an increased susceptibility to infection. Microatelectasis may result in ventilation and perfusion mismatching, causing hypoxia (usually with a normal or low CO_2). This can cause additional damage to the spinal cord.

During the period of spinal shock, when there is an absence of tone in all muscles below the level of the lesion, the distensibility of the ribcage and abdominal wall prevents the diaphragm from inflating the lungs in the most effective way. When the period of spinal areflexia is over, the reflexes return and the degree of tone in the intercostal muscles will, in general, improve the stability of the ribcage. It also provides some resistance in the abdominal muscles, thus rendering the action of the diaphragm more effective (Guttmann & Silver 1965, Silver & Moulton 1970).

The fall in vital capacity below the value that would be expected from the loss of motor power alone, and the rise which often occurs even in the absence of neuromuscular activity reflect the distortion of the ribcage and its later improvement as tone returns to the intercostal muscles and the ribcage joints stiffen (De Troyer et al 1983, Morgan & De Troyer 1984).

As a result of the paralysis of the respiratory muscles:

• The patient is unable to perform active, expulsive expiration.
• Total ribcage and lung inflation is impossible.
• The partial loss of inspiratory muscle function allows the pleural pressure generated by the diaphragm to distort the ribcage, which results in paradoxical motion. This can be seen in the absence of tone when the intercostal spaces are indrawn during inspiration. This increases the work of breathing and reduces the effectiveness of the action of the diaphragm.
• Without active abdominal muscles, the patient is unable to cough.
• The inability to inflate parts of the lung and to clear secretions tends to produce microatelectasis with subsequent fibrosis of lung tissue.
• Immediately after injury, small areas of collapse interfere with ventilation and may result in transient hypoxaemia.
• The reduction in available muscle power and the increased load placed on the remaining muscles of respiration increase the likelihood of respiratory muscle fatigue and failure (Morgan et al 1984).

EFFECT OF POSTURE ON RESPIRATION

In the supine position, the action of the diaphragm is aided by the weight of the abdominal viscera displacing the diaphragm cranially and assisting inspiration.

Paralysed abdominal muscles allow the abdominal viscera to fall downwards and forwards when the patient is erect. The diaphragm then descends lower into the abdominal cavity and may lie below the lower ribs at the start of inspiration. When the diaphragm contracts, the lower ribs are pulled inwards, reducing the lateral diameter of the lower chest instead of, as is usual, lifting the lower ribs and increasing the lateral diameter.

Research has shown that the vital capacity of the tetraplegic patient improves by 6% when the patient is tipped 15° head down from the supine position, and falls by approximately the same amount when the head is tipped up 15°. The vital capacity may fall as much as 45% when the patient is tilted towards the standing position.

The use of abdominal binders can lessen the change of vital capacity in the upright position.

Care must be taken that they do not restrict the movements of the ribcage (Goldman et al 1986).

GENERAL PRINCIPLES OF RESPIRATORY PHYSIOTHERAPY

Respiratory physiotherapy plays a significant role in the care of patients with spinal cord injury. When there is respiratory muscle paralysis, the inspiratory force and volume are reduced and the ability to produce a forced expiration with raised intrathoracic pressure may be absent. The vital capacity can be as low as 30% after injury and may fall further after the first few days, largely due to ascending oedema within the spinal canal (Ledsome & Sharp 1981). It then improves quite rapidly for the first 3–5 weeks, with further slow improvement up to 5 months. The improvement is due to resolving oedema, increased spasticity of the intercostal muscles reducing paradoxical movement, and possibly some reinnervation. Patients may also become hypoxic due to the reduced respiratory function and sputum retention. Respiratory muscle fatigue may occur. The principle of respiratory treatment is to replace the function of the paralysed respiratory muscles, and the aim is to maintain respiratory function by:

- promoting sputum mobilization and expectoration
- reducing airway obstruction
- improving ventilation and gas exchange.

It is important to maintain continuity with the patient by having one physiotherapist in charge of his care and, where possible, to educate and support helpers, medical staff and family in the patient's respiratory care.

Prophylactic treatment

Frequent respiratory assessment is essential for an effective treatment programme which needs to be constantly modified.

The assessment will include:

- history of present and relevant associated injuries

- past medical history, in particular respiratory or cardiovascular problems
- inspection of movement, using vision or palpation to assess paradoxical movement and diaphragmatic function
- strength and efficiency of cough
- auscultation, in particular listening for uniform air entry, crackles or wheezes in all lung areas
- vital capacity measurements (care should be taken not to tire the patient)
- blood gases
- chest X-rays.

Breathing exercises

Breathing exercises can be useful in maintaining lung expansion in all areas. Treatment should begin as soon as possible to minimize respiratory muscle-wasting. Apical, basal, lateral and diaphragmatic breathing exercises are usually taught twice daily. The emphasis is on relaxed comfortable breathing without excessive effort.

Training programmes for the respiratory muscles using various methods of resistance, e.g. incentive spirometry, are given in some spinal units. Biofeedback can also be used. The aim is to improve strength and endurance and to postpone fatigue. It is hoped that prophylactic training will increase respiratory reserve and enable the patient to deal more effectively with respiratory problems. This subject merits further investigation.

Positioning and postural drainage

The frequent repositioning to prevent prolonged pressure is also beneficial for respiratory care. Postural drainage, using gravity to free secretions from the peripheral airways, can be used if the patient's condition is stable, and where necessary the traction can be maintained. Padded head supports can be used when turning the patient from side to side to maintain alignment of the cervical spine.

Forced expiration

Patients with paralysis of their abdominal

muscles are unable to cough, and assistance to do so is required to prevent sputum retention and lung collapse.

Normal cough

A single cough consists of a rapid deep inspiration followed by a forced expiration against a closed glottis, which is followed by a sudden opening of the glottis with continued expiratory effort. The effectiveness of the cough depends on the linear velocity of the gas in the airways. At high lung volumes, the cough is effective in clearing secretions from the large airways. At low lung volumes, it becomes more effective in the small airways (Macklem 1974).

Spinal patients are unable to achieve high lung volumes. They are able, provided the vital capacity is not too severely affected, to bring sputum from the small to the large airways and they then need assistance with coughing to expectorate (Cheshire & Flack 1979). The forces generated in a cough are not due to active contraction of muscle but are the result of elastic recoil of the lung and thoracic tissue generated by the previous breath.

Assisted coughing

The patient with partial or complete paralysis of the abdominal muscles is unable to cough effectively. The therapist can replace the function of the paralysed abdominal muscles by creating increased pressure underneath the working diaphragm.

Methods of assisting the patient to cough. When the patient is supine, there are two main methods by which one therapist can assist the patient to cough:

• *Method 1.* One forearm is placed across the upper abdomen of the patient with the hand curved around the opposite side of the chest. The other hand is placed on the near side of the chest. As the patient attempts to cough, the therapist simultaneously pushes inwards and upwards with the forearm, stabilizing and squeezing with the other hand (Fig. 5.1).

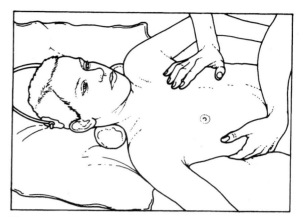

Figure 5.1   Assisted coughing. Method 1 using one therapist.

• *Method 2.* The hands are spread anteriorly around the lower ribcage and upper abdomen, and with elbows extended the therapist pushes inwards and upwards evenly through both arms as the patient attempts to cough (Figs 5.2a, b).

As it is essential for the effectiveness of method 2 that the therapist's arms are kept extended, this method may prove impractical when the patient is on a high bed. With the patient in the lateral position, method 1 may be preferable.

One therapist may not be able to give the necessary pressure to produce a cough, if, for example, the sputum is tenacious or the patient has a large thorax or is easily exhausted. In this case, two therapists working together are usually effective, using one of the methods described below:

• *Method A.* Standing on either side of the bed, the therapists place their forearms across the chest with the hands curved around the opposite side of the chest wall. The arms are placed alternately with the lowest arm across the diaphragm. When the patient attempts to cough, the therapists simultaneously squeeze the chest (Fig. 5.2c).

• *Method B.* Standing on either side of the bed, each therapist spreads his hands over the upper and lower ribs of the same side with the fingers pointing towards the sternum. When the patient

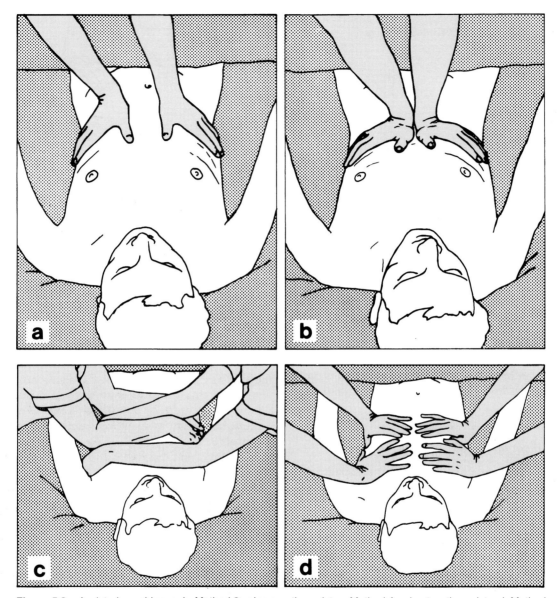

Figure 5.2 Assisted coughing. a, b: Method 2 using one therapist. c: Method A using two therapists. d: Method B using two therapists.

attempts to cough, the therapists simultaneously push on the chest wall (Fig. 5.2d).

Whichever method is used, the pressure must be even and firm with the weight of the therapist's body behind the 'push'.

The effectiveness of the cough depends on the simultaneous effort of the patient and therapist(s). For maximum effect, the pressure behind the push should be held until the very end of expiration and the force applied should be sufficient to deliver the sputum to the mouth. The sound of the cough produced is usually a good guide to the force needed.

It is essential to teach the techniques of assisted coughing to medical staff involved in the care of the patient, as well as to relatives, since the same techniques can be used if the patient is choking. Once up in his chair, the patient will need to be shown how to cough by himself or be assisted by another person.

Caution. Great care must be taken to avoid causing any movement or pain at the fracture site. Pressure on the abdominal wall alone must be avoided, as a patient with an acute lesion may have a paralytic ileus, internal damage or a bleeding gastric ulcer. Extreme care must be taken when assisting the patient to cough in the presence of any of these complications. The methods described above involving two therapists may be preferable under these circumstances.

Coughing in a wheelchair

To cough unaided, the patient himself must produce the pressure usually provided by the abdominal muscles. This can be done in the following ways:

• Hold one arm rest, press the other arm against the abdomen and lean well over it.
• Flex one elbow behind the chair back or chair handle; those with wrist flexors can hold the wheel. Press the other arm against the abdomen and lean over it (Fig. 5.3).
• Hold both armrests or flex the elbows behind the chair handles and lean over until the chest is pressing against the thighs (or abdomen if large) (Fig. 5.4).

To assist a patient to cough in a wheelchair. The therapist stands behind the chair and, linking her hands in front of the patient, pulls back against the upper abdominal wall and lower ribs (Figs 5.5 and 5.6). Should a second therapist be required, she stands in front of the patient and pushes on the upper thorax. If it is not possible to assist the patient from behind, the methods described on pages 35 and 36 may also be used with the therapist standing in front of the patient.

Caution. It is essential to stabilize the wheelchair when using these methods with the patient sitting, either by anchoring the rear wheels against a wall or with an assistant holding the chair from behind.

Frequency of treatment. It is important that the patient coughs several times a day to clear the throat even though the chest appears to be free from secretions. Patients with high lesions cannot clear the nose or throat unaided, and the normal amount of debris delivered daily from the lungs collects in the upper trachea. Although this will

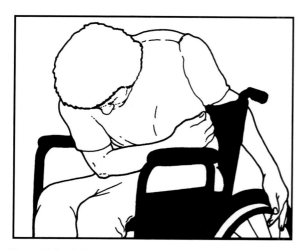

Figure 5.3 Independent coughing. Patient with a complete lesion below C7.

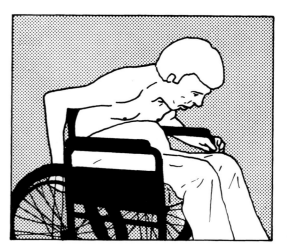

Figure 5.4 Independent coughing. Patient with a complete lesion below C6.

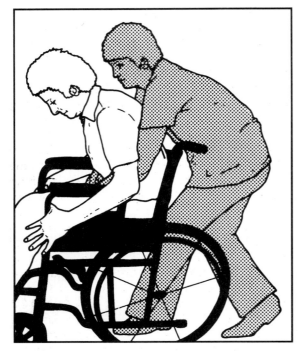

Figure 5.5 Assisted coughing in a wheelchair.

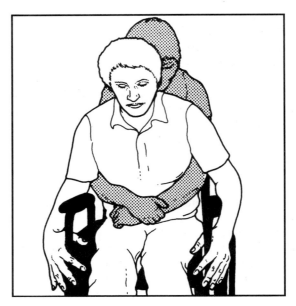

Figure 5.6 Assisted coughing in a wheelchair.

not cause distress for the first 2 or 3 days, towards the end of a week the patient will begin to experience some difficulty in breathing. Inspiration becomes slightly laboured and finally the debris is pushed down into the bronchial tree. At the end of the week, a patient with a previously clear chest may suddenly develop a high temperature and be found to have pneumonia or collapse of a lung.

This can be prevented by prophylactic treatment given three or four times a day for the first 2 weeks at least. Treatment is subsequently given once a day until the patient is up in a wheelchair and able to clear his secretions unaided. Tetraplegic patients also need prophylactic postural drainage at least once a day. If a mobile cervical patient with a lesion at or above C5 gets a heavy cold, he should return to bed for 24 hours. This prevents the nasal secretions dropping down into the chest and causing congestion. He will need assistance to blow his nose and clear his throat.

Physiotherapy for respiratory complications

Respiratory complications, such as retained secretions, collapse of lobe or segment, and infections, require careful and more frequent treatment. The frequency of treatment depends upon the severity of the chest infection. 'Little and often' is a good maxim. If the patient tires quickly and has copious sputum, it may be necessary to treat him every hour, day and night for 24 hours. For less severe cases, treatment at each turn will be sufficient.

Assessment

Treatment is directed at the particular area affected. Regular assessments are important to initiate or change treatment.

Oxygen therapy. If the blood gases are abnormal, e.g. low PO_2, oxygen may be required, which can be given via mask, nasal spectacles, minitrac or tracheostomy.

Humidification. Secretions may be thick and difficult to expectorate, and in addition there may be some difficulty with blocked nasal passages. Humidification can be given via ultrasonic or jet nebulizers with saline. It may be necessary to warm the saline.

Drug therapy. The effect of these complications can be reduced where appropriate by the use of drugs, e.g. bronchodilators, antibiotics or steroids for asthma and chest infections. Coordinating the time of treatment with therapy produces the best results.

Sputum mobilization

Chest mobilization. Shaking and vibration on expiration may assist in loosening secretions in peripheral airways to allow drainage to the main bronchus, provided the movement does not compromise the stability of the fracture.

Postural drainage. Gravity can also assist in the removal of secretions. Unless contraindicated, postural drainage may be given to any lesion. Care is taken to gain the correct drainage position for the area affected within the limits imposed by the hyperextended position and the type of bed in use. It is important to give postural drainage before as well as after the turn, and essential when treating high lesions. If both lungs are congested and the uppermost lung is not cleared before the turn, as the patient is moved secretions may drain into the trachea, completely blocking it and choking the patient. This can be prevented if the uppermost lung is cleared before the patient is moved. The therapist should wait whilst the patient is turned and treat him immediately in the new position, before the sputum has a chance to settle.

Continuous positive airway pressure (CPAP) and positive expiration pressure (PEP). CPAP may be useful in the prevention of alveolar collapse (Harvey & Ellis 1993). PEP may also be used.

Intermittent positive pressure breathing (IPPB). IPPB can also be used, the objectives being to open small airways, reduce airway collapse and improve ventilation and perfusion. Although improvements in lung volume during IPPB seem to be of sufficient magnitude to be of clinical value, the vital capacity changes immediately post-treatment are of such small magnitude that their clinical value would be less certain (Stiller

et al 1992). This area is yet to be evaluated. If, as the evidence from this study suggests, IPPB does not have a clinically significant sustained effect on lung volume, it may have to be given at frequent intervals to have any beneficial effect on respiratory function. Furthermore, if the inspiratory breath can be increased by using IPPB then the elastic recoil of the lung is increased and this can improve expiratory flow, assisting in the clearance of secretions (Jackson 1983). In stable tetraplegic patients, lung volume expansion alone has no major effect on lung function, and Rose et al (1989) suggest that it may be more useful in combination with respiratory muscle training. If the expansion of the ribcage is achieved by mechanical means, then full range of movement may be maintained by the remaining inspiratory muscle action. Loaded expiration or incentive spirometry may be useful in increasing the strength of the inspiratory muscles. IPPB should be used with care due to the potential hazards. Positive intrathoracic pressure can reduce venous return to the heart and can therefore reduce cardiac output. IPPB can generate high intra-alveolar pressure, which can result in damage to the lung and may cause an increase of bronchospasm in patients with asthma or similar conditions. Therefore, it should be used with care in patients with unstable cardiovascular systems and asthmatics and is contraindicated in patients with a pneumothorax (Webber & Proyer 1995). In view of this, treatment should not exceed 10 minutes in duration, including rest periods, but should be repeated several times a day. Severely ill patients may tire very easily and clear instructions to the patient and patience on the part of the therapist are vital for the success of this treatment.

Respiratory physiotherapy in ventilated patients

Despite efforts, some patients may require ventilation because of deterioration in their condition. The criteria for this are determined by the medical staff. Respiratory failure occurs especially in patients with high spinal injury who may become fatigued, have extensive secretions which may be difficult to remove, and have fractured ribs with flail segments. These patients will have blood gas and chest X-ray changes and their general condition will have deteriorated.

Assessment

It is important to establish whether or not the patient's cardiovascular system is stable.

Caution. Physiotherapy may be contraindicated when the cardiovascular system is unstable.

Bagging. Bagging is manually inflating the patient via a 2 L water bag, or, if the patient is on peak end-expiratory pressure (PEEP) whilst on the ventilator, an Ambu bag with an Ambu PEEP valve can be used. Bagging is used to stimulate a cough and to mobilize secretions by increasing the expiratory flow and lung expansion. Treatment should not exceed 15–20 minutes. The following techniques should be used to avoid precipitating bronchospasm: following a slow inspiration, given via the bag, the breath is held for a few seconds to allow the poorly ventilated parts of the lung to be aerated, and then the bag is released quickly and expiration occurs, producing a high expiratory flow rate which will help to move the secretions. Chest mobilizations are used on expiration to further assist in mobilizing secretions.

Drug therapy. It may be necessary for the patient to be sedated so that an effective treatment can be tolerated. Adequate pain control may also be required. If there is evidence of bronchospasm, bronchodilators or other drugs can be given prior to treatment.

Suctioning. To prevent bradycardia occurring during suction, it is best to preoxygenate the patient, to use catheters whose size should be no more than half the diameter of the endotracheal tube, and to be as quick as possible. Whilst suctioning the patient, the physiotherapist can use the assisted coughing technique to help mobilize the secretions by increasing expiratory flow.

Caution. Pharyngeal suction can excite parasympathetic nerves, e.g. the vagus nerve, and as this cannot be compensated for by increased

sympathetic activity, a profound bradycardia and even cardiac arrest may result. Atropine should be available by the patient's bed, to be given intravenously by the nursing staff or doctor. Atropine may cause secretions to become thicker and therefore more difficult to remove.

Tracheostomy

It may be necessary to perform a tracheostomy to maintain a clear airway. A tracheostomy reduces the respiratory 'dead space' by approximately one-half. In consequence, each breath becomes more effective in oxygenating the blood and removing carbon dioxide. It facilitates the removal of secretions from the lungs and the control of oxygen administration. Initially a cuffed tracheal tube is used, as this provides an effective seal for the lungs against secretions or inhaled substances and will readily connect with the tube from the ventilator. Overinflation of the cuff for long periods can cause excessive pressure on the tracheal mucosa and lead to necrosis, sloughing and in due course stricture. This is prevented by inflating the cuff just enough to make the seal and by deflating the cuff at regular intervals for a short time. The tube should be changed frequently as the lumen can become blocked by encrusted, dried secretions. Speaking tubes can be used prior to complete weaning off the ventilator. If the removal of secretions is the only problem and the patient does not require ventilation a mini-tracheostomy may be useful. A small bore tube is inserted into the trachea through the cricothyroid membrane, facilitating the removal of secretions (Gupta et al 1989).

Weaning. Once the patient's respiratory condition has stabilized or improved, weaning may be considered. Sedation is usually stopped, and the patient is disconnected from the ventilator for short periods several times a day. A spirometer can be used to measure tidal volume and vital capacity, and a graph to show time off the ventilator can be a useful incentive. During the weaning period, which may take several weeks, the patient will need a great deal of encouragement. As patients on ventilators cannot talk and communicate, all feel insecure. Anxiety and/or fear, sometimes amounting to panic, is experienced during treatment (Bergborn-Engberg & Haljamae 1989). These anxieties are exacerbated when the ventilator is being removed. The patient should be told exactly what to expect and be warned against being too disappointed when improvement is slow, or when there appears to be no improvement at all for a time. The ventilator should be replaced whenever the patient asks for it, otherwise he may become afraid of having it disconnected again. During these periods off the ventilator, the therapist encourages the use of the diaphragm and the accessory muscles of respiration. Initially, 5 minutes or less may be tolerated, but as the diaphragm becomes stronger, longer periods are gradually achieved. Sleeping without the ventilator is usually very difficult, a problem that can sometimes be due to fear alone, but this can gradually be overcome. CPAP and nasal intermittent positive pressure ventilation (NIPPV) can offer useful respiratory support during this period.

Long-term ventilation

Patients with high cervical lesions, e.g. lesions above C4, may require long-term ventilation. For the patient to have some mobility and independence, all the necessary equipment, such as ventilator unit with a back-up system, mobile suction equipment, manual hyperinflation bag, suction catheters, gloves etc., must be attached to the chair and easily available at all times. Close liaison with those providing care in the community is essential if these patients are to be safely discharged to the home (see Ch. 13).

Diaphragmatic pacing

The development of the phrenic nerve stimulator has given some patients, who would otherwise be totally dependent on a life support system, a new independence (Collier & Wakeling 1982). A paralysed diaphragm may be electrically stimulated if the lower motor neurones in the phrenic nerve are intact and the cell bodies in the C3, 4 and 5 segments are viable. Some or all of the phrenic nerve cell bodies or lower motor

neurones may have been destroyed. The viability is first established by percutaneous stimulation of the phrenic nerve. Contraction of the diaphragm is estimated by X-ray screening, ultrasound or palpation. Surface electrodes in the lower intercostal spaces may be used to measure the phrenic nerve conduction time. If the results are satisfactory, electrodes are placed on the phrenic nerve, in either the neck or the thorax, and connected to a receiver embedded in the skin of the anterior chest wall. A radio transmitter is placed on the skin surface over the receiver and the phrenic nerve is stimulated (Glenn et al 1984). The aim is to enable the patient to breathe via the stimulator initially during the day, and eventually, for 24 hours if possible.

Patients with diaphragmatic pacers are discharged from hospital earlier, are able to communicate more naturally and are better at manipulating the power drive wheelchair than patients on mechanical ventilation (Esclarin et al 1994).

OTHER CONDITIONS AFFECTING RESPIRATORY FUNCTION IN THE SPINAL PATIENT

Patients with spinal cord injury may have associated injuries or conditions and treatment must be adapted accordingly.

Paralytic ileus and gastric dilation

The initial signs of this complication, often first noticed by the physiotherapist, are distension of the abdomen and/or complaints by the patient of difficulty in breathing. This can be particularly dangerous for the tetraplegic patient with his already compromised respiration. Assisted coughing must be given with great care to avoid regurgitation, vomiting or aspiration. If such a patient is likely to vomit, he is turned from side to side only until the danger is past.

Head injuries

Physiotherapy may have to be adapted to prevent a further increase in intracranial pressure in patients with head injuries, e.g. turning, tipping, bagging, coughing and suctioning. Priorities in treatment must be discussed with the medical staff. The failure of the patient to understand or cooperate with treatment may cause problems. Sedation may depress respiration.

Fractured ribs

Special care must be taken when treating patients with fractured ribs to avoid further damage to the chest, including pneumothorax. A flail segment of rib may cause paradoxical movement of part of the chest wall.

Fat embolus

A fat embolus can follow a long limb fracture and is diagnosed by increased confusion, altered blood gases, petechial rash and retinal haemorrhages. Oxygen therapy and steroids are used in treatment.

Adult respiratory distress syndrome

Spinal patients can develop adult respiratory distress syndrome. Careful consideration is required as to whether physiotherapy should be given in such cases because of the pulmonary oedema.

Other respiratory complications

Underlying respiratory pathology may be present in patients who receive a spinal cord injury. Such problems may increase with a cervical injury, e.g. the symptoms of asthma. Prophylactic management may be required.

Cardiovascular conditions

Any circulatory problem can be complicated further by a spinal cord injury and treatment should be altered accordingly.

6

Pressure – effects and prevention

Ida Bromley   Lone Rose

The direct cause of pressure sores is pressure. It cannot be overemphasized that pressure sores are caused in bed or in the chair through prolonged pressure, which prevents adequate circulation to the area.

Contributory factors in patients with spinal cord injury

Loss of sensation and voluntary movement

The loss of sensation prevents the patient from receiving warning of long-standing pressure. He is not only unaware of the discomfort normally felt, but due to his immobility he is unable to shift his position to relieve it.

Loss of vasomotor control

The impairment of the circulation produces a lowered tissue resistance to pressure. Ischaemia due to local pressure therefore occurs more readily. The vasomotor paralysis is most extreme immediately after injury, and severe sores can be produced very rapidly. Although the vasomotor system is never subsequently normal, some improvement does occur when reflex activity returns to the isolated cord.

Effect of posture

Sores develop mainly over bony prominences which are exposed to unrelieved pressure in the lying or sitting position. The most vulnerable areas are the sacrum, trochanters, ischial tuberosities, knees, fibulae, malleoli, heels and fifth metatarsals. The occiput and elbows are also at risk in patients with cervical cord lesions. If the patient is placed in a plaster cast, sores may also develop over the ribs, spinous processes and anterior and posterior superior iliac spines. Pressure sores also readily occur under splints, plasters, calipers and braces applied over paralysed areas.

Pathology

The pathology may be summarized briefly as follows.

First stage

There is transient circulatory disturbance producing erythema and slight oedema. When pressure is relieved, this inflammation disappears within 48 hours.

Second stage

There is permanent damage to the superficial layers of the cutaneous tissues. Vascular stasis occurs, and reddening and congestion of the area do not disappear on digital pressure. The breakdown of skin or the development of blisters is followed by superficial necrosis and ulcer formation.

Third stage

There is penetrating and frequently extensive necrosis with destruction of subcutaneous tissue, fascia, muscles and bone. If the infection extends to the bone, periostitis and osteomyelitis will develop, which may result in the destruction of joints and the formation of ectopic bone. If unchecked, these major lesions may lead to general septicaemia and death.

Development of bursae. A bursa can develop, frequently over the ischial tuberosity, due to prolonged sitting. The surrounding tissues are rapidly involved if infection occurs, and a very small skin opening may be the only visible sign of a deep cavity reaching down to the infected bursa, and usually to the bone.

PREVENTION OF PRESSURE SORES

As Sir Ludwig Guttman used to say, 'Where there is no pressure, there will be no sore.'

Prevention therefore depends primarily upon the frequent relief of pressure in conjunction with the correct positioning of the patient (see Ch. 4).

Turning the patient

Patients are turned every 3 hours, day and night, using the supine and side-lying positions. Besides preventing the effects of prolonged pressure, regular turning also aids renal function by preventing stagnation in the urinary tract. The most susceptible areas, i.e. where bony points are close to the skin, must be kept free of any pressure by adjusting the pillows accordingly. At each turn, all such areas are inspected, the skin is checked and all wrinkles and debris are removed from the bed linen. Any evidence of local pressure, however minor, is an urgent warning. Redness that does not fade on pressure, septic spots, bruising, swelling, induration or grazing indicate an impending pressure sore. All pressure must be relieved from any area thus affected until it is healed. For example, if the sacrum shows signs of redness, the left and right lateral positions only should be used until the mark has completely disappeared.

At the National Spinal Injuries Centre, the Egerton–Stoke Mandeville 'electrical turning and tilting bed' is currently used to facilitate the 3-hourly turning of patients. This bed is divided longitudinally into three sections. On pressing a button, two of these sections elevate to 70°. The remaining third can be slightly raised to maintain the patient in position. The head and foot of the bed will tilt down to 15°. The Guttmann head traction unit is applied when skull traction is required. This unit enables constant cervical traction to be maintained when turning the patient. A face-piece supports the head in the lateral position. The senior nurse organizes each turn and ensures that correct spinal alignment is maintained whilst the patient is moved.

If the Egerton bed is not available, the patient can be positioned on a bed with sorbo-rubber packs. The space between the packs is altered to suit the position and stature of the patient, so that the bony prominences are free from pressure. The prone position is particularly useful for the non-acute lesion if the sores are on the sacrum, trochanters or ischia, or on all three sites. In this position, care must be taken to ensure that the toes, knees, iliac crests and genital areas are clear of pressure (Fig. 6.1). Support to the back is given by sandbags when in the side-lying position.

If sorbo packs are not available, pillow packs can be used. These are made by tying five or six pillows tightly together.

Body support systems are constantly being developed to facilitate the healing of pressure sores. The type of bed used has to meet the needs of the individual patient.

Care of the skin

The emphasis is on cleanliness and dryness. Intact skin is kept clean by the normal use of soap and water. No local applications of methyl alcohol etc. are used. Dead epithelium tends to collect, through disuse, on the soles of the feet and palms of the hand. It can be prevented and removed by thoroughly washing and towelling these areas and then rubbing in lanolin.

POSTURE AND SEATING

Any wheelchair user needs a well-fitting wheelchair with an effective cushion if the dangers of prolonged pressure and poor posture are to be minimized. Even the most sophisticated cushion cannot work optimally if it is not adequately supported by the wheelchair. It is therefore essential when assessing a wheelchair user that the wheelchair and cushion are considered as one unit.

The purpose of the seating is to offer the user a stable and comfortable base from which he can function at his full potential with maximum efficiency and minimum effort. It should also promote a symmetrical posture and provide adequate skin protection.

Posture

Most patients with a recent spinal cord injury will need some encouragement and support to adopt the correct position in the wheelchair, i.e. with the trunk and head symmetrical and all four limbs resting in normal alignment, the weight distributed evenly over as wide an area as possible and the anatomical curves of the

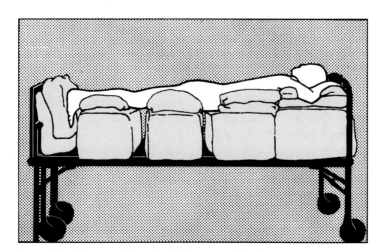

Figure 6.1   Prone position of patient on a pack bed.

spine maintained. For this to be achieved, the wheelchair and cushion must be the correct size for the patient.

The width of the seat should allow a hand to slide down between the hips (at the widest point) and the edge of the seat. The length of the seat must support the whole length of the thighs to within 5 cm (maximum) of the popliteal fossa. The backrest should be high enough to give adequate support without interfering with the shoulder girdle and upper limb function. A rough guide would be to have it no higher than the inferior angle of the scapulae and no lower than the level of sensation.

The footplates must be adjustable to allow the thighs to be in contact with the full length of the cushion. If armrests are used, they should allow the forearms to rest comfortably with the shoulders relaxed.

Assessment

The assessment of the seating requirements of a spinal patient is an ongoing process, as his needs will often change as rehabilitation progresses and after he returns home.

Due to the lack of, or altered, sensation below the level of the lesion, the patient will not receive the normal sensory input to tell him when he is adopting a normal posture in the chair. He needs time to learn to recognize when he is positioned correctly by using the sensory input from the unaffected parts of the body. To achieve this, it is crucial that this sensory stimulus is that of normal postural alignment from the first day out of bed, and this should be carried on throughout the 24 hour period, not just when the patient is up in the wheelchair. Attention to detail and a consistent approach to positioning in the early days of rehabilitation will soon show the benefit. The therapist needs to take a very active role in guiding and supporting not only the patient but also all other professionals involved with positioning the patient, whether in the wheelchair or in bed. This is particularly the case with patients who have high tone or patients with asymmetrical neurological deficit or incomplete lesions.

After the prolonged period of bedrest, the postural muscles unaffected by the spinal cord injury will inevitably be weak. It is beneficial if static neck and back extension exercises can be initiated during the last couple of weeks prior to getting up and carried on during the initial rehabilitation phase.

If the patient is struggling to maintain an upright and symmetrical posture, a body brace may be used (cf. three-point brace, p. 57). This is usually only necessary in the short term for patients undergoing initial rehabilitation. For some patients with established postural problems, it may be an effective long-term solution.

Once a postural problem has been identified, it is essential to establish whether it is fixed or correctable as this will determine the appropriate intervention.

Pressure and its measurement

Poor posture in the wheelchair will not only affect the patient's function and comfort, it will also affect the distribution of pressure and thereby increase the risk of pressure problems.

Apart from meeting the patient's need for postural support, the cushion must also be able to distribute the pressure over as wide an area as possible. The more the cushion can conform to the body's contours, the better it will achieve this. Measurements of pressure in sitting can be taken using a pressure transducer system. Capillary occlusion and tissue necrosis result from 13 to 34 mmHg of unrelieved pressure. The length of time that an individual can withstand a certain pressure over bony prominences varies greatly from person to person. (A guideline is given by Reswick & Rogers 1983.) If shearing forces, e.g. through bad posture or transferring, as well as vertical pressure are applied to the tissue, the process of tissue necrosis will be accelerated.

Interface pressures can be assessed by using either simple hand-held pressure transducer systems as described by Rothery (1989) and Dover et al (1992) or more sophisticated (and more accurate) computerized systems as described by Bar (1991), Henderson et al (1994) and Bogie et al (1995). Single cell transducers can help to identify peak pressures. However, interface pressure monitors which are able to map the entire seating area via a series of interconnected cells will give a more complete impression of the distribution of pressure. The cushion should distribute the pressure evenly throughout the contact area with no peaks and troughs. The *pattern* of distribution is of primary interest, not merely the absolute value of pressure measured at a certain point. Whatever system is used, it is important that the therapist takes into consideration the degree to which the pressure pad itself may interfere with the pressure-distributing properties of the cushion being assessed. Interface pressure measurements are an extremely useful adjunct to a full clinical assessment, but as most only demonstrate the pressure distribution at the moment of use, they should never be used as the sole indicator of a cushion's suitability.

Cushions

A wide variety of cushions is available worldwide. No one cushion will be appropriate for every patient. When selecting a cushion, the therapist will need to examine and assess not only the patient's posture and skin care needs, but also comfort, the method of transfer, the patient's balance and stability in sitting and his degree of independence. Some cushions, for example, may cause difficulties when transfer-

ring, may be too heavy for the patient or relatives to handle, or may not be available in the appropriate size. The user and anybody involved in his care after discharge need to understand how the cushion works and how to look after it. Where the user has more than one wheelchair, it is important that the cushion can be used in both. This also applies to any special back supports which may be used. Trial periods with more than one cushion may be necessary.

Cushions are made from different substances, including foam and gel emulsion. Some are a combination of a shaped, firm foam base with a fluid-filled (Flolite) pad on top, such as the Jay (Fig. 6.2), and some are air-filled, e.g. the Roho dry flotation cushion (Fig. 6.3). Many cushions are now designed to lower the ischial tuberosities into the cushion and to lift the distal end of the femur, promoting a more upright position of the pelvis (Green & Nelham 1991). Those cushions that have a divide between the right and left sides will offer the greatest postural control. The Jay 2 and Jay Medical cushions have several options for modifications (Fig. 6.4) which can be employed either for assessment or for permanent use. Depending on the material of the cushion and the way it is used, it may last for anything from 6 months to several years. The user must know the likely life span of the cushion, how to assess the wear and how to organize a replacement. Most cushions come supplied with an

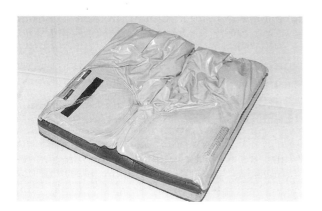

a

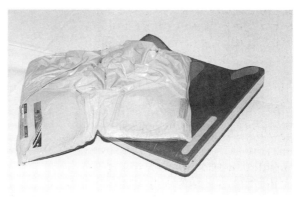

b

Figure 6.2   a: Jay 2 cushion without external cover. b: Jay 2 base and Flolite pad separated.

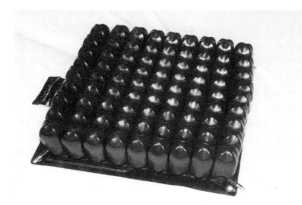

Figure 6.3 Roho Quadtro cushion. It has four intercommunicating compartments, allowing for greater stability and postural control.

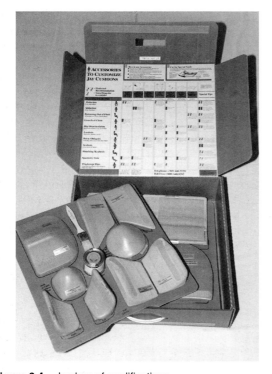

Figure 6.4 Jay box of modifications.

outside cover. Although the cover needs to be well-fitting, it must not detract from the conforming properties of the cushion, as the user will then be supported by the cover rather than the cushion itself. This is a common problem with PVC-type covers. The best material for a cover is a two-way stretchy cotton material, e.g. terry towelling.

Posture and seating clinics

The value of using posture and seating clinics as an integral part of the rehabilitation programme is well documented (Noble 1981, Rothery 1989, Dover et al 1992). They serve not only to facilitate early identification of problems through continual assessment of the individual seating needs of the patient, but also to create an important focus for education on matters relating to skin care and posture for patients as well as carers and staff. Patients usually attend for an initial assessment for wheelchair and cushion, and advice on posture and pressure prevention, as soon as they are out of bed. The patients continue to be seen regularly whilst in hospital and after discharge at follow-up outpatient attendances. Attempts are made to evaluate the quality of life of each patient, as social and psychological factors influencing behaviour inevitably have an effect on the incidence of pressure sores (Macleod 1988, Rothery 1989).

The long-term effects of ill-fitting seating should not be underestimated. It will reduce the user's function and increase pain and discomfort. The function of the inner organs may be compromised. The risk of contractures and deformities will increase as will the risk of pressure sores. If a sore develops, the cost to the patient can be catastrophic in terms of social isolation, poor psychological well-being and financial hardship, as prolonged enforced bedrest may put his employment at risk.

PRESSURE CONSCIOUSNESS: RE-EDUCATION IN SELF-CARE OF THE DESENSITIZED AREAS

Whilst the patient is in bed, the prevention of pressure sores is the responsibility of the medical team. As soon as he is mobile, this responsibility must be transferred to the patient if he is to remain free from pressure sores in the future.

Pressure relief

To allow adequate circulation to be maintained in the areas of maximum pressure, relief of pressure at regular intervals is essential, regardless of the type of cushion used. In the upright sitting position, maximum weight is taken on the ischial tuberosities. Therefore as soon as the patient sits in the wheelchair, the therapist must teach him the most practical method of pressure relief – by 'lifting', leaning side to side or leaning forward.

The ability to lift depends primarily upon the level of the lesion, although other factors, such as overweight or associated fractures of the arms, will obviously influence it.

Various methods of lifting for patients with lesions at different levels are shown in Figure 6.5. The position of the hands and trunk and the use of the head will vary considerably in patients with cervical lesions.

The simplest lift is achieved by pushing down on the armrests or the top of the rear wheel, straightening the elbows and depressing the shoulders (Fig. 6.5e–h). Lifting and repositioning should be done slowly and carefully. Patients with cervical lesions may only be able to lift one side at a time (Fig. 6.5a–d), and those without triceps need to hyperextend the elbows (Fig. 6.5c).

Often, patients are instructed to relieve pressure every 10 minutes for 10–15 seconds. However, recent studies of transcutaneous oxygen flow carried out at the National Spinal Injuries Centre, Stoke Mandeville Hospital, indicate that the oxygen levels take a lot longer to recover than 10–15 seconds. By placing an oxygen sensor over the ischial tuberosity with the patient in side-lying, a baseline reading of transcutaneous oxygen is established, as described by Bogie et al (1995). The sensor stays in place while the patient is transferred to the wheelchair and cushion currently being used and adopts his usual posture. As the ischial tuberosity is now weight-bearing, the effect of loading on the transcutaneous oxygen levels can be monitored. As the level of oxygen displayed on the monitor is visible to the patient, the educational benefit of this procedure is considerable. Inevitably the oxygen level will drop during loading. While carrying out pressure relief, the patient is encouraged to time how long it takes for the oxygen to return to unloaded levels. Usually this takes between 1.5 and 2 minutes. Few patients at the early stages of rehabilitation will have the strength or stamina to perform the traditional lift on the wheels or armrests for that length of time.

Different methods of pressure relief can be tried to find the one that is most effective and comfortable. For most patients, leaning forward is the most practical, either onto the elbows (Fig. 6.6a) or completely forward with the chest resting on the knees (Fig. 6.6b). For those patients unable to relieve pressure independently, leaning forwards may be the most suitable method, as a helper can easily provide the necessary assistance (Fig. 6.6c). The helper can stand either by the side or in front of the patient. If the patient is unable to tolerate leaning forwards or is anxious in this position, leaning sideways may be an alternative.

None of these methods may be practical for patients who have a lot of pain or who are ventilated. An alternative may be to tilt the chair backwards as long as the tilt is sufficient ($65°$), although this is not as effective as leaning forwards (Henderson et al 1994). To minimize the strain on the person assisting in this method, the assistant should be seated behind the patient with the wheelchair tilted back, resting against the knees. At each assessment, the method of pressure relief is reviewed. To give the patient more choice in adopting the most appropriate method in any given situation, he will be taught several methods if possible.

All patients are instructed to relieve pressure for 1.5–2 minutes once every half-hour, including during mealtimes and when out socially, e.g. visits to the cinema. In many cases the interval will gradually extend to once every hour. Pressure relief will eventually become second nature and the patient will do it automatically. Until that time, he will need to be frequently reminded and encouraged. If required, various pressure gauges with alarm systems are available to assist the patient to remember to lift.

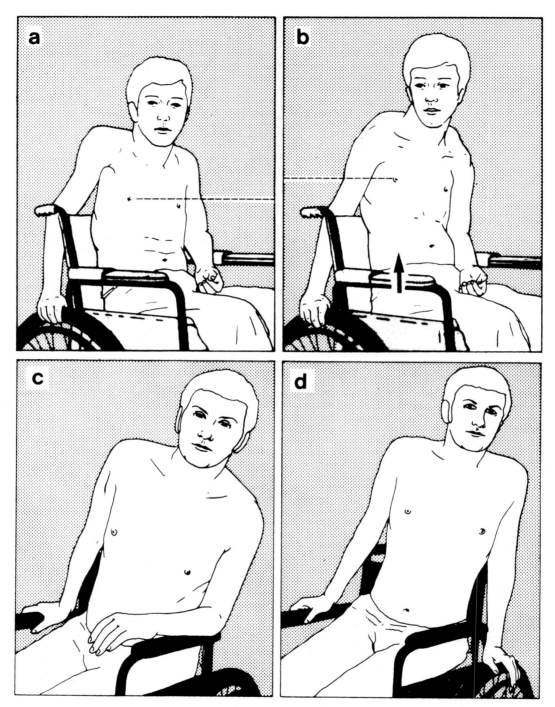

Figure 6.5 a, b: Patient with a complete lesion below C5. c: Patient with a complete lesion below C6 without triceps. d: Patient with a complete lesion below C7 with wrist control only.

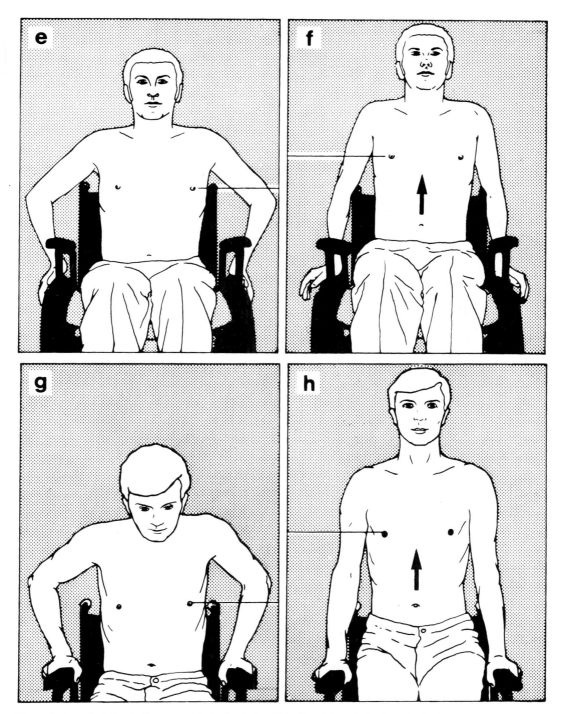

Figure 6.5   e, f: Patient with a complete lesion below C7 with wrist control only. g, h: Patient with a complete lesion below T5.

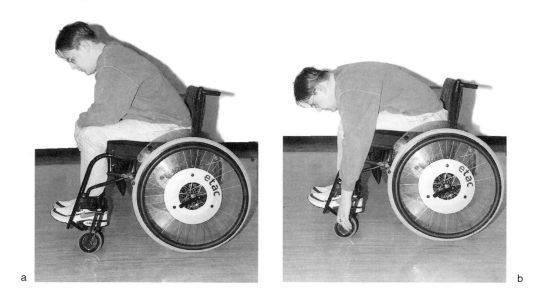

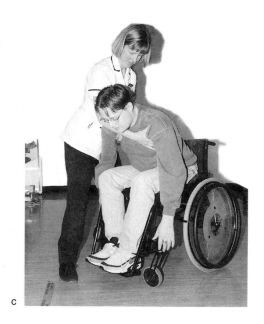

Figure 6.6 a: Forward lean onto elbows. b: Full forward lean. c: Assisted forward lean.

Some common problems and their possible causes

When the area most at risk of pressure is the sacrum or spinous processes, usually associated with a slouched posture/sacral sitting

• The backrest may be too high, pushing the top of the trunk forwards. This gives the user the feeling of falling forwards. To compensate, the hips are pulled forwards, causing posterior tilt of the pelvis.

• The backrest may be too low and the patient may extend over it, levering the hips forward and thereby allowing the pelvis to tilt posteriorly. A temporary back extension may help until the patient's balance and postural control have improved.

• The backrest is too upright. If there is a natural increase in the thoracic kyphosis, a straight back will force the trunk forwards when the hips are placed right back in the seat. The user will have no horizontal vision. A tension adjustable backrest (p. 94) can be adjusted to maintain control of the pelvis across the sacrum and lumbar spine but slackened off in the upper part to accommodate the kyphosis.

• If a lumbar cushion is used without the patient having adequate mobility in the lumbar spine and the ability to maintain the lumbar lordosis, it may gradually push the patient forwards and the posterior tilt of the pelvis will return. A tension adjustable backrest may provide a more effective and comfortable way of giving lumbar support.

• If a reclined position is needed, 90° at the hips must be maintained (unless hip flexion is limited) by wedging the front end of the cushion. This will prevent the patient constantly sliding forwards, which causes shearing across the sacrum. Alternatively, use a chair where the rear of the seat can be lowered, creating a tilt-in-space effect.

• The footplates are too low, which drags the user forward.

• The seat is too long, making it impossible for the user to place his hips right back in the chair.

• Footplate angle – if the footplates are angled away from the chair, this may pull on the hamstrings, effectively forcing the pelvis to tilt posteriorly.

• Prominent spinous processes, due to a gibbus, scoliosis or other spinal deformity, may cause pressure from contact with the backrest. A sheepskin or padding attached to the backrest may help to protect the vulnerable areas. A special fat-pad dressing may be used on the area itself.

• Other causes not related to seating may be long sitting in bed, poor transfer technique, inadequate mattress or lying supine for too long, tight-fitting clothes or pulling on the waist band of the trousers during an assisted transfer.

When the area most at risk of pressure is the one ischial tuberosity (unilateral), usually associated with a tilted posture, with one side of the pelvis lower (obliquity) and often with secondary scoliosis and rotation of the pelvis

• Sagging seat canvas. Most cushions are designed to sit on a flat surface. By placing it on a curved surface, the cushion itself will curve. It is very difficult to place the two ischial tuberosities horizontally on a curve. The sag can be eliminated by a solid seat insert made of wood, plastic or shaped foam positioned underneath the cushion.

• The seat is too wide, allowing the pelvis to 'float' to either side.

• Bad habits, e.g. hooking the same arm round the handle of the chair; low armrests; always leaning to the same side; working sideways from the same side of the chair. Education of the user plus some adaptation of the workstation may be needed. Improved stability within the chair may reduce the need for hooking the arm behind.

• Ossification of one hip may force one side of the pelvis up. This can be accommodated for in some cushions. Uneven muscle bulk or swelling can have the same effect. Asymmetrical neurology, both sensory and motor, can cause the user to adopt an asymmetrical posture. Early re-education is essential.

When the area most at risk of pressure comprises both ischial tuberosities (bilateral)

- The cushion is not sufficiently supportive and the user is sitting through it – 'bottoming out'.
- The footplates are too high. The weight will be concentrated over a smaller contact area, causing increased pressure at the back.
- A sagging seat canvas combined with a sagging back canvas can create a space between the back rest and the seat where the cushion is unsupported. A ridge of high pressure will be created where the slack is taken up, usually under the ischial tuberosities. Seat and back canvasses need replacing regularly to avoid this problem. A wooden base or other solid seat insert may prolong the life of the canvas.

When the area most at risk of pressure comprises the greater trochanters (uni/bilateral)

- the chair is too narrow, causing pressure at the hips
- inadequate support from the mattress on the bed
- infrequent turning at night
- tight clothing.

Turning at night

The patient must also become responsible for the prevention of pressure occurring during the night. He must learn to turn himself regularly in bed, to reposition the pillows between the legs and to ensure as far as possible that he is not lying on any creases in the bed linen. The interval between turns will depend on the condition of the skin and the type of mattress used.

Inspection of the skin

Care of the desensitized and paralysed areas of the body must form an integral part of the patient's daily life. He must learn to inspect his skin night and morning for pressure marks, abrasions and septic spots. Special attention should be given to the most vulnerable areas, i.e. the sacral, ischial and trochanteric areas, plus the knees, malleoli and toes. A mirror is used to inspect any areas the patient cannot view directly. Those patients who are unable to inspect their own skin must be responsible for requesting that this is done. If a mark is discovered, the cause of it must be determined in order to prevent it happening again.

The paralysed limbs

Great care must be taken in lifting the limbs whenever the patient transfers. A bruise sustained by knocking the malleolus against the footplate, for example, can become a deep sore and take weeks and even months to heal. Bruises devitalize the overlying skin and should be treated as pressure marks. As the vasomotor system does not allow adjustments of the circulation, care must be taken also to ensure that the desensitized areas are protected from excessive heat or cold.

Do's and don'ts

The patient is taught the following list of simple do's and don'ts when he first gets out of bed:

- *Do* relieve pressure in the chair for 1.5–2 minutes every half hour.
- *Do* lift the paralysed limbs when transferring.
- *Do* use a mirror for detection of marks, abrasions, blisters and redness on buttocks, back of legs and malleoli.
- *Do* watch for marks on the penis from the sheath.
- *Do* protect the limbs against excessive cold.
- *Do* have the bath water ready and not too hot.
- *Don't* open the hot tap when having a bath in case hot water drips on the toes.
- *Don't* have a hot water bottle in bed.

- *Don't* expose the body to strong sunlight; tetraplegic patients must wear a hat.
- *Don't* knock the limbs against any hard object.
- *Don't* carry hot drinks on the lap.

- *Don't* rest the paralysed limbs on hot water pipes or radiators.
- *Don't* sit too close to the fire.
- *Don't* leave the legs, particularly the feet, unprotected against car heaters.

7

Initial physical re-education

As soon as the spine has consolidated and the general condition permits, the patient is allowed to sit up in bed prior to sitting in a wheelchair. A support is usually worn for 2 or 3 weeks to prevent acute flexion until the spinal musculature becomes stronger. A padded, metal-framed brace with three-point support on the pelvis, the sternum and the midpoint of these two at the back is used for patients with thoracic lesions (Fig. 7.1). If a firmer support is required, a corset made from polypropylene is supplied by several firms. Those with cervical lesions use an anterior collar, which holds the neck in the anatomical position. Both thoracic and cervical supports can be made-to-measure or obtained commercially.

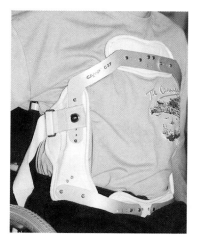

Figure 7.1   Three-point brace.

Programme for patient's activities

Once out of bed the patient, relevant members of the rehabilitation team and the ward sister liaise to work out a programme of increasing activity according to the patient's individual needs. For rehabilitation, the patient needs to wear loose clothing that is comfortable and easy to clean, and flat, lace-up shoes.

Initially the patient will attend the physiotherapy and occupational therapy departments for only a short period, approximately 1 hour in each department. Gradually, as the patient is able to stay up for longer, the programme is increased. As always, this will depend upon the patient's age, general state of health and previous medical history.

Assessment for a suitable wheelchair and cushion is undertaken as soon as possible.

IMPORTANT PHYSICAL FACTORS INFLUENCING THE RESTORATION OF INDEPENDENCE

As with all patients, age, sex, medical history, current associated problems and previous lifestyle play a part in successful rehabilitation. The majority of patients incurring injuries to the spinal cord are young males, for whom expectations for the achievement of independence should be high.

Previous employment and leisure activities inevitably affect the existing strength of shoulder and shoulder girdle muscles. A coal miner will have greater strength in the shoulders and be more used to using his muscles than an office worker. Similarly, a trained athlete, horseman or squash player has greater coordination and visuospatial appreciation than a patient who has never used his body in these ways.

The degree of motor function, the amount of spasticity present and the height and weight of the patient inevitably influence the restoration of independence. It is thought that the length of the arms in relation to the length of the trunk is also a factor.

Motor function

The degree of motor function, which depends upon the level of the lesion, is obviously a crucial factor in determining the independence finally achieved: 'Very considerable variations exist in the segmental supply of muscles which may influence the clinical presentation' (*Gray's Anatomy* 1995). An easy reference guide to the major segmental innervation of the most important muscles of the upper and lower limbs is provided in Appendices 3 and 4.

A rough guide to the amount of functional control of the joints of the upper and lower limbs at different segmental levels is given in Appendix 5.

A chart of progressive attainment in the four broad areas of daily living activities – personal independence, wheelchair manoeuvres, transfers and gait – is given in Appendix 6. Each activity is listed at the highest segmental level at which it is currently attainable.

Physical proportions of the patient

The physical proportions of the patient influence the ease and speed with which independence can be achieved. Height, weight and the length of the arms in relation to the length of the trunk appear to affect the rehabilitation of all patients with spinal cord injury, but particularly those with lesions complete below C6.

The most intrepid patients having led the way, therapists have gradually come to expect a greater degree of independence for these patients (Yarkony et al 1988). Achieving it, however, is expensive in effort and time for both the patient and the therapist and may incur extended hospitalization.

In order to identify those patients most likely to benefit from extended rehabilitation, it is necessary to determine the factors that differentiate between the successful and unsuccessful groups.

Physical ability in relation to anthropometric measurements in persons with lesions at C6

A study was undertaken at the National Spinal Injuries Centre in 1985 (Bergström et al 1985) to assess which anatomical and anthropometric characteristics of the patient with tetraplegia complete below C6 could be of value in predicting which patients would learn to transfer independently.

The 36 chronic patients were restricted to those with a transverse spinal cord syndrome complete below C6 where extensor carpi radialis was present and the triceps muscle was absent or graded 2 or less on the Oxford scale. There were 33 males and 3 females and the ages ranged from 18 to 52 years. 23 anatomical and anthropometric variables were selected in order to give as complete a picture of the patient as possible. Spasticity, although difficult to quantify, was included, as it was felt that, if severe, it could prevent patients from transferring independently. Two groups of patients were defined: those who could transfer independently from a

wheelchair to a surface of similar height (T) and those who could not (NT).

Table 7.1 shows the results for the total group of 36 patients, and for the subgroups representing transfer and non-transfer ability. It is interesting that the data does not show the 'monkey syndrome' (long arms and a short trunk) to be statistically significant for the ability to lift, although this is the subjective impression of therapists working in this field. Although not significant, functional arm length was greater in the T group.

The largest significant difference between the two groups was in the base triangular measurement. This measurement was devised to obtain an impression of how much the subject leans forward in sitting and lifting (Fig. 7.2). The 'triangle' was formed from:

Table 7.1 Means and standard deviations of all the measured and predictor variables for the total group and the subgroups (T, NT). The Student's *t*-value and its level of significance for the difference between NT and T groups are also shown

Variables	Units	Total group $n = 36$		NT group $n = 25$		T group $n = 11$		*t*-value	Level of significance
		$\overline{X}$	SD	$\overline{X}$	SD	$\overline{X}$	SD		
Age	years	28.4	7.9	29.1	9.0	26.7	4.8	1.0	ns
Weight	kg	65.7	14.3	68.4	15.0	59.6	11.0	2.0	ns
Stature	cm	176.1	9.2	176.3	9.3	175.5	9.4	0.2	ns
Sitting height	cm	93.1	4.5	93.4	4.3	92.2	5.0	0.7	ns
Cervicale to datum*	cm	66.3	3.6	66.6	3.3	65.8	4.2	0.5	ns
Right shoulder flex	cm	10.6	1.8	10.3	1.6	11.1	2.1	1.1	ns
Left shoulder flex	cm	9.9	1.7	9.7	1.5	10.5	1.9	1.3	ns
Biacromial width	cm	38.5	2.5	38.4	2.5	38.9	2.6	0.6	ns
Bitrochanteric width	cm	34.4	2.4	38.8	2.1	33.5	2.7	1.4	ns
Functional arm length†	cm	60.6	3.8	60.3	3.4	61.1	4.5	0.5	ns
Acromion to floor static	cm	59.0	4.2	59.1	3.5	58.8	5.7	0.2	ns
Acromion to floor lifting	cm	59.0	3.9	59.2	3.4	58.4	4.9	0.5	ns
Triangular base static	cm	12.5	5.6	11.6	4.0	14.4	8.1	−1.1	ns
Triangular base lifting	cm	13.0	5.4	11.0	4.3	17.1	5.4	−3.3	P<0.005
Head circumference	cm	57.9	1.8	57.8	1.8	58.1	1.8	−0.4	ns
Spasticity	Grade	4.6	0.6	4.5	0.7	4.7	0.4	−1.3	ns
Σ4 – skinfolds	mm	44.1	23.4	50.3	25.1	30.0	9.3	3.5	P<0.001
Fat (% of body weight)	%	17.9	6.6	20.1	6.3	12.9	4.1	4.1	P<0.001
Fat mass	kg	12.3	6.5	14.2	6.7	8.0	3.5	3.6	P<0.001
Fat free mass	kg	53.4	9.4	54.2	10.0	51.6	8.2	0.8	ns
Functional arm length/stature	Ratio	0.3	0.01	0.3	0.01	0.3	0.01	1.3	ns
Functional arm length/sitting height	Ratio	0.7	0.03	0.6	0.03	0.7	0.04	−1.4	ns
Functional arm length/cervicale to datum	Ratio	0.9	0.05	0.9	0.05	0.9	0.05	−1.3	ns

ns = not significant.
* C7 to ischium.
† Anterior aspect of head of humerus to base of palm.

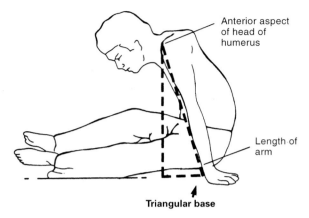

Figure 7.2 Triangular base.

- the perpendicular from the anterior aspect of the head of the humerus
- the distance along the floor to the hand
- the length of the arm.

The subjects with transfer ability leaned further forwards when lifting. This gives greater mechanical advantage as it balances the body more accurately over the acromial point which is the fulcrum for the lift.

There was a significant difference between the two groups in the data on total body fat. This indicates that additional weight as fat is detrimental when attempting to lift and transfer.

The NT group had considerably broader hips. This forces the subject to place the arms further away from the sides, which effectively reduces arm length and minimizes any mechanical advantage. Morphologically, females have narrower shoulders and broader hips than males. This data confirms the clinical impression that tetraplegic women do not lift as well as men and that fewer can transfer.

As 23 variables were considered to be too many for practical use, an analysis was carried out on these variables to assess the extent to which a smaller number of anatomical and anthropometric data could predict the final ability to transfer. Nine variables were finally selected:

- biacromial width
- body weight
- cervicale to datum
- fat percentage
- head circumference
- shoulder flexibility
- sitting height
- spasticity
- triangular base lifting.

Using these variables, it is possible to predict into which group (T or NT) a patient will fall with an accuracy of 90%.

However, this result is tentative due to the small size of the sample. Data needs to be collected from a further sample of patients, and the present results used to classify patients into the T or NT group, in order to assess the validity of the process.

Spasticity

There is no doubt that severe spasticity is one of the most incapacitating complications of spinal cord injury and can seriously curb rehabilitation, in some cases preventing even a minimal degree of self-care. Early positioning of acute lesions has a great influence on the development of reflex patterns of spasticity in both complete and incomplete lesions. With adequate early treatment, the majority of patients are left with a degree of spasticity which is useful to them in many ways and which does not inhibit daily life. Some patients, however, develop incapacitating spasticity in spite of treatment.

The problems arising from severe spasticity are dealt with in the relevant sections of subsequent chapters.

AIMS OF TREATMENT

The ultimate aim of rehabilitation is to achieve the highest degree of fitness, independence, balance and control which the patient's lesion permits. This is to be achieved by re-education and the fullest possible use of each muscle over which the patient has voluntary control. The immediate aims of treatment therefore are:

- readjustment of vasomotor control
- re-education of postural sensibility

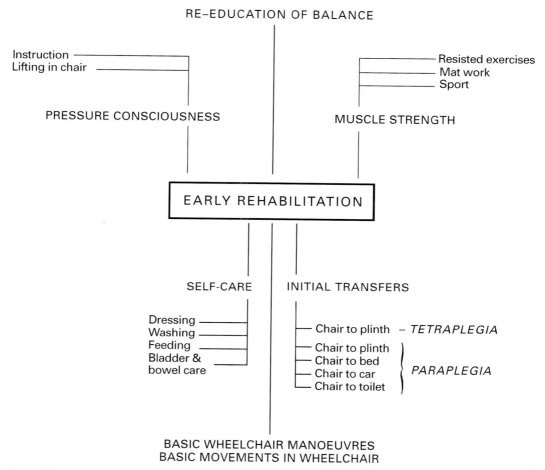

Figure 7.3   Early physical rehabilitation.

- the re-education and hyperdevelopment of the normal parts of the body to compensate for the paralysed muscles; the fulfilment of these aims is the foundation for restoring independence (Guttmann 1946a) (Figs 7.3 and 7.4)
- the education of the patient in self-care of the desensitized areas (see Ch. 6).

Those patients who have had some form of surgical intervention and spend less time in bed will follow the same overall programme of rehabilitation. Certain elements may have to be curtailed initially and progression will vary depending upon the procedure undertaken.

VASOMOTOR DISTURBANCE

Postural hypotension is particularly common in patients with cervical or high thoracic lesions. This is due primarily to loss of vasomotor control in the splanchnic area. The blood vessels in the viscera are unable to constrict when the body is raised from the horizontal to the vertical position. The vasomotor control that is lost cannot be regained, but the patient can overcome this by developing other vascular reflexes which are still intact.

The reflexes are trained in a variety of ways, by means of deep breathing exercises, tilting exercises in bed, frequent changes of position and

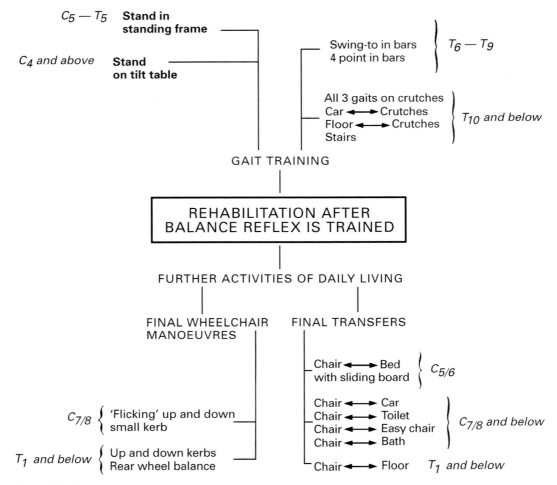

Figure 7.4 Independence expected according to the level of the lesion.

graduated balance exercises in the sitting and standing positions.

Before sitting out in the wheelchair, the patient is tilted in the bed. Gradual progression is made from the initial 30° until the patient can sit at 90° without feeling faint. Deep breathing exercises are given in each position. The time in the tilted position is lengthened gradually from 10 to 15 minutes to 3 hours over approximately a week. The skin over the ischia and coccyx is not accustomed to weight-bearing. Constant inspection is necessary as a pressure sore can easily develop.

Whilst sitting, the paraplegic patient should practise lifting his body weight on his hands. He can either push down on the bed or use wooden lifting blocks if available. This exercise helps to establish the vascular reflexes, increases the strength of latissimus dorsi and relieves pressure on the buttocks.

When vasomotor control is established in the bed, training is commenced in the wheelchair, initially for a few moments at a time. The process of gradually and regularly extending the time is repeated.

Active rehabilitation in the various departments commences when the patient can tolerate 1.5 hours in the wheelchair. At first the patient will need to be pushed to the departments. As he has not experienced motion of any kind for several weeks, even relatively slow speeds will seem alarmingly fast. As soon as possible, the patient should push himself and be responsible for keeping his own appointments.

Fainting

As fainting can occur, it is advisable not to leave the patient alone during the early days of vasomotor training in the wheelchair.

If the patient complains of feeling faint or dizzy, has blurred vision or appears white and sweaty, the legs must be elevated immediately and the chair tipped onto its rear wheels. Deep breathing is encouraged by giving pressure during expiration over the lower ribs and upper abdomen. Should loss of consciousness occur with no signs of recovery within a minute, the patient should be placed flat.

The vasomotor problem must be explained to the patient. Instructions should be given on how to aid the circulation when feeling faint by brisk movements of the arms and deep breathing. Encouragement is essential, as once a patient has fainted, fear of a recurrence may inhibit his activity.

POSTURAL SENSIBILITY

The patient with a complete spinal cord lesion has lost not only sensibility to touch, pain and temperature, and motor power of the trunk and limbs, but also his postural or kinaesthetic sense, below the level of the lesion.

Kinaesthesia is the perception of the position and movement of one's body parts in space. It also includes perception of the internal and external tensions and forces tending to move or stabilize a joint (Rasch & Burke 1971).

In complete lesions above T12 where postural sensibility in the hip joints is abolished, the patient has difficulty in keeping his balance in the unsupported upright position. The development of a new postural sense is a major objective in the rehabilitation of these patients. It is the foundation for all daily living activities.

Postural control is achieved largely through those muscles which have a high innervation and low distal attachment. These muscles form a bridge between the normal parts of the body, including of course the brain, and the paralysed areas. The most important of these muscles is the latissimus dorsi. It has a high segmental supply (C6, 7, 8) and an extensive attachment to the spine and pelvis. Therefore, in all lesions below C7, it bridges the paralysed and non-paralysed parts of the body and allows patients with high thoracic and low cervical cord lesions to regain a high degree of balance and control.

Proprioceptive impulses arising from any movement of the pelvis are transmitted centrally along the afferent nerve fibres of these normally innervated muscles and thus reconnect the insensitive part of the body with the cerebral and cerebellar centres promoting appropriate efferent postural responses to the paralysed area…. Eventually a new pattern of postural sensibility develops along the nerve supply of the trunk muscles. (Guttmann 1976)

Latissimus dorsi is important both in the restoration of the paraplegic's upright position and in future gait training. The function of this muscle is greatly assisted by other trunk and shoulder girdle muscles, particularly trapezius, because of its dorsal attachment as low as T12, and the abdominal muscles with their insertion on the pelvis.

The patient develops his new postural sense primarily by visual control. He performs exercises sitting in front of a mirror where he can see the position of his body and limbs. This visual–motor feedback helps him gradually to develop more acute sensory impressions, i.e. interpreting the muscle stretch sensations of the latissimus dorsi and other trunk muscles, and a new sensorial pattern becomes established. He will then perform movements without the aid of a mirror, and eventually functional activity without conscious effort to balance.

Balance exercises in the sitting position

These exercises are primarily carried out sitting on the plinth in front of the mirror, though some patients may need to begin their exercises sitting in the wheelchair (see p. 65).

Position of the patient

- The patient sits on a low plinth in front of a long mirror. A pillow is placed under the buttocks to guard against excessive pressure.
- The thighs and feet are well supported so that a right-angle is formed at the hips, knees and ankles.

Role of the therapist

- The therapist stands behind the patient so that she can watch his movements in the mirror and have control should he lose balance.
- Her hands initially support the patient either over the shoulders or around the thorax. Her hands should be visible to the patient. Should she put them where he cannot feel, he will be unaware of the support and lose confidence.
- Assurance is given that the therapist will not move away. The fear of falling, especially backwards, is very marked. The therapist should never leave her position unless the patient has some form of support, as he can easily overbalance and fall off the plinth. The position is obviously more dangerous for those with severe spasticity.
- The therapist can, to a large extent, control the speed of the patient's activity by her voice and her general handling of the situation. Her voice should be quiet and confident and, most important of all, unhurried since all exercise involving balance must be performed slowly.
- She should give constant direction and encouragement.
- When the patient overbalances, the therapist should allow a gross movement to occur before restraining him, otherwise he may not be aware of the movement that has taken place.

Progression of exercises

Self-supported sitting. Watching himself in the mirror, the patient learns to support himself in as upright a position as possible, with his hands first on the plinth at his sides and then on his knees. If the lesion is high and the arms are short in relation to the trunk, it may help to have a pillow at each side of the patient to support the hands. Time and trouble should be taken to teach the patient to hold the correct sitting position before commencing exercises involving motion.

Single arm exercises. Always watching himself closely in the mirror, the patient raises one arm first sideways, then forwards and lastly upwards whilst supporting himself with the other hand on his knee. A small degree of movement of the head and trunk to the side of the supporting hand will be necessary to compensate for the weight of the moving arm. Single arm exercises are not found to be helpful for patients with lesions at C6 or above, since without triceps the supporting arm is ineffective.

Bilateral arm exercises. Larger compensatory movements of the head and trunk will be necessary when moving both arms in the unsupported sitting position. The patient first tries to lift the hands from the knees to the arms bend position and then progresses to raising both arms sideways, forwards and upwards (Fig. 7.5).

The sideways stretch position presents little difficulty since the centre of gravity is barely altered.

In the forwards stretch position, the patient must lean his head and body backwards to counteract the line of gravity which would otherwise fall in front of the hip joints.

The upwards stretch position is particularly difficult for patients with high lesions, since the centre of gravity is raised and the patient has no abdominal muscles to help him to maintain his equilibrium.

Bilateral arm exercises without the mirror. When the patient has mastered the basic positions and exercises, bilateral exercises are performed without the mirror and with the eyes closed.

Other exercises. Balance can be further improved by, for example, asymmetrical work, altering the rate of movement, resisted trunk exercises, stabilizations and ball throwing.

Duration and frequency of treatment

These exercises are physically and mentally exhausting. Treatment is given daily for only

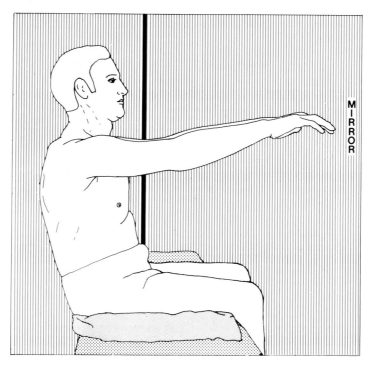

Figure 7.5   Balance position of a patient with a complete lesion below T6.

5–10 minutes initially, progressing gradually to half an hour. Frequent rests should be given during treatment by allowing the patient to lean back against the therapist for a few moments. Tetraplegic patients need to rest the head to allow the neck extensors to relax. Balance training requires constant practice and it is valuable to treat patients with thoracic lesions twice daily.

Balance in the wheelchair

Balance exercises are commenced in the wheelchair for the following reasons:

- Poor posture when sitting on the plinth. This occurs:
  - with high cervical lesions, C5 or above, where the head pokes forward and the patient is unable to extend the neck
  - with some thoracic lesions where the trunk is flexed due to weak extensor muscles. It may be necessary for such patients to concentrate on back extension exercises for

a week, balancing only in the wheelchair. When the general muscle tone has improved the patient can return to balance exercises on the plinth.
- General debility. The patient may not be fit to be moved in and out of the chair.
- Recently healed sores. The scar tissue may be delicate. Movement in and out of the wheelchair may constitute a potential danger until the scar tissue becomes stronger.

Exercises in the wheelchair are carried out in front of the mirror as described above, first leaning against the back of the chair and progressing to sitting away from the back rest. As soon as possible, balance on the plinth should be commenced or resumed.

Posture

Although the aim is to achieve as upright a position as possible, this will vary according to the level of the lesion.

The low thoracic lesion (with abdominal muscles) should have a straight back.

The upper thoracic lesion (without abdominal muscles) has a typical posture with increased kyphosis and lordosis.

The low cervical lesion usually has a good, straight posture providing trapezius is strong and the patient has not been allowed to sit on his sacrum for several weeks or months, producing a long kyphosis.

The high cervical lesion may have a poor posture with poking head and flexed spine or, where the neurological deficit is asymmetrical, a scoliosis.

Sport

Archery and table tennis are useful activities in training postural control.

MUSCLE RE-EDUCATION

To establish a satisfactory compensatory mechanism to cope with the paralysed limbs, all innervated muscles need to be as strong as possible (Guttmann 1976a). For patients with complete lesions, it is particularly important where possible to hypertrophy the following:

- latissimus dorsi
- shoulder and shoulder girdle muscles, particularly adductors
- arm muscles
- abdominal muscles.

The choice of technique for strengthening these muscles belongs to the individual patient and therapist. Methods currently used include:

- manual resistance, including proprioceptive neuromuscular facilitation (PNF) techniques (Knott & Voss 1968)
- spring and sling suspension therapy
- weights – tetraplegic patients can use weighted cuffs round the wrists
- weights and pulleys, including all types of multigym
- sport.

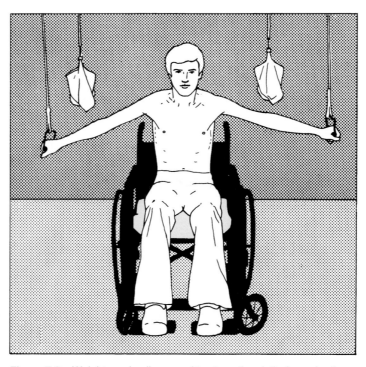

Figure 7.6 Weights and pulleys used to strengthen latissimus dorsi.

PNF is particularly useful for:

- patients with incomplete lesions with very little spasticity
- strengthening the trunk muscles
- strengthening the arms of patients with cervical lesions.

In the absence of more sophisticated systems, bilateral strengthening exercises for latissimus dorsi and the pectoral muscles can be carried out by paraplegic patients using a simple system of weights and pulleys (Fig. 7.6). With the pulley handles at shoulder level, the patient pulls down to the chair wheels keeping the elbows straight. If the elbows are allowed to flex, triceps will be strengthened and not latissimus dorsi as desired.

Body weight is useful as resistance in free exercises such as press-ups and lifting up on blocks.

Progression

In all exercise programmes, progression must be carefully graded both for strength and endurance and for the effect on cardiorespiratory function. It is often helpful for patients to watch in a mirror when performing exercises so as to have some visuospatial feedback.

Biofeedback can be useful in muscle re-education. It assists the patient to strive for maximum effort and enables him to measure his achievement.

8

Personal independence

Close cooperation between the occupational therapist and the physiotherapist is essential in planning the patient's rehabilitation programme. The work of the two disciplines complement one another and in many areas overlap.

All but those with the highest lesions need to learn to dress, and in addition tetraplegic patients must learn to eat and drink, brush their hair, clean their teeth, and wash and shave. All need to be able to instruct others as to how to undertake those tasks they cannot do for themselves. For all practical purposes, patients without finger movement can be divided into four groups: those with lesions at C1–3, C4, C5 and C6.

PATIENTS WITH LESIONS AT C1–3

These patients have varying degrees of head control and no other movement. They can use a computer and specially adapted environmental system with chin, breath, head or combined breath and head control. Although voice-activated computers are useful, they cannot be accessed by voice, and so have their limitations.

PATIENTS WITH LESIONS AT C4

These patients are without any muscle power in the upper limbs. By means of appropriate mouth sticks with a dental bite (Fig. 8.1h), they can learn to use a computer, word processor, calculator and dictaphone, turn the pages of a small paper or magazine, type, paint and play board games where the pieces have been suitably adapted.

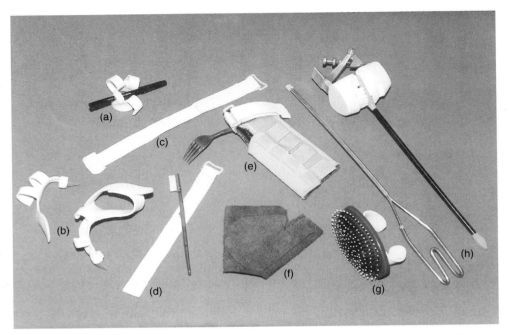

Figure 8.1 a: Finger splint to hold pen. b: Rubber tipped finger splints for using computer. c: Strap with slot for holding gadgets. d: Strap with slot and toothbrush. e: Wrist support with strap for fork. f: Pushing glove. g: Hairbrush. h: Mouthsticks, with dental bite and without.

PATIENTS WITH LESIONS AT C5

These patients have good functioning deltoids and biceps but no muscle control at the wrist. A light cock-up splint is used to stabilize the wrist joint. This contains a slot in the palmar surface to hold simple gadgets such as a spoon, fork or typing stick (Fig. 8.1e). With practice, most patients with lesions at this level learn to eat, type, move papers and operate a computer using a stick with a rubber cap, and to play games such as draughts, chess and dominoes with specially adapted pieces.

Mobile arm supports may be of use to patients with weak shoulder and/or elbow muscles.

Functional electrical stimulation (FES) in the upper limb

The neurocontrol 'Freehand system' is an upper extremity neuroprosthesis using FES to increase hand function for patients with spinal cord injury at C5. It was designed at Case Western Reserve University, Cleveland, Ohio in 1987 (Keith et al 1989). A programme was started in 1995 at the Salisbury district hospital, which is the European Training Centre for Neurological Control. Six patients have been fitted successfully with the neuroprosthesis (Kilgore et al 1996).

The system is designed to provide the patient with two hand grasps: the palmar or power grasp, where the fingers flex towards the abducted thumb, used for holding a glass and picking up large objects; and a lateral prehension grip, where the thumb adducts to the flexed fingers, used for small objects such as a key. The ability to open and close the hand allows the patient to have more control over everyday tasks such as eating, writing, using a telephone and inserting a computer disk.

A pacemaker-type stimulator is implanted in the upper chest on the side of the hand to be controlled, and from it electrodes control eight muscles in the hand, enabling the fingers to flex and extend and the thumb to abduct and adduct with the fingers in flexion.

An external transmitter is placed over the chest implant and connected to a microprocessor which can be attached to the wheelchair. A small, light metal stick with a ball-bearing joint at one end and a disc at the other (a joystick) is fixed to the upper sternum. The disc end is located on the shoulder on the opposite side to the hand to be controlled. Signals pass from the joystick via the microprocessor to the external transmitter over the implant site. Small movements of elevation, depression, protraction and retraction of the shoulder then control the opening and closing of the hand. The grasp can be locked and unlocked by a strong, quick movement into elevation at the shoulder so that the grasp can be maintained as long as required.

To enhance the usefulness of the implanted system, the patient may also have the posterior fibres of deltoid transplanted into triceps to provide elbow extension and extend the range of movement of the arm. Both surgical procedures, implanting the neuroprosthesis and transplanting the muscle, can be carried out at the same time.

As with all FES systems, the team approach is essential and the surgeon, clinical engineer and occupational therapist need to be involved from the outset. A comprehensive assessment of the patient, including both physical and psychological aspects, is also essential if the patient is to be successful (see p. 153). It is important that the patient identifies his goals for having the system implanted and these can be used subsequently to judge its success.

A training programme involving surface stimulation for the muscles to be used is undertaken by the patient prior to operation. Postoperatively the patient has his arm in plaster for 2–4 weeks, and after that a phased programme to use the system is commenced.

So far, the components of the Freehand system have demonstrated excellent reliability. Only one failure in 60 implants has necessitated further surgery.

Transplants on their own may be useful for some patients, e.g. fibres from deltoid to triceps for patients with lesions at C6 in order to increase the ability to transfer.

Handmaster

The handmaster is a device for improving hand function (Uzerman et al 1996). It may be useful for patients with lesions at C5 who have shoulder and elbow movement. It uses non-invasive functional electrical stimulation with a wrist and forearm support, not only to exercise muscles but also to restore some function to the hand. To date, it has been used with patients who have stroke and head injury more than with patients who have spinal cord injury.

PATIENTS WITH LESIONS AT C6

These patients have an active extensor carpi radialis and are able to pick up objects by using the wrist extension grip. Patients with lesions at C7 without finger movement can be included in this group, although the active elbow extension and wrist flexion give greater dexterity in all activities. As a weak grip can be sustained, these patients can achieve a measure of independence in the wheelchair.

The grip is practised and the patient is taught to pick up everyday objects of different sizes, to manipulate paper and to turn the pages of books and magazines. A small leather or webbing strap with a slot in the palmar surface is used to hold various implements for daily living (Fig. 8.1c). The strap is both light and unobtrusive and the patient can put it on unaided. After the initial period of training, most of these patients become so skilful at using their hands that gadgets are rendered unnecessary.

A number of wrist/hand orthoses are available to increase the function of weak wrist muscles and produce grip. The flexor hinge splint, which utilizes extensor carpi radialis to produce a pincer grip, can be a useful asset to some patients, especially those who return to work. Modular kits are available which enable the splint to be fitted and in use within a few days.

Curtin (1994) suggests that research is needed to further develop appropriate assessment tools for hand function and to determine which splints are the most useful.

Activities for patients with lesions at C6

Feeding

Patients start to eat by using the strap to hold the fork or spoon and by extending and relaxing the wrist. After some practice the strap is usually discarded and the fork held by balancing it over the thumb and against the palm of the hand or over the little finger. A plate guard may be helpful initially.

Drinking

A cup or mug with a large handle is held by hooking the thumb through the handle and extending the wrist. A glass without a handle can be lifted by sliding the fingers and thumb around the glass with the wrist extensor relaxed and then extending the wrist to produce the necessary grip.

As the hands are insensitive and the movements slow and clumsy, insulated mugs are preferred whilst training. Standard cups are used later by most dexterous patients.

Cleaning the teeth

The toothbrush is used in the strap (Fig. 8.1d) or laced between the fingers. To unscrew the cap from the toothpaste tube, the cap can be held by the teeth whilst both hands rotate the tube. The teeth can also be used to squeeze out the paste. Toothpaste dispensers can be obtained from companies specializing in products for disabled people.

Brushing the hair

Most patients find a shampoo brush with a wide handle easy to use (Fig. 8.1g).

Shaving

To enable the patient to shave unaided, a soft leather jacket can be sewn around the electric shaver and a strap attached to fit over the dorsum of the hand. Many patients learn to use the razor without the jacket. The patient manoeuvres the razor into position between the fingers and palm of the right hand, with the head of the razor projecting between the thumb and first finger. He then places his left hand round the other to strengthen the grip. By pressing the two hands together the grip is maintained.

Bladder, bowel and skin care

The care of the bladder and bowels is dealt with in Chapter 2 and re-education in self-care of desensitized areas in Chapter 6.

Computers

Computers and word processors can be used for both work and leisure activities. Most patients use a small, rubber-tipped stick on an extension splint on the first or second finger (Fig. 8.1b). Where possible, both hands are used.

Dressing

Dressing training is commenced as soon as the spine is stable. Upper extremity dressing refers to the ability to put on and remove clothing over the upper limbs. Lower extremity dressing refers to the ability to put on and remove clothing over the lower limbs. Total dressing refers to the ability to achieve both the foregoing.

Although most paraplegic patients will finally achieve total dressing both in bed and in the wheelchair, they are initially taught to dress in bed. Tetraplegic patients need to gain some sitting balance before attempting to dress, and it is usual to begin with upper extremity dressing in the wheelchair. Each patient, having learnt the basic methods, will find an individual way which best suits his requirements and daily schedule. Dressing techniques are described later.

Caution. Training is delayed where there is:

- instability of the spine at the site of the injury
- a need to avoid rotation after surgical intervention
- delicate scar tissue which might easily break down during rolling or through friction.

Clothing. All clothing should be loose-fitting. The trousers need to be at least a size larger than normally worn to accommodate the urinal and avoid trauma due to friction. Zips in a side seam of the trouser leg are also helpful if wearing a urinal or calipers. A wrap-over skirt and rubber pants with a front fastening may be helpful for female patients who find difficulty in removing clothing for toilet purposes.

Shoes that are ½–1 size larger than those worn prior to the paralysis are usually required to avoid pressure sores and accommodate for any oedema or spasticity. They should have smooth inside seams, must remain in position when the legs are lifted and should be selected according to the patient's needs.

For tetraplegic patients, zips or Velcro fastenings are the most easily managed. Since the thumb is used as a hook on many occasions, loops or split rings on the zipper pulls may be helpful. Brassières should have stretch straps and should not be boned, because of the danger of pressure marks.

Loose woollen socks are easier to put on initially. Progression can be made to nylon socks later if desired. Clip-on ties may be useful for some patients with cervical lesions.

Level of lesion in relation to dressing. Total dressing should be achieved by patients with lesions as high as C7, i.e. patients with active flexion and extension of elbows and wrists.

Total dressing may be achieved by patients with lesions at C6 both with or without triceps, but lower extremity dressing for these patients, though useful in emergency, is usually so costly in time that it is not practical. Upper extremity dressing should be achieved by patients with lesions at C5–6 except for the following activities:

- putting on a brassière
- tucking the shirt tails into the trouser band
- fastening buttons on cuffs and shirt fronts.

Patients without finger movement cannot usually manage to put on the urinal.

As always, these objectives are only possible within the limits imposed by the previous medical history, age and physical proportions of the patient.

Using the telephone

A telephone can be adapted to allow the patient with an ultra-high lesion to make independent calls. If these adaptations are not available the receiver can be mounted on a retort stand and a simple wooden bar with a firm handle placed across the receiver rest. A mouth stick can be used to dial and to remove and replace the wooden bar. Some environmental control systems have the facility to use a phone, as for the higher lesions.

Writing

Several gadgets are available for use with a pen or pencil. Small splints supporting finger and thumb can easily be made for the individual patient (Fig. 8.1a). Some tetraplegic patients give up the gadget in time and either lace the pen through their fingers or hold it in one hand, putting the other hand on top to reinforce the grip.

Housework

Both low tetraplegic and paraplegic patients prepare for their return to housekeeping in the occupational therapy department kitchen and in the ward. They dust, cook, wash up, make their own beds and do their own laundry. They have the opportunity to discuss ways and means to overcome individual problems in the home and in this way gain the necessary confidence to return to their family responsibilities.

Dressing techniques

In most movements, two actions are involved:

- moving the garment
- moving the body, i.e. wriggling into or out of the garment.

Balance

Those tetraplegic patients who can lift in the chair during dressing should put the stronger hand towards the back of the armrest, with the forearm braced against the backrest support and the weaker hand towards the front of the armrest. This arrangement gives more stability anteroposteriorly and allows wriggling movements forwards and backwards as well as from side to side.

Patients who have difficulty in maintaining balance whilst using both arms are more stable if the buttocks are brought a few inches forward in the chair.

Spasticity

Increased tone may be an advantage in flexing and extending the lower limbs. Uncontrollable muscle spasm in the lower limbs may render independent dressing impossible. Sitting cross-legged for 15–20 minutes may help to reduce severe extensor spasticity before attempting to dress.

As it is easier to achieve, the tetraplegic patient is taught to undress first. However, for clarity, in the following section the method for putting the garment on is described first. This procedure is usually reversed when taking it off.

Dressing in the wheelchair

Upper extremity dressing in the wheelchair

As upper extremity dressing provides no problem for low lesions, i.e. those with abdominals, reference in this section is to patients with cervical and high thoracic lesions.

Putting on a garment of soft material with or without a front fastening. This method can be used for blouses, vests, sweaters, skirts and dresses that open down the front. If it is found easier and the garment is large enough, the buttons can be left fastened. Many tetraplegic patients without a grip can learn to fasten buttons by using a button hook.

1. Position the garment on the thighs, with the neckline towards the knees.
2. Put both arms under the back of the garment and through the armholes.
3. Push the garment past the elbows.

4. Using the wrist extension grip, hook the thumbs under the garment and gather the material up from the neck to hem.
5. Using adduction and lateral rotation of the shoulders and flexion of the elbows and neck, pass the garment over the head.
6. Relax the shoulders and wrists and remove the hands from the back of the garment. Most of the material will be gathered up at the back of the neck and under the arms.
7. There are several ways in which the garment can be worked down into place:
   a. shrug the shoulders and/or elevate and laterally rotate the shoulders with the elbows extended to get the material down across the shoulders
   b. hook the wrists into the sleeves and pull the material free at the axilla
   c. using two hands pull down on each side of the front
   d. hook one hand in the material at the neck, lean on the opposite forearm on the armrest and pull the garment down.

Taking the garment off.

1. Hook the thumb in the back of the neckline, extend the wrist and pull the garment over the head, turning the head towards the side of the raised arm. Maintain balance by either:
   a. leaning on the opposite forearm
   b. pushing the thigh with the extended arm.
2. Hook the thumb in the opposite armhole and push the sleeve down the arm. Pull the arm out of the garment.

Putting on a jacket.

1. Put the weaker arm in the armhole and push the sleeve up the arm.
2. Maintain balance by leaning on and over the forearm resting on the armrest.
3. Put the other arm in the armhole behind the back.
4. Elevate the arms and shrug the shoulders to get the jacket over the shoulders.

Removing a jacket. Reverse the above procedure.

Putting on a brassière with fastening at the back.

1. Powder under the breasts and round the chest wall, especially if subject to sweating attacks.
2. Place the bra on the knees, inside out and upside down, i.e. with the lower edge of the bra towards the knees.
3. Balance on the weaker elbow. Hold the middle of the bra with the strong hand, take behind the back and bring the fastening to the front.
4. Fasten the hooks or Velcro at the front. It may help to lift slightly on the forearms.
5. Wriggle the bra round to the back. Powder again if necessary.
6. With the thumbs in the strap pull up over breasts.
7. Place one arm at a time in the appropriate shoulder strap. Hook the thumb under the bra strap, lean to the opposite side and put the strap over the shoulder. Repeat for the other arm.
8. Look in the mirror to see that the bra is not wrinkled.
   (Note: adjust the length of the straps when the bra is off)

Taking off the brassière.

1. Hook the thumb under the opposite strap, and push down whilst elevating the shoulder.
2. Pull the arm out of the strap.
3. Repeat on the other side.
4. Push the bra down and turn it round to bring the fastening to the front.
5. Undo the fastening.

Lower extremity dressing in the wheelchair

When dressing the lower extremity, the socks should be put on before the trousers to avoid catching the toes and causing trauma.
   Putting on and removing socks and shoes. Whether in the chair or on the bed, maximum control is achieved when putting on and taking off socks and shoes by crossing one ankle over the opposite knee. The tetraplegic patient uses the wrist extension grip and the palm of the hands in a patting movement to pull on the socks.

Putting on trousers

1. Lift the right leg with the right wrist behind the knee and the forearm on the armrest. Put the trouser leg over the foot. Repeat with the left leg.
   Alternatively, cross the right ankle over the left knee, put the trousers over the foot and pull up to knee height. Replace the right foot on the footplate. Repeat with the left leg.
2. Pull the trousers well up over the knees and under the thighs, lean on the left forearm and lift the right knee with the left wrist to pull the trousers up the thigh.
3. Hook the right fingers or thumb inside the back of the waistband, lean over to the left and lift on the left hand and forearm. Repeat from side to side. At each lift, wriggle forwards and backwards whilst the buttocks are in the air.

Alternative method to pull the trousers over the buttocks for paraplegic patients

1. Lean forward on the forearms on the armrests, depressing the shoulders and lifting the buttocks, and pull the trousers up.
2. Lean well back taking the weight on the top of the backrest, wriggle the buttocks forward and at the same time pull up the trousers.

Dressing on the bed

Upper extremity dressing on the bed

This presents no real problems for paraplegic patients. Tetraplegic patients have more stability for upper extremity dressing in the wheelchair and rarely do it on the bed.

Lower extremity dressing on the bed

Putting on trousers

1. Put the trouser legs over the feet as for the socks.
2. Flex the knee with the hand, wrist or forearm and pull the trousers up over the thighs. Lean on the elbows if necessary.

3. Repeat for the other leg.
4. Lean to the right on the right elbow, and pull the trousers over the left buttock.
5. Lean to the left and pull the trousers over the right buttock. Repeat this as often as necessary.

A monkey pole may be necessary for patients with high thoracic lesions to lift onto the side at the commencement of training.

The trousers may be removed by reversing the procedure.

Alternative method for putting on trousers for tetraplegic patients

1. Sit up, hook the right hand under the right knee and pull the knee into flexion.
2. Put the trousers over the right foot.
3. Repeat for the left foot. It may help to have both legs slightly flexed and laterally rotated at the hips.
4. Work the trousers up the legs by alternately flexing the knees and using a patting sliding motion with the palms of the hands.
5. Lie down and pull the right knee onto the chest.
6. Stay supine and hold the right knee with the left forearm or roll into left side-lying. Throw the right arm behind the back, hook the thumb in the waistband or belt loops, or the hand in the trouser pocket, and pull the trousers over the right buttock.
7. Repeat for the other side. These steps may need to be repeated several times until the trousers are in place over the hips.
8. Fasten the trouser placket by hooking the thumb in a loop on the zipper pull.

If the patient cannot cross one ankle over the other, the trousers, socks and shoes have to be put over the feet in long-sitting. This is more difficult since the heels are resting on the bed.

ACCOMMODATION

The two major practical problems in resettlement are obtaining suitable accommodation and employment. Paraplegic patients, except for those handicapped by age or other illness, are usually able to return to live independently in the community. The majority of tetraplegic patients do return to their own homes, although often with maximum support from the social services and the family.

The home may need to be adapted or to have an extension, or it may be totally unsuitable, in which case the only solution is for the patient to be re-housed in a flat or bungalow.

Accommodation for patients who are unable to return home may be found in young chronic sick units, Cheshire homes, geriatric units, voluntary institutions and hostels with sheltered workshops.

Adaptations

The need for adaptation to the home varies considerably in relation to the level of the patient's lesion and to his age and sex. Those adaptations most frequently necessary are to the bathroom facilities, which are usually too small, and to the kitchen. Access for the wheelchair to the toilet and bath or shower is necessary for those patients capable of independent transfer. To cook without unnecessary danger may necessitate adaptations to cupboards, cooker and working surfaces in the kitchen.

Free access to the house from outside is essential and those able to drive will need a garage wide enough to accommodate the wheelchair beside the car for independent transfer.

Equipment

Some patients will need very little, if any, special equipment in the home; others may need a great deal. A bed, special mattress, hoist, and home nursing equipment, as well as a telephone and environmental control system, may all be necessary for a patient with a high cervical lesion.

EMPLOYMENT

Future employment is discussed with the patient as early as possible. Many patients are unable to return to their former employment as most are manual workers. Unemployment rates amongst registered disabled persons are higher than in the working population as a whole. Assessment at an industrial rehabilitation unit may be necessary, followed by retraining at a day or residential training establishment for disabled people. Para-plegic patients have been retrained in a variety of occupations, and others, already in professions or business, have returned to all types of work. The internet is proving a great asset to many who find travelling to work difficult.

9

Basic functional movements

MOBILIZATION AND STRENGTHENING OF THE TRUNK AND LIMBS

Some degree of stiffness in the trunk will result from the weeks of immobility in bed. In addition, there will be some shortening of the hamstring muscles. If the activities of daily living are to be mastered, good mobility is essential.

Therefore, mobilization of the trunk in all directions and stretching of any tight muscle groups form an essential part of early rehabilitation. Active assisted, active and resisted work are given as indicated for trunk, shoulders, shoulder girdle and head. The use of the head and shoulder girdle in flexion and rotation is essential in many functional activities, especially for patients with cervical or high thoracic lesions.

Caution. As the fracture is recently healed, mobilization of the trunk must be undertaken very gradually and with extreme care. Forced movements, particularly forced flexion, must be completely avoided. Initially only free active flexion is given.

PRELIMINARY TRAINING FOR FUNCTIONAL ACTIVITIES

To give the patient confidence, these activities need to be undertaken on a wide plinth.

Lifting the buttocks by pushing on the arms is the basis of most of the activities of daily living. An effective lift depends upon balance and strength and upon knowing exactly where to place the hands and how to hold the head, shoulders and trunk. The following comments apply primarily to patients with cervical and high thoracic lesions. Where the abdominal muscles are innervated, trunk control will be adequate and all lifts will be relatively easy.

Basic principles

In order to maintain balance whilst moving, the first principle of body mechanics must be observed, i.e. the line of gravity must remain inside the base of support. To achieve this in the sitting position with no muscle power around the hips, the head and shoulders must be kept forward of the hip joints. When lifting the trunk with the hands just in front of the hip joints, the head, trunk and hips *must be flexed as much as possible*. This position gives a mechanical advantage so that the same strength achieves a higher lift. An optimum degree of flexion will be reached beyond which the lift becomes impractical for those without triceps, because the elbows will be flexed.

All patients start lifting themselves with extended elbows. Many patients with triceps later progress to lifting with the elbows flexed, when the mechanical advantage increases as the degree of hip flexion increases.

In all movements the head acts as a weight to assist or resist any movement. When the arms are short or when there is extra weight around the hips, lifting is more difficult (see Ch. 7).

The following manoeuvres provide the basis for functional activities such as dressing, turning in bed and transfers:

- lifting and moving
- moving the paralysed limbs
- sitting up and lying down
- rolling prone and turning onto the side.

The therapist is behind, at the side of or in front of the patient as required to assist or resist each component of the movements involved. Clear instructions should be given at every step. Initially assistance will be necessary to maintain sufficient flexion of the head and trunk as patients generally feel that they need to extend

the trunk in order to lift. The therapist should never try to assist the patient in functional activities by lifting under the axillae. This action entirely negates any effort by the patient to lift by depressing the shoulders.

LIFTING

The therapist

The therapist is behind the patient and, as well as maintaining the necessary flexion, may need to aid the lift with her hands under the buttocks. Later, where possible, stabilizations are given in the lifted position.

Action of the patient

1. To balance in long-sitting, flex the head, shoulders and trunk so that the line of gravity is kept in front of the hip joints. With the arms close to the sides, place the hands on the plinth slightly forward of the hips and preferably with the palms flat and fingers extended. Where triceps is paralysed, lateral rotation of the arms assists stability at the elbows.
2. Lean forward with the head and shoulders bent over the knees. A greater degree of flexion is needed by tetraplegic patients. When innervated, the abdominal muscles will flex the trunk and the movement of the head and shoulders becomes less important.
3. With the elbows extended, push down on the hands.
4. Depress the shoulders and lift the buttocks off the plinth. At the moment of lift, raise the head. This will prevent the trunk collapsing forward.

To lift and move sideways

The therapist

In addition to the factors already mentioned, the therapist may need to encourage rotation.

Action of the patient

1. Place the right hand on the plinth close to and slightly in front of the hip.

2. Place the left hand at the same level but approximately a foot away from the body. This distance will depend on the length of the arm in relation to that of the trunk. The elbows are extended and the forearms supinated, or in mid-position (Fig. 9.1a).
3. Flex further forward over the knees and lift the buttocks. At the same time twist the head and shoulders to the right, bringing the left shoulder forward and the right shoulder back (Fig. 9.1b). Where latissimus dorsi is innervated, it will pull the pelvis forward towards the arm which is away from the side.

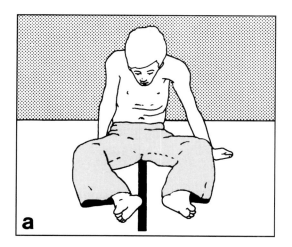

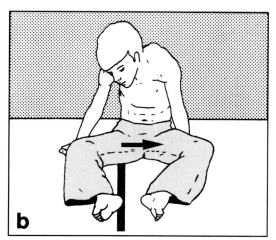

Figure 9.1 Lifting sideways. Patient with a complete lesion below C6 without triceps and with the clavicular portion of pectoralis major only.

To lift and move forward

The legs need to be in lateral rotation and free to flex at the knee:

1. Lean well forward, with the head over the knees (Fig. 9.2a).
2. Place the hands on the plinth a little in front of the hip joints and close in to the sides. The elbows are extended and forearms supinated.
3. Lift the buttocks (Fig. 9.2b).
4. Keep the head flexed and the buttocks will move forward. Once beyond the point of balance, the patient will collapse forward (Fig. 9.2c).

MOVING THE PARALYSED LIMBS

In order to perform the activities of daily living, the patient will need to lift and move his paralysed limbs.

The paraplegic patient will accomplish this quickly and easily, almost automatically. The tetraplegic patient will need intensive training and practice, and must not be disheartened if success is delayed.

It is necessary to be able to:

- move the legs along the plinth
- cross one ankle over the other
- cross one ankle over the opposite knee
- flex the leg in sitting and side-lying.

A method for tetraplegic patients to flex and lift the leg is described on page 86.

Balance can be maintained whilst moving the legs by leaning forward on one or both elbows. This position leaves the hands free to lift, push or pull the leg. The pelvis must be straight and the patient leans a little to one side, as well as forward, to keep the body weight over the static leg.

SITTING AND LYING

These movements can be achieved without any equipment or using a monkey pole.

To sit from the supine position without using a monkey pole

Action of the patient

1. In one brisk movement throw the right arm

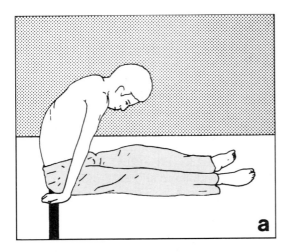

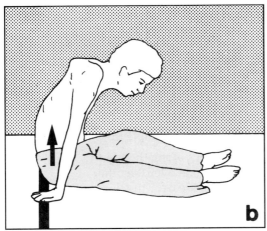

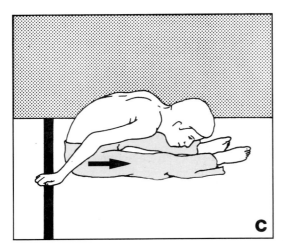

Figure 9.2 Lifting forwards. Patient with a complete lesion below C6 without triceps and with the clavicular portion of pectoralis major only.

over to the left, flex the head and shoulders and twist them to the left. This will rotate the upper part of the trunk (Fig. 9.3a & b).
2. Balance on both elbows (Fig. 9.3c).
3. Take the weight on the right elbow and bring the left elbow closer to the trunk.
4. Balance on the left elbow and, holding the head forwards and protracting the shoulders, transfer the right arm to the right side of the body and balance on both elbows (Fig. 9.3d).
5. Lean over on the left elbow, outwardly rotate the right arm and extend it behind the body (Fig. 9.3e).
6. Adjust the position until the weight can be taken on the right arm and extend the left arm in a similar manner (Fig. 9.3f).
7. Slowly bring the hands forward alternately, a few inches at a time, until the weight is over the legs (Fig. 9.3g).

Where possible, step 4 can be omitted.

Alternative method for steps 1–4
1. With the arms in pronation by the sides put the wrists under the buttocks.
2. With the elbows on the plinth strongly extend the wrists.
3. Flex the head, protract the shoulders, and with the elbows as the pivot-point pull the weight of the head and upper trunk onto the elbows.
4. Move each elbow backwards a few inches at a time.

Continue as in the previous method, steps 5, 6 and 7. If the patient finds difficulty with the hands under the hips, the thumbs can be hooked in the trouser pockets initially to enable him to get the feel of the movement.

Alternative method from step 2
From the position where the weight is on both elbows (Fig. 9.3c), the patient can 'walk' on his forearms along the plinth to achieve the sitting position (see Fig. 15.1).

To lie down from the sitting position

1. Keeping the head flexed and shoulders protracted, lean over to the right and drop the weight onto the right elbow (Fig. 9.3h).

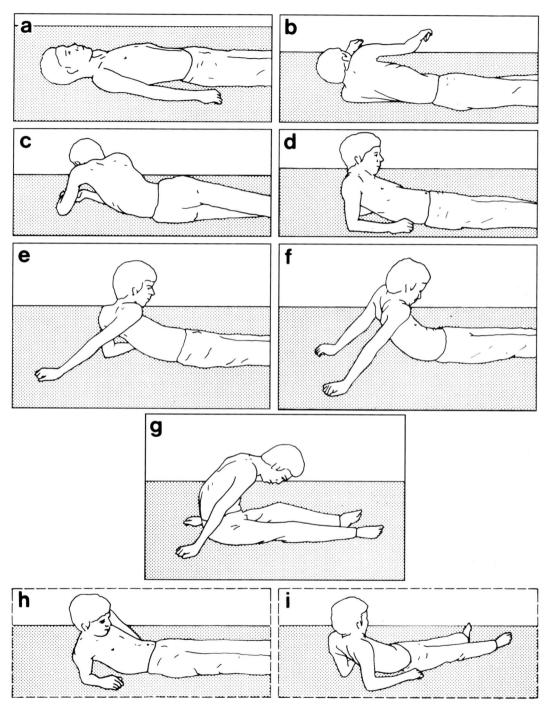

Figure 9.3   a–g: Sitting up. h, i: Lying down. Patient with a complete lesion below C6 without triceps and with the clavicular portion of pectoralis major only.

2. Balance on the right elbow.
3. Flex the left arm and transfer half the weight onto the left elbow.
4. Still keeping the head and shoulders forward (Fig. 9.3i), straighten one arm at a time until lying flat.

To sit from the supine position using a monkey pole

Position of the monkey pole

The point of suspension for the monkey pole is over the midline of the body or slightly beyond midline towards the side of the supporting arm and approximately level with the xiphisternum. The handle should be just within the reach of the patient's extended wrist.

Action of the patient

To lift onto one elbow:

1. Extend the right arm and hook the extended wrist over the monkey pole (Fig. 9.4a).
2. Pull the body towards the monkey pole and lean on the left elbow (Fig. 9.4b).
3. Flex the right elbow over the monkey pole and hold the body weight whilst bringing the left elbow closer to the trunk.
4. Support the body weight on the left elbow (Fig. 9.4c).

To get up on two extended arms, proceed with either of the following methods.

Method 1
5. Lean on the left elbow.
6. With the elbow flexed flick the right arm into lateral rotation and hold the wrist against the monkey pole chain (Fig. 9.4d).
7. Hold the body weight with the right arm, outwardly rotate the left shoulder and extend the arm behind the body (Fig. 9.4e).
8. Lean well over the left arm, release the monkey pole and extend the right arm behind the body.
9. Move the hands forward alternately, a few inches at a time, until the weight is over the legs (Fig. 9.4f).

Method 2
5. Lean well over to the left and balance on the left elbow.
6. Take the right arm out of the monkey pole, outwardly rotate the shoulder, and extend the arm behind the body.
7. Transfer most of the weight onto the right arm and push the left arm straight.
8. Move the hands forward alternately, a few inches at a time until the weight is over the legs.

Patients without pectoral muscles, or with the clavicular head of pectoralis major only, may find method 1 to be the easier of the two. Patients with good hand function grasp the monkey pole with one hand and lift onto the opposite elbow. From there, the procedure is the same as method 2.

Occasionally a paraplegic patient may need to use a monkey pole for one of the following reasons: age, overweight, ossification around the hip joints or a previous medical history of heart or lung disease.

To roll prone from the supine position

To roll to the right:

1. Flex the head and shoulders and fling the arms over to the left, so that the necessary momentum can be gained in step 2 (Fig. 9.5a).
2. In one brisk movement, flex the head and shoulders and fling the arms from left to right. As this movement is completed, the right shoulder is pulled back as far as possible (Fig. 9.5b).
3. The momentum of the arms is transferred to the trunk and legs and the lower half of the body will roll prone (Fig. 9.5c).
4. Place the left forearm on the plinth and take the weight on it.
5. Pull the right shoulder back and take the weight on both forearms (Fig. 9.5d).
6. Lie flat and put the arms by the sides.

To turn onto the side

Action of the patient

1. Sit up with or without the monkey pole as described.

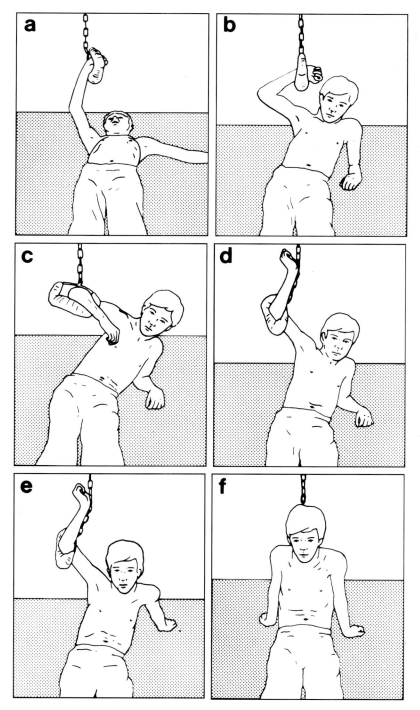

Figure 9.4 Sitting up using a monkey pole. Patient with a complete lesion below C6 without triceps and with the clavicular portion of pectoralis major only.

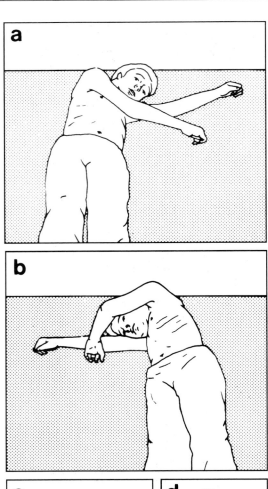

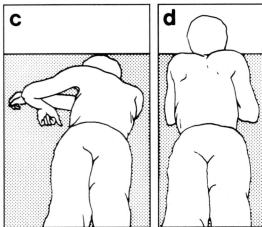

Figure 9.5 Rolling. Patient with a complete lesion below C6 without triceps and with the clavicular portion of pectoralis major only.

2. Lean on the left extended arm.
3. Hook the extended right wrist under the right knee and flex the leg.
4. Facing the left, lean down on the left elbow and at the same time pull the right leg into further flexion and cross the right knee over the left leg.
5. Place the right forearm on the plinth and take the weight on it.
6. Lower the trunk into side-lying.

To turn in bed

When the patient is able to turn on the mat and to move and position his legs, progression is made to turning in bed.

The patient turns from supine to right side-lying and positions the leg pillow.

Action of the patient

To sit up, either of the two ways already described can be used, or the patient can sit up using a bed loop. The loop is attached to the end of the bed and is just long enough to hook on the forearm:

1. Put the left forearm through the loop and flex the right elbow, extending the wrist to 'grip' the edge of the mattress (Fig. 9.6a).
2. Pull on the loop with the left arm and transfer the weight onto the right elbow (Fig. 9.6b).
3. Release the strap (Fig. 9.6c).
4. Extend the left arm behind the body and take the weight on it (Fig. 9.6d).
5. Extending the right arm take the weight on both arms. Move the hands forward until the weight is over the legs (Fig. 9.6e).

To position the pillow:

6. Flex the left knee with the extended left wrist and push the pillow under the knee (Fig. 9.6f).
7. Keeping the weight well over the right hip, lift the lower leg onto the pillow with the right arm (Fig. 9.6g). Adjust the position of the pillow and legs.

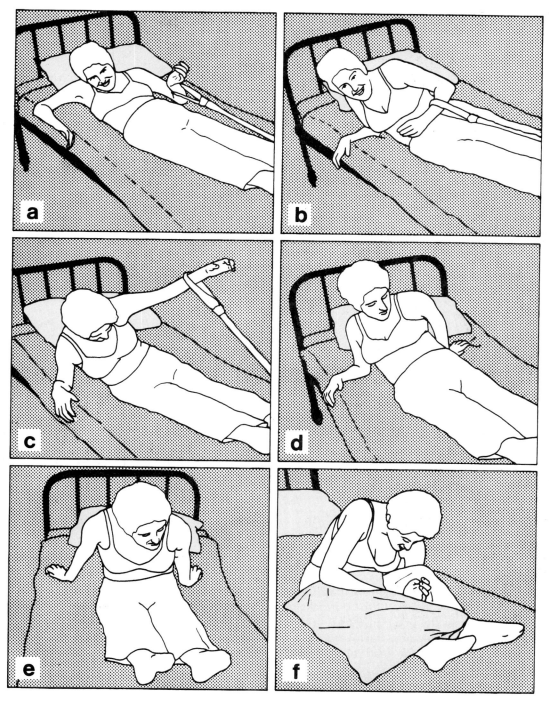

Figure 9.6   a–f: Turning in bed. Patient with a complete lesion below C7 with wrist control only.

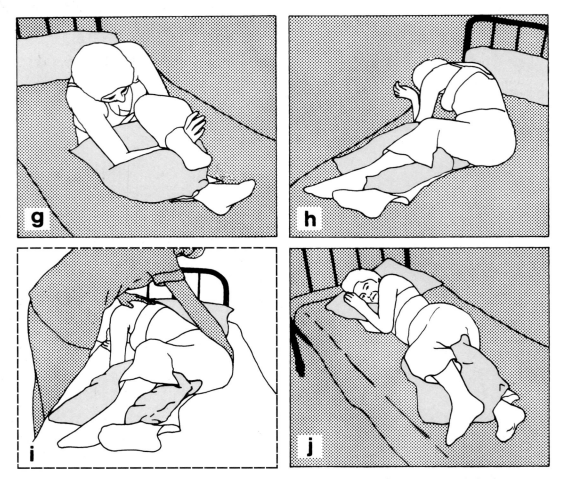

Figure 9.6 cont'd g–j: Turning in bed. Patient with a complete lesion below C7 with wrist control only.

8. Turn the upper trunk to the right and take the weight firstly on the right and then on both elbows.
9. Lean forward and take the maximum weight on the left elbow and forearm. Rock onto the left elbow and pivot the buttocks backwards across the bed (Fig. 9.6h).
10. When adequate movement backwards has been achieved, adjust the head pillow for individual comfort.
11. Take the weight onto the left elbow and lower the weight onto the right shoulder, lying down on the side (Fig. 9.6j).

Initially the therapist may need to assist the patient to achieve the rocking movement by pressing down over the patient's left shoulder girdle with one hand and lifting under the right buttock with the other (Fig. 9.6i).

When the patient can turn himself in bed and position the pillows correctly he will be encouraged to take responsibility for turning himself at night with supervision from ward staff.

10

Wheelchairs and wheelchair management

TYPES OF WHEELCHAIR

Hand-propelled folding transit chair: standard and junior models

Most firms make the two main sizes of wheelchair: standard (or adult) and junior. The difference between these is usually 5 cm in seat width and 5 cm in overall height. There is very little difference in weight. In general, there are also two sizes for children. It is often possible to put a larger seat and backrest onto the largest of the children's chairs to adapt for the growing child. On all chairs, the footrests need to be swinging and detachable to allow easy access for transfers. For the same reason, the armrests need to be detachable.

The angle of incline of the backrest should not be more than 5°. The diameter of the wheels varies from 18 to 24 inches (wheels are measured in inches in the UK, the USA and other parts of the world). The larger the wheels, the less effort is involved in pushing the chair. The 8 inch castors are preferred to the 5 inch ones, as they are easier to push over carpets, kerbs and other small obstacles.

Wheels

Large wheels at the back and small ones at the front allow the patient to remain supported by the backrest whilst pushing the chair.

Pneumatic rear and solid front tyres give the best combination for function and comfort. Pneumatic front tyres are used when the patient's predominant need is to push over rough ground. They give less vibration but are harder to push.

Footplates

The footplates need either heel loops or a calf strap to prevent the feet slipping backwards off the footplates and becoming entangled in the front wheels. Heel loops are easier if the footplates are constantly being removed for transfers, etc. If the patient is excessively spastic in the lower limbs, both may be necessary.

The approximate weight of the standard chair is 25 kg.

The standard lightweight chair

A lightweight chair is made by most firms in the standard models. It is approximately two-thirds the weight of the standard model. Some patients who are constantly putting the chair into a car prefer this type.

A semi-reclining back chair

A wheelchair in which the backrest can be angled to 30° from the vertical is made by several firms. This chair allows patients with high cervical lesions to balance and breathe more easily. It is obviously heavier than the standard model and the overall length is greater, making it more difficult to manoeuvre in a small area. This chair is commonly used for the ultra-high lesion.

The transit chair

This chair is attendant propelled, having small wheels at the front and rear. It is approximately the same weight as the lightweight chair. It is a necessity for the patient using a power-drive chair and useful for the patient with a semi-reclining chair. The various components of the power-drive chair are heavy and it is time-consuming to dismantle it for transport.

The power-drive chair

The power-drive chair is manufactured in both

standard and junior sizes. There are three means of control:

- arm or hand control
- breath control
- head, chin or mouth control.

The weight of the chair with the batteries is approximately double the weight of the standard chair. It is used by patients who are unable to push a wheelchair.

A control box can transform a manual chair into an electrically driven wheelchair. The unit is light enough to be easily mounted on and removed from even an ultra-light wheelchair. Several models are available.

The stand-up chair

This chair (Fig. 10.1) enables the patient to raise himself to the standing position to perform an activity and to sit down again independently. The seat of the chair is raised slowly to the

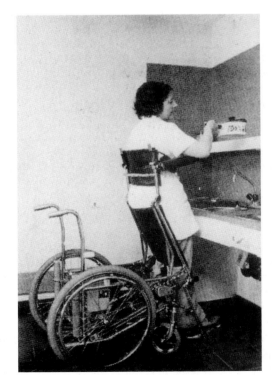

Figure 10.1 Stand-up chair.

required height by pressing a simple switch. The movement can be interrupted or reversed at will. Several models and mechanisms are available.

The chair with variable seat height

Some firms manufacture a chair in which the seat, with backrest, footrests and armrests, can be raised 25.5 cm. This can be particularly useful for children.

Sports chair

An ultra-lightweight chair weighing under 12 kg has been designed for use in rigorous wheelchair sports. The frame can be dismantled and stowed in a kitbag.

High performance wheelchairs (HPWs)

The development of a more manoeuvrable and durable wheelchair for the sportsman led to the design of a high performance wheelchair for everyday use. The construction of these chairs is fundamentally different (compare Figs 10.2 and 10.3). Although some have rigid and some folding frames, they all have quick release hubs allowing the wheels to be removed. The chairs fold either vertically or horizontally. The wheels are angled in towards the top of the frame, improving direction stability, and they can also be placed in several positions on the frame, thereby lengthening or shortening the wheelbase. Lighter materials, aluminium and titanium, have reduced the weight of the chair to between 10 and 12 kg. In addition, there is an extensive choice of sizes and accessories.

The options provided through the design of this chair allow it to be adjusted to fit the user more accurately than the standard wheelchair. Postural stability, efficiency of propulsion and manoeuvrability are all increased, facilitating the use of the chair, e.g. in rear wheel balance, which is the key to mobility in the environment. Some patients with low cervical lesions can go up and down kerbs and transfer to the floor, whilst some skilled patients with lower lesions can ascend and descend small flights of steps. Removable wheels and the lighter weight of this chair make it easier to handle for both user and carer.

The abilities, circumstances and priorities of the user need to be considered when selecting a chair and it is essential to try it out in circumstances he will encounter in daily life, e.g. pushing on different surfaces, transferring and getting the chair in and out of the car. With the number of options and the continuing development of these chairs, expert advice is required to select an appropriate chair for each individual.

Outdoor wheelchairs/vehicles

A range of battery-driven wheelchairs are produced for use both indoors and outdoors, e.g. the 'Mobility 2000' which goes up and down kerbs and in which the seat can be raised, or outdoors only, e.g. the 'Countryside Buggy' for use over rough country. The manual wheelchair fits in the buggy.

WHEELCHAIR ACCESSORIES

There are various accessories which can be obtained with most models when necessary.

Anti-tipping levers

These levers are designed to prevent the chair and patient overbalancing backwards. They can be adjustable and are removable, and it is possible to mount small kerbs with them in situ, thus increasing independence for children and patients with cervical lesions.

Armrests

There are several models, all detachable:

- standard
- desk arms – the front upper quarter is cut away to allow the chair to be wheeled closer to a desk or table
- height adjustable
- lift-up
- swing-away tubular.

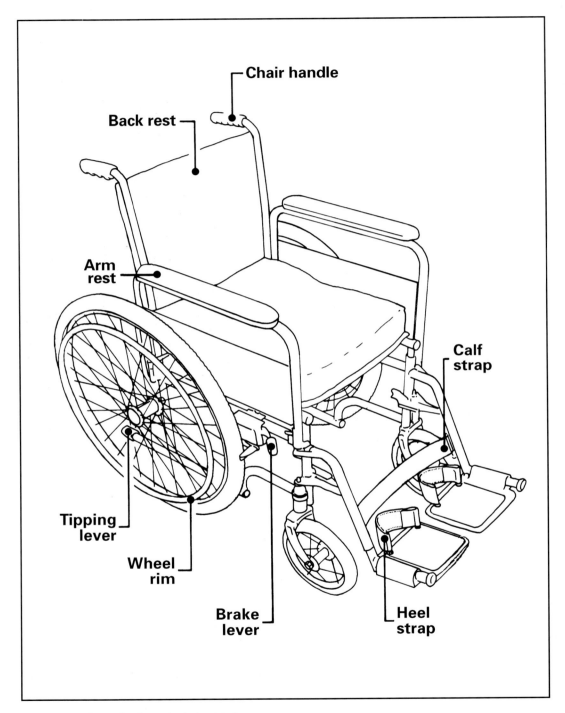

Figure 10.2 Example of standard wheelchair.

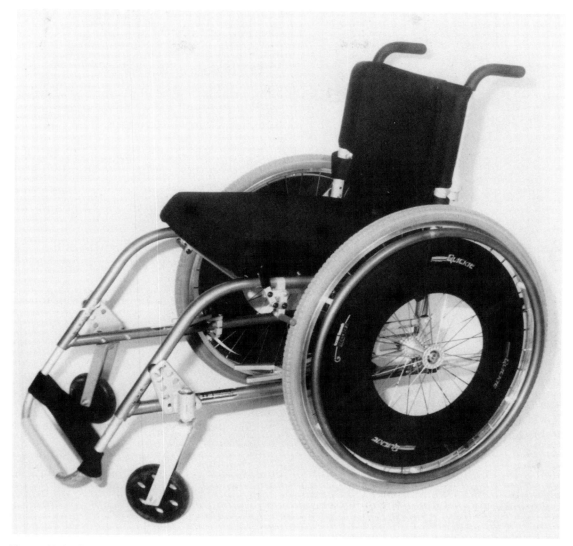

Figure 10.3   Example of high performance chair.

Most detachable armrests have automatic locking devices.

Backrests

These are available in a number of sizes to provide sufficient support without impeding mobility. The angle of the backrest is adjustable, which permits patients, particularly those without abdominal muscles, to recline a few degrees from the vertical, allowing greater freedom to use the arms.

Tension adjustable backrest. The tension adjustable backrest consists of adjustable bands between the two upright struts. These are adjusted by means of Velcro so that the spine can be supported wherever the support is needed (Fig. 10.4).

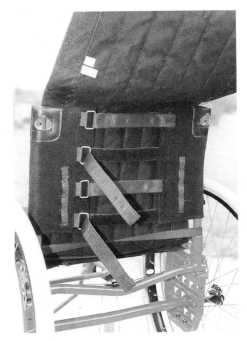

Figure 10.4 Tension adjustable backrest.

Brake extensions

These are sometimes necessary to enable patients with cervical lesions to reach the brakes without falling forward.

Capstans

Capstans are rubber-capped projections spaced at regular intervals around the rim of the wheel. These help some patients with high cervical lesions to get a purchase on the wheels when pushing the chair.

Friction-coated hand rims increase the effectiveness of the push for weaker users.

Carrying bag

This receptacle will suspend under rigid or folding HPW chairs to hold personal belongings.

Castors

Several sizes of castors and castor forks are available. The castors can be solid or pneumatic for indoor or outdoor use.

Castor locks contribute to sideways stability of the chair for transfers.

Crutch or walking stick holder

This consists of a small platform attached to the tipping lever and a strap on the upper part of the backrest to carry the crutches.

Cushions

See Chapter 6.

Elevating leg rests

These increase the overall length of the chair by 4–5 inches and its weight by approximately 1 kg. They are useful for:

- patients with high lesions with vasomotor problems
- any patient with a leg injury.

Footplates

Rigid, flip-up, swing-away and detachable footrests are available. All are adjustable and some models permit adjustment of the angle of the footplate.

The footplate hanger attaches the footrest to the chair. It is not adjustable but its angle to the vertical can be selected from a limited range.

Guards

Side guards. The intrinsic stability of the chair is high, so that even patients with cervical lesions may not need armrests. In this case, side guards may be required to protect the clothes.

Spoke guards. Guards on the outside of the wheels protect the fingers, especially of patients with cervical lesions.

Head extension

This can be attached to the backrest to increase its height and give added support when necessary.

Kerb climber

This device enables kerbs of up to 13 cm to be mounted in a power-drive chair.

Mobile arm support

A splint supports the weight of the arm and pivots allow maximum performance from minimum motor power.

Restraining or safety strap

This is attached to the supports for the backrest on each side and fastens with Velcro across the abdomen. All patients with cervical lesions use them when first mobile, and those with lesions at C4–5 and above continue to use them.

Seat

Differing widths and depths are provided.

Tray

The tray clips on to the armrests and provides a useful surface for many activities. It is also useful, when well padded, as a support for the arms for patients with high cervical lesions.

Tyres

High pressure, pneumatic and solid tyres are available.

Wheels

There is a range of sizes from 12 to 26 inches in diameter.

Zipper backrest

This can be fitted to standard and junior chairs and permits entry and exit from the rear of the chair.

THE POSITION OF THE PATIENT IN THE WHEELCHAIR

The majority of patients are apprehensive and unstable when first sitting up in a wheelchair.

They are unwilling to release their grasp on the armrests and sit afraid to move. Gradually the patient becomes aware of the correct posture to be adopted and learns to relax in the chair. This can only occur if the chair is:

- of a suitable type for the patient
- adjusted to support him correctly.

The correct position of the patient in his wheelchair is important if pressure sores and deformities are to be avoided and if the patient is to have maximum stability for independent activity. The posture should be as symmetrical as possible, weight being distributed through both ischial tuberosities and the whole of the thighs and buttocks (see Ch. 6).

WHEELCHAIR MANOEUVRES

The basic movements within the wheelchair and the initial wheelchair manoeuvres described below are written for tetraplegic patients without a grip. The basic safety measures, such as holding on with one elbow or wrist, become progressively unnecessary as the level of the lesion descends. The advanced wheelchair manoeuvres are divided into sections, since some activities are unsuitable for patients with cervical lesions. Adaptations in technique may have to be made for chairs with minor differences in construction, e.g. in the type of brake lever.

BASIC MOVEMENTS WITHIN THE WHEELCHAIR

- To manipulate the brakes
- To remove the armrest
- To pick up objects from the floor
- To reach down to the footplates
- To lift the buttocks forward in the chair.

Whenever the patient prepares to move within the wheelchair or to move into or out of it, he must first position the wheelchair itself. To give maximum stability, the small front wheels must point forward, as this prevents the chair tipping onto the footplates, and the brakes must be applied. If the patient is going to lean out of the chair in any direction, the buttocks must be well back in the seat.

To manipulate the brakes

To reach the right brake:

1. Hook the left elbow behind the left chair handle.
2. Lean forward and to the right, allowing the left biceps to lengthen as the trunk movement occurs.

To release the brake, use flexion of the elbow and shoulder to push the lever forward with the palm of the hand or the lower part of the supinated forearm (Fig. 10.5a). To apply the brake, pull the lever back using the right biceps and either the extended wrist (lesion at C6, Fig. 10.5b) or the supinated forearm (lesion at C5).

To remove the armrest

To remove the right armrest:

1. Release the catch by pushing down with the base of the thumb over the catch (Fig. 10.5c).
2. Hook the right elbow behind the right chair handle.
3. Place the left hand at the front and the right hand at the back of the right armrest. Using the wrist extension grip, lift the armrest out of its sockets with both hands (Fig. 10.5d).
4. Hold the armrest with the left hand and balance it on the supinated forearm (Fig. 10.5e).
5. Place the armrest on the floor beside the rear wheel, or hook it over the left chair handle.

To pick up objects from the floor

Objects are picked up by leaning sideways out of the chair, and not by leaning forward over the footplates; the forward position is unstable and therefore dangerous.

To lean to the left

Position the chair sideways in relation to the object. Hook the right elbow behind the right chair handle and lean over the left armrest. To avoid excessive pressure on the rib cage, maintain this position for only a few seconds at a time. The armrest can be removed to allow shorter patients the necessary reach.

To regain the upright position, pull up with the right elbow. When triceps is innervated, the extended wrist can be used under the outer rim of the armrest to maintain balance and regain the upright position.

To reach down to the footplates

This position will be necessary to adjust the footplates, to empty the urinal or for adjustments when dressing:

1. Lean forward on the elbows on the armrests.
2. Change the position of the arms one by one and lean on the forearms on the thighs.
3. Put one hand at a time down to the feet, leaning the chest on the thighs.

To regain the upright position, patients without triceps must (1) throw the stronger arm back over the backrest and hook the extended wrist behind the chair handle, and (2) pull the trunk upright by strongly extending the wrist and flexing the elbow.

Patients with good functioning triceps pull the trunk upright by hooking one or both extended wrists underneath the upper, outer edge of the armrest(s).

To lift the buttocks forward in the chair

Patients with cervical lesions without triceps

This manoeuvre is described in detail in Chapter 11.

Patients with cervical lesions with triceps

To lift the right buttock forward:

1. Lean over the left forearm, which is placed well forward on the armrest.
2. Lift with the right hand on the armrest.
3. At the same time, throw the head back and wriggle the right buttock forward (Fig. 10.6).

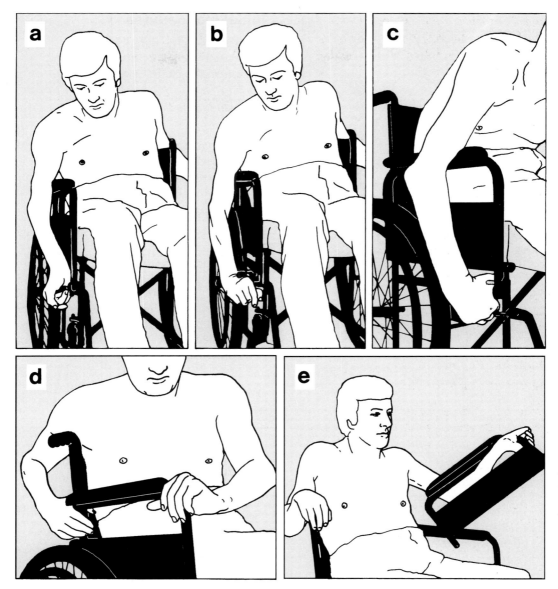

Figure 10.5   a, b: Manipulating the brakes. c–e: Removing the armrest. Patient with a complete lesion below C6 without triceps.

Repeat this procedure to lift the left buttock forward.

Patients with paraplegia

1. Lift on both armrests.
2. Extend the head and shoulders and 'throw' the buttocks forward.

INITIAL AND ADVANCED WHEELCHAIR MANOEUVRES

When putting the wheelchair in motion in any direction, the position of the head and shoulders is important. They are used to reinforce the action of the arms, whether to gain greater momentum or to act as a brake.

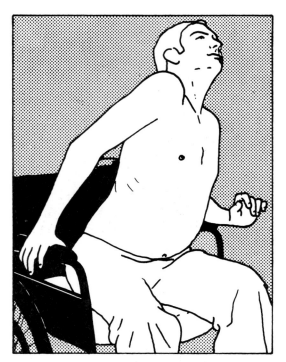

Figure 10.6 Lifting the right buttock forward. Patient with a complete lesion below C7 with wrist control only.

Patients start moving the chair by pushing on the tyres. Paraplegic patients may progress to using the wheel rims, particularly outside, but many patients with tetraplegia continue to use the tyres because they find the purchase easier and the push more effective. Pushing gloves (see Fig. 8.1f) are used by tetraplegic patients to protect the skin from callus formation and abrasions due to friction or injury. Temporary capstans, using rope or rubber tubing wrapped around the wheel, may help older patients with lesions at C5 to learn to push the chair.

Many of the initial wheelchair manoeuvres can be taught in a group where patients learn from and encourage each other. Competition over slalom courses where the obstacles include ramps and turns in narrow confines is also useful. Penalties are given for touching as well as moving any of the marker buoys.

Initial manoeuvres

- To push on the flat
- To use the chair on sloping ground
- To turn the chair.

To push on the flat

When wheeling on the flat, the push forward with the arms is reinforced if accompanied by strong flexion of the head and shoulder girdle. Momentum is gained because there is a general thrust forward with the upper part of the body.

To reverse on the flat

1. Put both arms over the backrest between the chair handles.
2. Place the hands on the wheels with the elbows extended and shoulders elevated.
3. Leaning backwards, depress the shoulders and thrust downwards, with as much weight as possible over the arms. Slopes can be ascended in reverse in this way if the patient is unable to push up forwards.

To use the chair on sloping ground

To push up a slope

1. Leaning forward, place the hands towards the back of the top of the tyre (Fig. 10.7a).
2. Push forward using flexion of the elbows and flexion and adduction of the shoulders (Fig. 10.7b). The chair can be held on a slope by turning the wheels across the incline.

To slow down when going down a slope

Extend the head and shoulders and brake either with both hands towards the front of the tyres or with the first metacarpals under the wheel rims and the wrists extended (Fig. 10.7c).

To turn the chair to the right

1. Place the right hand towards the back of the tyre with the arm over the backrest, behind the chair handle.
2. Laterally rotate the right arm and with the body weight over the hand push backwards on the inner side of the wheel (Fig. 10.7d).
3. Push forward with the left hand.

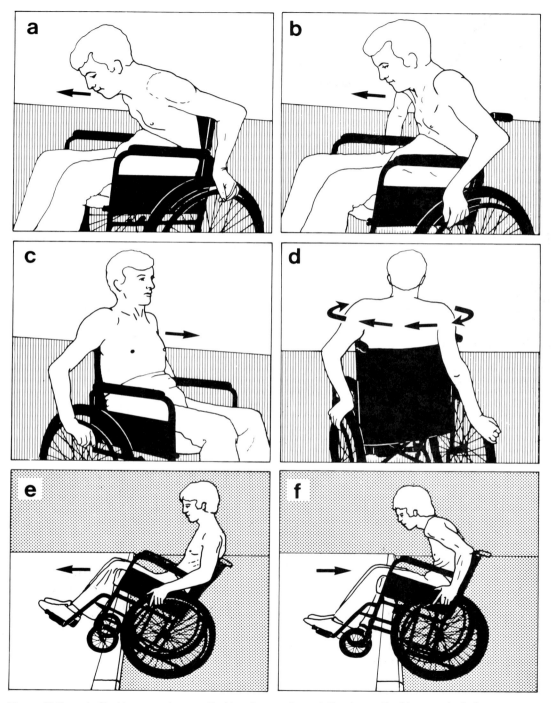

Figure 10.7 a, b: Pushing up a slope. c: Pushing down a slope. d: Turning. e: Pushing up a kerb. f: Descending a kerb. a–d: Patient with a complete lesion below C6 without triceps. e, f: Patient with a complete lesion below T8. This can be achieved by a patient with a complete lesion below C7 in a high performance wheelchair.

Advanced manoeuvres: tetraplegic patients

To push the chair over a 5 cm step

This manoeuvre can be accomplished by patients with lesions at C6 without triceps, and may be necessary to get over a draft excluder or similar obstacle:

1. Place the palms on top and to the outer side of the tyre with the fingers down over the rim and the thumb between the rim and the tyre.
2. Push the chair backwards, then
3. Push briskly forward, leaning the body weight forward at the same time.

Advanced manoeuvres: paraplegic patients

- To mount and descend a kerb
- To balance on the rear wheels
- To 'jump' the chair sideways
- To mount and descend a flight of stairs in a high performance wheelchair
- To transfer a wheelchair into a car.

To mount and descend a kerb

This activity can be accomplished by patients with a normal grip, i.e. those with lesions at T1 and below.

To push up a kerb

1. Tilt the chair onto the rear wheels.
2. Push forward until the front wheels hang over the kerb (Fig. 10.7e) and lower them gently.
3. Leaning forward, push forward forcefully to bring the rear wheels onto the pavement.

If the patient is unable to tilt the chair onto the rear wheels, he should 'flick' the front wheels high enough to mount the kerb. The flick up is achieved in the same way as the tilt but requires less strength and balance. Patients with lesions at C7–8 with good hand function may mount kerbs in this way and some patients with lesions at C6 in a high performance wheelchair may also be able to do it.

To descend a kerb

With the back to the kerb, lean well forward and push slowly backwards until the rear and then the front wheels roll down the kerb (Fig. 10.7f).

To balance on the rear wheels

Balance and movement on the rear wheels are useful to facilitate independent travel over rough ground, e.g. over grass, sand or shale, and also in negotiating kerbs or a step. This technique is safe only for patients with a good grip, i.e. for patients with lesions at T1 and below. In a HPW, patients with lesions at C7/8 may also manage it. Anti-tipping levers are used initially. There are three manoeuvres involved:

- To tilt the chair onto the rear wheels
- To balance the chair on the rear wheels
- To move and turn the chair on the rear wheels.

Action of the therapist. The therapist always stands behind the patient in step-standing, with the thigh of the forward leg ready to support the chair if control is lost. She holds the chair handles loosely (Fig. 10.8d). Assistance is given to tilt the chair by pressing down on the chair handles, and to find the balance point by giving pressure in each direction as necessary.

The therapist's hands must be very sensitive to the movement of the chair, correcting it only when the patient is out of control. She must allow enough scope for the patient to be really aware of each movement that occurs, so that the patient can become familiar with the 'feel' of the chair in the balance position.

Caution

The therapist's hands must remain on the chair handles until the patient has complete control, as it is all too easy for the patient to overbalance backwards and injure himself. Much practice will be needed. Not until the therapist is entirely satisfied that the patient is utterly competent should he be allowed to balance without her behind him as a safeguard.

Action of the patient
To tilt the chair onto the rear wheels

1. Place the hands on the wheels approximately

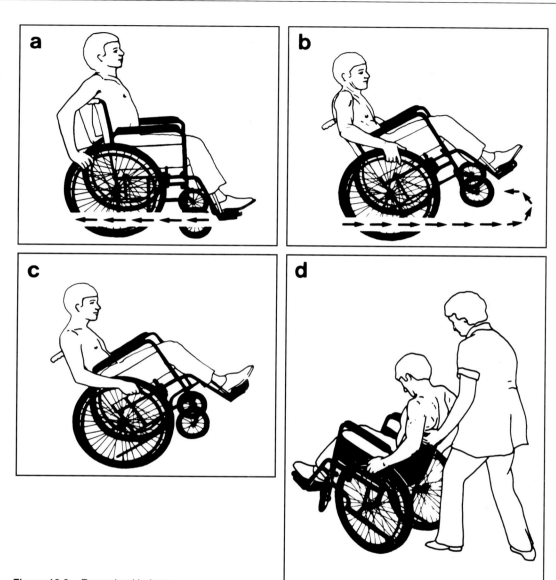

Figure 10.8 Rear wheel balance.

in the 10 o'clock position, holding the tyre and the rim or the tyre only, whichever is most comfortable.

2. Slightly extend the head, and put pressure on the wheels as though moving backwards (Fig. 10.8a).
3. Push forward quickly and forcefully, and the front wheels will lift off the floor (Fig. 10.8b). The height of the lift depends upon the force of the push.

To balance on the rear wheels

The balance point is much further back than most patients realize. It is found by playing the wheels forwards and backwards and using the head and shoulders as a counterweight. When overbalancing forwards, push the wheels forward. When overbalancing backwards, push the wheels backwards. Control may be easier when holding the rims or the wheel and rim.

To move and turn on the rear wheels

Once balance is achieved, it is not difficult to move on the rear wheels. The technique is the same as with the front wheels down.

To 'jump' the chair sideways

This manoeuvre can be useful when turning into a doorway from a narrow passage:

1. Apply the brakes.
2. Lean away from the back of the chair.
3. Grip the highest point of the wheel rims.
4. Lift the buttocks off the chair.
5. Quickly lift the wheels up and sideways before the buttocks descend again to the seat.

To mount and descend a flight of stairs in a high performance wheelchair

To go up and down a flight of stairs, each step must be deep enough to accommodate the weight-bearing section of the wheel. Within normal limits, the height of the step is not a limiting factor. This manoeuvre is only taught to patients who have already mastered all other activities in the wheelchair and who are willing to undertake the risks involved in learning the procedure.

To go up a flight of stairs with the rail on the right

Action of the therapist.

The therapist can assist using either of two methods:

• Stand behind the patient, holding the chair handle with one hand and grasping the stair rail with the other to anchor both herself and the patient (Fig. 10.9a).

• Stand on one side of the patient and control the twist of the chair by holding the wheel on the step whilst the patient alters the position of his arms to pull up the next step (Fig. 10.9b). Should assistance continue to be required this method can be taught to relatives or friends to enhance mobility in the community.

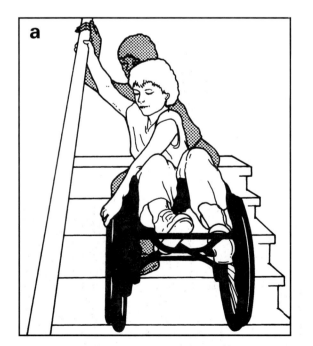

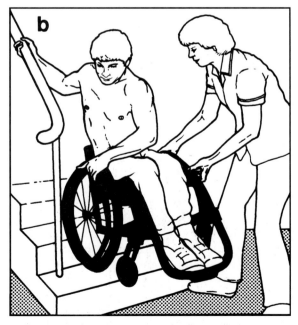

Figure 10.9 a: Ascending a flight of steps with assistance from behind. Patient with a complete lesion below T10. b: Ascending a flight of steps with assistance from below. Patient with a complete lesion below T12.

Action of the patient

1. With the chair close to the rail and the rear wheels against the step, stretch the right arm back and grasp the stair rail (Fig. 10.10a).
2. Lean back and balance on the rear wheels.
3. Grasp the right wheel rim with the left hand as far down the wheel as the patient can reach.
4. Pull the arms towards each other and ascend the step (Fig. 10.10b).
5. Hold the right wheel firmly against the next step with the left hand and slide the right hand up the rail.
6. Move the left hand down the wheel.

Repeat 4–6 to ascend each subsequent step.

To go down a flight of stairs

The steps are descended backwards.
Method 1 (using a rail on the left)

1. Position the chair close to the rail.
2. With the left hand, grasp the rail approximately level with the shoulders.

3. With the right hand, grasp the top of the right wheel and/or wheel rim.
4. Lean forwards and allow the chair to move backwards down the step, controlling it with the right hand (Fig. 10.11).
5. As the wheel descends onto the step, sit a little more upright and stabilize the chair. Lower the left hand on the rail and repeat 4 to go down the next step. (The footplates may bump onto the upper step as the chair descends.)
6. The left arm moves gradually down the rail with the chair. There is a tendency for the chair to twist as it descends.

Method 2 (using a rail on the right). Those patients who are both exceptionally skilled and strong may descend steeper steps in the following way:

1. With the left forearm held close to the chest, grasp the rail with the left hand.
2. Rotate the upper trunk and grasp the rail approximately midway between the top and next step with the right hand (Fig. 10.12a).

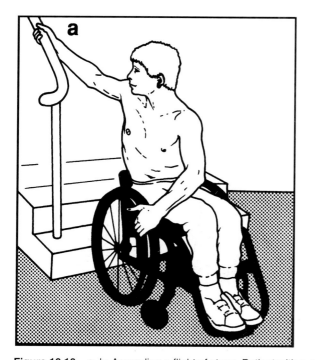
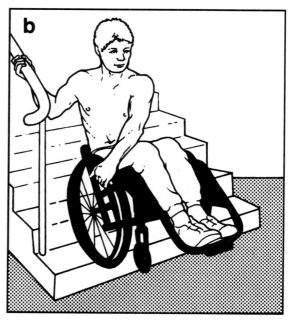

Figure 10.10   a, b: Ascending a flight of steps. Patient with a complete lesion below T12.

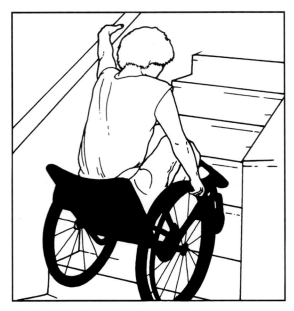

Figure 10.11 Descending a flight of steps holding rail and wheel. Patient with a complete lesion below T10.

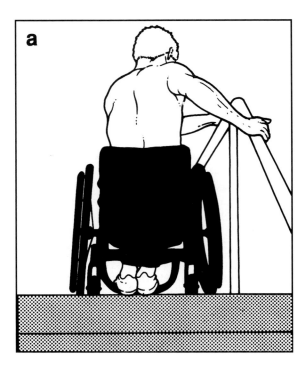

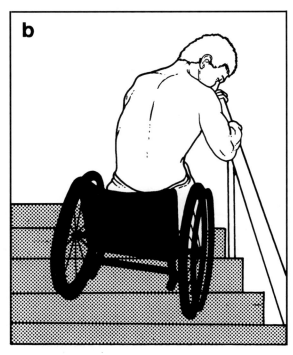

Figure 10.12 a–c: Descending a flight of steps holding only the rail. Patient with a complete lesion below T12.

3. Lean on the rail to take some of the body weight; great care must be taken not to pull the body out of the wheelchair.
4. In quick succession, let first one wheel and then the other descend the step. The chair twists during this manoeuvre and it is difficult to hold it with only one wheel on the step (Fig. 10.12b & c).

In either method, the therapist stands behind the chair, controlling its descent as necessary.

To descend shallow steps in a high performance wheelchair

Tip the chair onto the rear wheels and lower the chair onto the next step as in going down a kerb. Stop on each step to ensure continued control (Fig. 10.13).

To transfer the high performance wheelchair into the car

Action of the patient:

1. Move the driver's seat as far back as possible and recline the back of the seat.

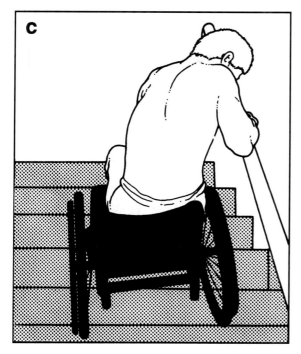

Figure 10.12c

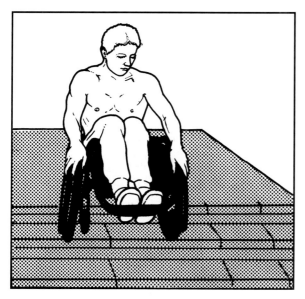

Figure 10.13 Descending shallow steps without a rail in a high performance wheelchair.

2. With the rear wheels towards the driver, tip the chair onto the front wheels (Fig. 10.14a).
3. Rest the top of the backrest against the open door.
4. Remove the left wheel (Fig. 10.14b).
5. Pull the chair towards the car and remove the right wheel (Fig. 10.14c).
6. Turn the chair until the seat faces the driver.
7. Grasp the front of the seat with the right hand and hold the top of the backrest with the left hand (Fig. 10.14d).
8. Lean against the back of the car seat and lift the chair across the body and into the back of the car (Fig. 10.14e & f).

Reverse the procedure to take the chair out of the car.

To transfer wheelchairs without removable wheels into a car

Patients can transfer the wheelchair into the car through the front passenger door. The chair is accommodated either in front of or behind the seat, which is adjusted accordingly.

Method 1

1. Transfer into the car through the passenger door.
2. Fold the wheelchair, leaving the brakes off.
3. Lift the front wheels of the chair into the car.
4. Transfer to the driver's seat.
5. Pull the chair into the car.

Method 2. Alternatively, after step 2 of method 1:

3. Transfer to the driver's seat.
4. Lean across the passenger seat and tip the chair onto its rear wheels.
5. Pull the chair, rear wheels first, into the car.

The efficiency of either method depends largely upon the physical proportions of the patient, and the best way should be found by trial and error. To get the chair out of the car, the procedure is reversed. It is easier to push the chair out when the rear wheels are adjacent to the door, i.e. using method 1.

Some cars can be adapted with a sliding door in place of the passenger door, and a hoist for loading the wheelchair.

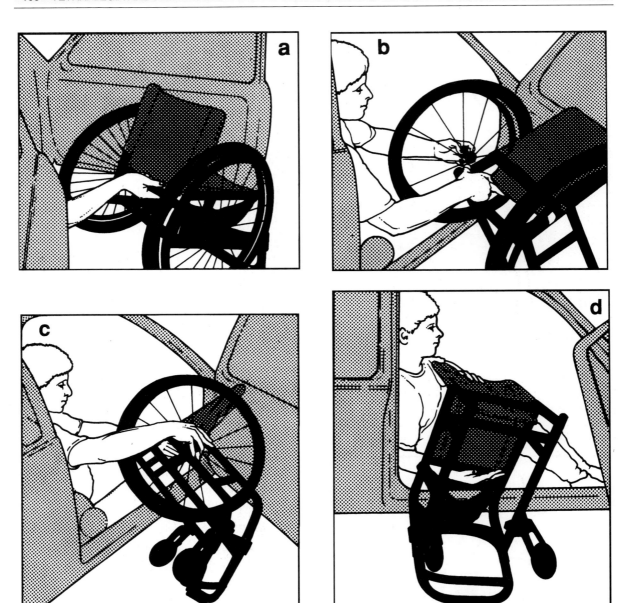

Figure 10.14   a–d: Transfer of a high performance wheelchair into a car. Patient with a complete lesion below T12.

TRANSPORT

Both paraplegic and tetraplegic patients have their own cars converted to hand controls. A patient with a lesion as high as C6 without triceps can drive a car providing it has automatic transmission. Adaptations for patients with special needs, e.g. those with incomplete lesions, are developed on an individual basis. Patients with paralysis of both lower and one upper limb can drive (Dollfus et al 1983).

Many spinal units have facilities for driving assessment. Most patients learn to drive through national organizations.

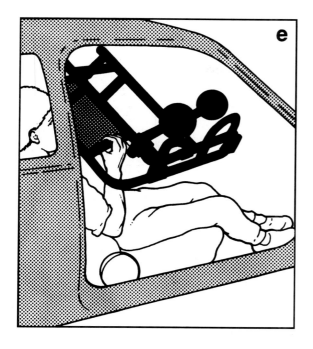

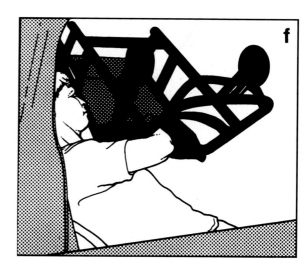

Figure 10.14 cont'd.   e,f: Transfer of a high performance wheelchair into a car. Patient with a complete lesion below T12.

Some makes of cars and vans can be adapted with a ramp or hoist to give access to the driving position for the patient in his wheelchair. This is particularly useful for those who are able to drive but unable to transfer, e.g. those in electrically powered chairs.

Some car rental firms have adapted vehicles for disabled users. Automatic rented cars can be quickly adapted to accommodate a paraplegic driver, enhancing the possibilities of independent travel (Dollfus et al 1983).

11

Transfers

For patients with spinal cord injury, transfers fall broadly into three groups:

1. those in which the feet are lifted and the trunk moves horizontally, e.g. transfer to plinth or bed
2. those in which the feet are at floor level and the trunk moves horizontally, e.g. transfer to toilet or easy chair
3. those in which the feet remain on the floor and the trunk moves vertically, e.g. transfer to bath or floor.

The first group is the most stable. The second requires skilled balance. The third requires considerable strength.

These factors explain the division of the transfers into initial and advanced for both tetraplegic and paraplegic patients. All patients commence with the transfers in group 1. Tetraplegic patients without triceps progress only to the easiest of those in group 2. To lift without triceps, the patient must have a strong deltoid to hold the shoulder joint in three planes, an elbow joint capable of being locked in hyperextension, and sufficient mobility in the wrist joint to allow weight to go through the arm with the palm on a flat surface. As can be seen in the following list, advanced transfers for the most active tetraplegic with triceps and wrist control only reach group 3 with the bath transfer, whereas advanced transfers for paraplegic patients are in group 3 exclusively.

For patients with tetraplegia

- *Initial transfers*

–chair to plinth
–removal of footplates
* *Advanced transfers*
–chair to bed
–chair to car
–chair to toilet
–chair to easy chair
–chair to bath.

For patients with paraplegia

* *Initial transfers*
–chair to plinth or bed, sideways and forwards
–chair to car
–chair to toilet, sideways and backwards
–chair to easy chair
* *Advanced transfers*
–chair to bath
–chair to floor.

TECHNIQUE

The techniques described are those most commonly used for the various transfers. Slight variations will occur depending upon the individual height, weight, agility and age of the patient, and the level of the lesion.

All transfers, except for that from the chair to the floor, are described for the tetraplegic patient. It is a simple matter to adapt the transfer for a patient with a lower lesion. The patient is always to lift, and not drag, his body to avoid knocking his limbs on the furniture or his buttocks on the wheel.

Whilst transferring the buttocks, the head, shoulders and trunk must be flexed with the head well forward over the knees. It is essential that the plinth be the same height as the wheelchair for transfer training, and, ideally, all surfaces should be at the correct height. Tetraplegic patients will achieve a transfer only under these conditions, but after training, most paraplegic patients will transfer to any surface without difficulty.

To prevent damage through shear forces, an orthoplast shield can be made to fit over the upper quadrant of the wheel during transfers. This can be useful for patients, particularly those with cervical lesions, who find difficulty in learning to transfer.

The chair

In all cases, the chair must be in the position of maximum stability. It may slip during the transfer if the tyres are worn or the floor is slippery, or if the patient pushes horizontally instead of vertically. If possible, the footplates are removed but this will depend upon their design. This is not necessary for independent transfer to the plinth or bed. It is dangerous to pull up the footplates without swinging them out, since they may catch on the malleoli and cause bruising or damage to the skin.

TRANSFERS BY THE THERAPIST

When *one* therapist transfers a patient who can give little or no assistance, the therapist must take great care to position herself and the patient correctly in order to avoid undue strain.

To transfer from chair to plinth with the patient moving to his right

Position of the chair. The chair is angled at approximately 30° to the side of the bed.

Position of the patient
1. Bring the buttocks forward in the chair until the feet are on the floor.
2. Flex the trunk and hips until the patient is lying over the therapist's right shoulder (Fig. 11.1a). The therapist always has her head turned in the direction of the movement (Fig. 11.1b).

Action of the therapist

1. Brace the feet and knees against the outside of the patient's feet and knees.
2. Flex the hips, keep the back straight and hold the patient under the buttocks.
3. Rock the patient against the knees and move him across to the plinth (Fig. 11.1c & d).

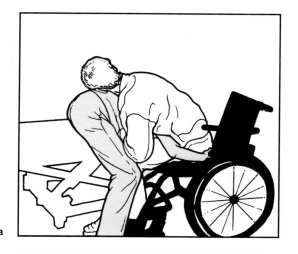

a

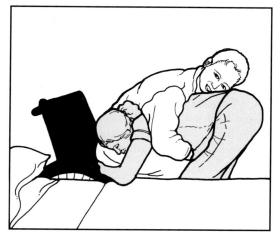

b

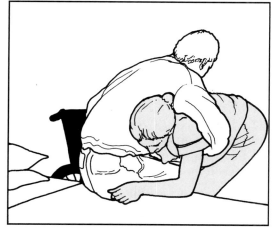

c

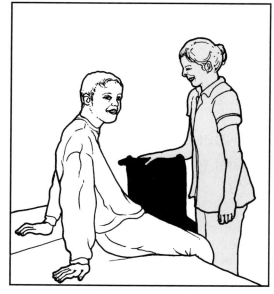

d

Figure 11.1 Transferring a patient with a lesion above C5.

If preferred, a transfer belt can be used instead of holding the patient under the buttocks. The belt is made of reinforced strong webbing. It has three or four loops or holding straps along its length. The belt is fastened securely round the patient's waist. The therapist grasps either one of the loops or the bottom of the belt on each side.

A sliding board can also be used to assist in the transfer. Boards are available in a variety of shapes, e.g. straight when the board has to be placed in front of the rear wheel, or horseshoe-shaped when the board fits around the wheel.

The 'cervical lift' using two therapists

Where other methods of transferring the patient are not possible and mechanical equipment is not available, this method is considered the safest for both patient and therapists. The lift can be used to transfer a patient to and from the bed, a second chair or from the floor in an emergency.

Transfer from bed to chair

The chair is angled at approximately 30° to the side of the bed.

Position of the patient. The patient is in long sitting with the head and trunk flexed and the arms folded across the lower ribs.

Position of the therapists to transfer the patient to the left. Operator 1 stands behind the patient with one leg on each side of the right rear wheel. She holds the patient around the thorax, grasping the patient's folded arms. The therapist must grip the lower thorax with her forearms to prevent the upper spine from elongating as the patient is lifted.

Operator 2 is in step-standing facing the bed. She grasps the legs with one arm high up under the thighs and the other under the lower legs. The heavier the patient, the higher up the legs the grasp needs to be (Fig. 11.2a).

On a prearranged signal, both operators lift together, operator 1 taking a step sideways and operator 2 a step backwards. The patient must be lifted high enough to avoid knocking the buttocks against the rear wheel or the spine against the chair handle or backrest support (Fig. 11.2b).

INDEPENDENT TRANSFERS

To transfer to the plinth (moving to the right)

This transfer consists of three manoeuvres:

- to bring the buttocks forward in the chair
- to lift the legs onto the plinth
- to transfer the trunk onto the plinth.

Position of the chair

Line the chair up with the plinth at an approximate angle of 20°. With the buttocks forward in the chair, this small angle allows the transfer to occur in front of the rear wheel. An orthoplast shield or a pillow is placed over the rear wheel to prevent injury should the buttocks knock against it during training.

The therapist

The therapist stands in front of the patient, ready to encourage flexion of the head and trunk and to

assist or resist the individual movements as necessary.

Action of the patient

To bring the buttocks forward in the chair

1. Extend the right wrist and flex the forearm under the right armrest.
2. Using the right arm, pull the trunk a little to the right and insert the left wrist behind the left hip. If wrist extension is strong, the forearm is pronated; if it is weak, the forearm is supinated (Fig. 11.3a).
3. Push on the right elbow on the back of the armrest. Flex the left elbow and push the left hip forward and at the same time extend the head and lean backwards. The cushion will slide forward with the leg (Fig. 11.3b). Repeat to bring the right hip forward. Figure 11.3c shows an alternative method for bringing the hips forward by pushing with both hands behind the hips at the same time. Two further methods are given in Chapter 10.

To lean forward over the legs, place both hands on the rear wheels and at the same time flex the head, protract the shoulders and thrust forward on the hands (Fig. 11.3d).

To lift the legs onto the plinth

1. To maintain balance, hook the right forearm round the right chair handle.
2. Put the left wrist under the right knee and lift the leg by flexing the elbow (Fig. 11.3e). Pull the knee up to the chest by pulling the trunk upright with the right arm and leaning back in the chair.
3. Rest the left wrist on the right armrest and bring the right arm forward onto the plinth (Fig. 11.3f).
4. Change the position of the arms so that the right wrist holds the knee, with the forearm supported on the armrest. The supinated left forearm moves down to support the lower leg (Fig. 11.3g).
5. Push the heel onto the plinth. Remove the right armrest as described on page 96.
6. Lift the left knee as for the right and hold the hip and knee in as much flexion as possible.

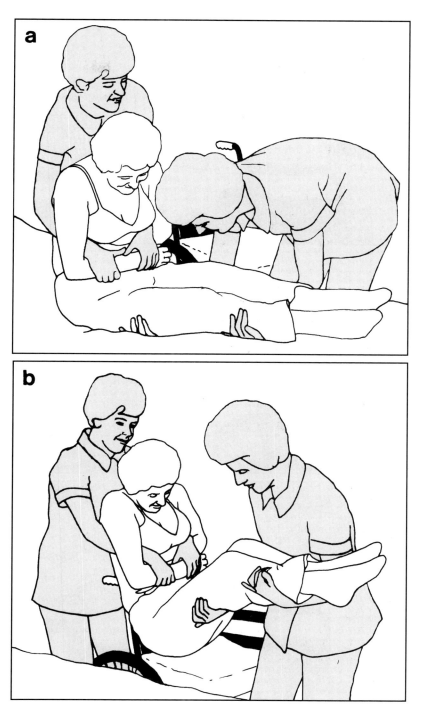

Figure 11.2 Transfer using two therapists.

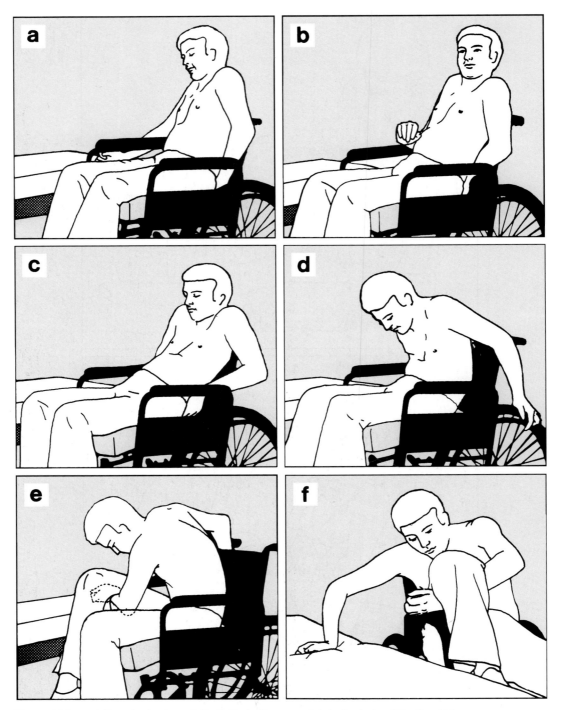

Figure 11.3 a–f: Transferring to a plinth. Patient with a complete lesion below C6 without triceps.

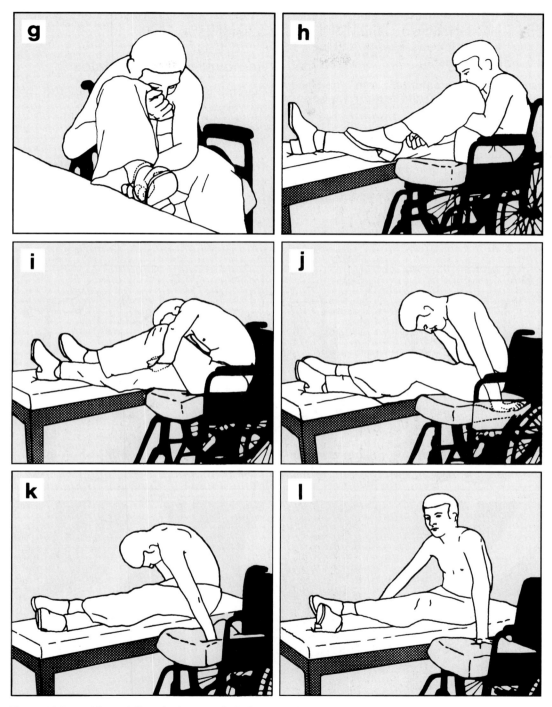

Figure 11.3 cont'd. g–l: Transferring to a plinth. Patient with a complete lesion below C6 without triceps.

7. Maintaining balance on the left elbow, lift the lower leg with the right wrist (Fig. 11.3h).
8. Lean over to the right and cross the left leg over the right (Fig. 11.3i).

To transfer the trunk onto the plinth. The basic technique for this activity is the same as for lifting sideways on the mat:

1. Place the right hand on the plinth level with the upper thigh and the left hand on the cushion (Fig. 11.3j), or on the armrest where possible.
2. With the head and trunk flexed, lift upwards and then to the right (Fig. 11.3k).

3. Several lifts will be necessary to complete the transfer (Fig. 11.3l).

Removal of the footplates

Depending on the type of chair the footplates may need to be removed.

To remove the right footplate

Transfer the right foot to the left footplate or to the floor

1. Balance is maintained with the left hand on the armrest if the patient has a lesion at C7, or

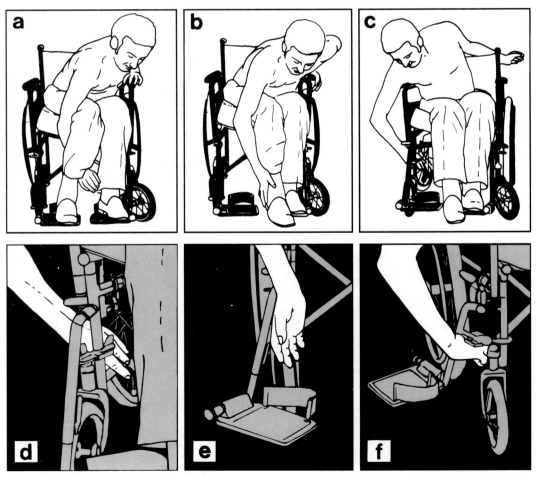

Figure 11.4 Tetraplegic patient removing the footplate.

with the left elbow or wrist hooked around the left chair handle if triceps is paralysed.
2. With the right wrist extended under the lower leg (Fig. 11.4a), flex the elbow and lift the foot over to the left footplate (Fig. 11.4b).

Remove the footplate (Fig. 11.4c–f)

1. With the wrist extended, release the lever by pushing it forward with the dorsum of the hand (Fig. 11.4d).
2. Swing back the footplate using extension of the wrist (Fig. 11.4e).
3. Lift the footplate off the bracket using the dorsum of the hand and wrist extension (Fig. 11.4f).

To transfer to the car (moving to the left)

Some patients with lesions at C6 without triceps, and those at C7 with no hand function, may find that a sliding board facilitates this transfer. The most useful dimensions of the sliding board have proved to be 60 × 20 × 1.5 cm tapered at both ends. A notch at the end facilitates the handling of the board, and a loop may be necessary for some patients to enable them to remove the board after transfer.

Position of the chair

The chair is angled at approximately 30° to the side of the car. Remove both footplates or, if preferred, only one (the left in the case of Fig. 11.5).

Action of the patient

1. Lift the feet into the car as for transferring to the plinth. Remove the armrest.
2. Place a sliding board under the left thigh.
3. Lift using the left half of the sliding board and the right armrest or chair seat (Fig. 11.5a), keeping the head and trunk well flexed.
4. Repeat the lift as often as necessary, moving the hands a little to the left each time (Fig. 11.5b). The head and trunk must remain flexed with the nose almost touching the steering wheel during the later lifts (Fig. 11.5c).

5. Remove the sliding board from the right and adjust the legs in the sitting position (Fig. 11.5d).

To transfer to the toilet (moving to the right)

Position of the chair

Place the chair at an angle of between 50 and 90° to the toilet seat. Many patients find the lift easier with the chair at right angles, because this position brings the armrest furthest from the toilet, closer to the handrail. Remove the footplates if necessary.

Position of the therapist

The therapist stands in front of the patient, bracing the patient's knees and feet and holding under the buttocks or in the trouser band. As the patient's proficiency increases, the therapist gradually withdraws her support.

Action of the patient

1. Check the position of the feet to see that they are flat on the floor and vertically beneath the knees so that the weight is over them. Remove the right armrest.
2. Keep the head and shoulders flexed throughout the transfer.
3. With the left hand on the armrest and the right on the rail, lift to the right (Fig. 11.6a & b).
4. With the left hand on the wheel and the right hand on the rail, lift further back onto the toilet (Fig. 11.6c).

To transfer back to the chair reverse the procedure.

In the absence of a wall rail, the experienced paraplegic patient can lift with his right hand on the toilet seat.

To transfer to the toilet through the back of the chair

This method can be used when spasticity is severe. For example, the patient may be at risk

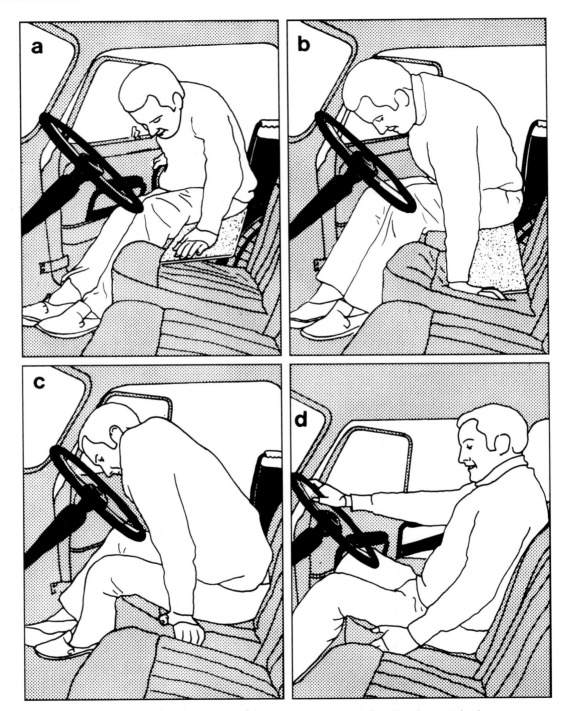

Figure 11.5 Transferring to a car. Patient with a complete lesion below C7 with wrist control only.

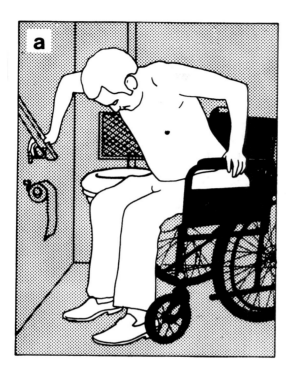

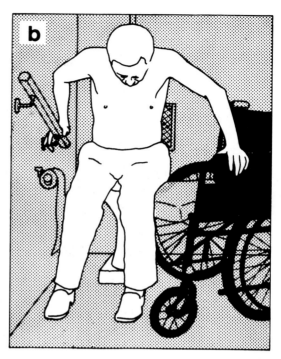

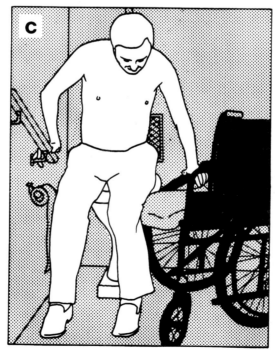

Figure 11.6   Transferring to a toilet. Patient with a complete lesion below C7 with wrist control only. (Note back support on toilet.)

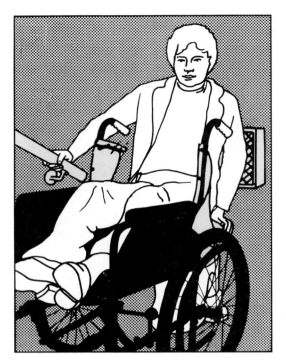

Figure 11.7 Backwards transfer.

transferring sideways when there is a combination of hip extension and knee flexion spasticity.

The normal backrest can be replaced by one which opens throughout its length by means of a zipper. The patient lifts backwards as shown in Figure 11.7, with one hand on the rail and the other on the toilet seat. Relaxation of the extensor spasticity may be obtained by flexing one or both legs before lifting backwards.

To transfer into an easy chair

This transfer is basically the same as the sideways transfer to the toilet, the arm of the easy chair being used instead of the wall rail. The wheelchair is positioned at right angles to the easy chair, with the front edge of the seat approximately halfway along the seat of the easy chair. This position brings the two lifting points closer together.

To transfer to the bath

The bath is filled with water before entering and drained before leaving. Bath transfer can be accomplished by patients with lesions at C7 and below.

To transfer over the bath end

Action of the patient

1. Position the chair so that the feet almost touch the bath.
2. Lift both legs onto the edge of the bath (Fig. 11.8a).
3. Swing away the footplates (Fig. 11.8b).
4. Wheel forward until the chair is adjacent to the bath (Fig. 11.8c).
5. Lift the buttocks forward in the chair.
6. Continue lifting forward with the right arm on the bath edge and the left arm on the armrest (Fig. 11.8d).
7. Transfer the left hand to the bath and lift onto the edge of the bath with the trunk almost fully flexed (Fig. 11.8e).
8. Maintaining the flexion, move the hands along the bath sides and lift, lowering the body into the bath as gently as possible (Fig. 11.8f & g).

To get out of the bath, reverse the procedure, flexing the legs before commencing to lift. Those patients who are unable to lift the whole depth of the bath can use a low wooden bath seat as an interim step. The edge of the seat must be padded and care taken to ensure that the skin is not damaged during the lift.

To transfer over the bath side

Position the chair either sideways at an angle of 30° to the bath or facing the bath:

1. Lift the legs into the bath.
2. Lift onto the bath edge.
3. With one hand on each side of the bath, turn to face the bath (Fig. 11.9).
4. Lift and lower gently into the bath.

Where there is a ledge behind the bath, a combination of these two methods can be used.

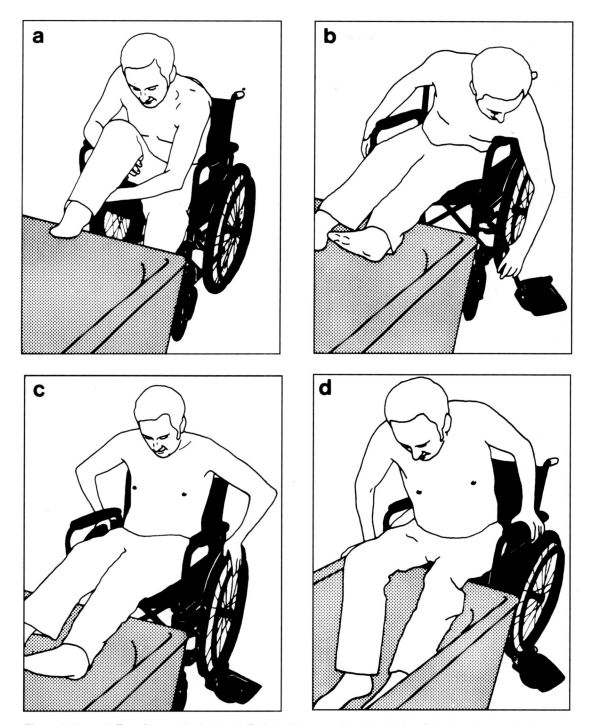

Figure 11.8   a–d: Transfer over the bath end. Patient with a complete lesion below C7 with wrist control only.

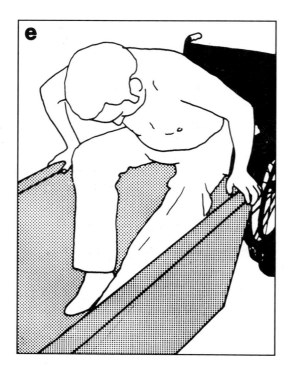

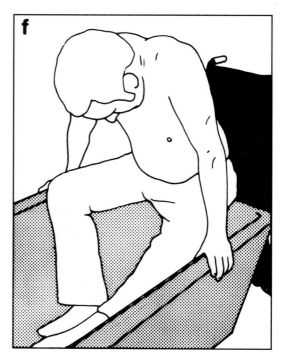

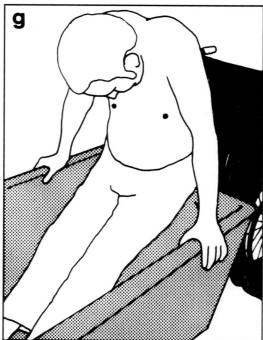

Figure 11.8 cont'd e–g: Transfer over the bath end. Patient with a complete lesion below C7 with wrist control only.

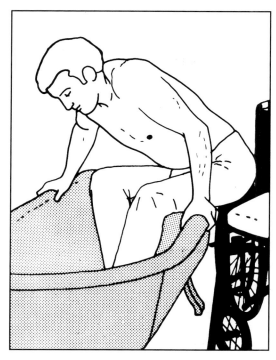

Figure 11.9 Transfer over the bath side. Patient with a complete lesion below C8.

First, transfer over the side onto the ledge, where the patient is more stable, and from there into the bath, as in Figure 11.8.

To transfer to the floor

The therapist

The therapist stands in front of the patient, correcting his position and assisting him to maintain balance as necessary.

Action of the patient

1. Remove the armrests.
2. Lift with the left elbow on the backrest and the right hand on the wheel, and pull the cushion out with the left hand (Fig. 11.10a).
3. Remove the footplates and place the cushion between the front wheels for protection when sitting on the floor (Fig. 11.10b).

4. Gripping the front of the seat supports, lift the trunk (Fig. 11.10c) and allow the buttocks to slip forward over the edge of the chair (Fig. 11.10d).
5. Gradually lower the weight to the floor (Fig. 11.10e).

Patients without abdominal muscles will need to extend the head and shoulders to tip the buttocks forward off the chair at step 4. The extension is maintained to prevent the patient pitching forward whilst lowering the trunk.

To lift back into the chair

Sitting with the back to the chair:

1. Either place both hands on the front of the seat supports or replace one footplate and place one hand on the top of the footplate fitting.
2. Lift strongly, extending the head and neck (Fig. 11.10f).
3. Contract the abdominals, if present, and depress the shoulders to pull the pelvis back onto the seat (Fig. 11.10g).
4. Lift the feet onto the footplates.

To replace the cushion

Double the cushion and place it between the wheel and the hip (Fig. 11.10h). Lift on both wheels and the cushion 'springs' into place under the buttocks (Fig. 11.10i).

Alternative method for patients without abdominals. Replace the armrests. Double the cushion and place it low down between the back and the backrest. Lift on both armrests and the cushion 'springs' into position.

In both methods, the position of the cushion may need final adjustment.

To transfer forward onto the bed

The forward transfer may be useful for the very young or for those who are overweight or severely spastic:

1. Lift the feet onto the bed.

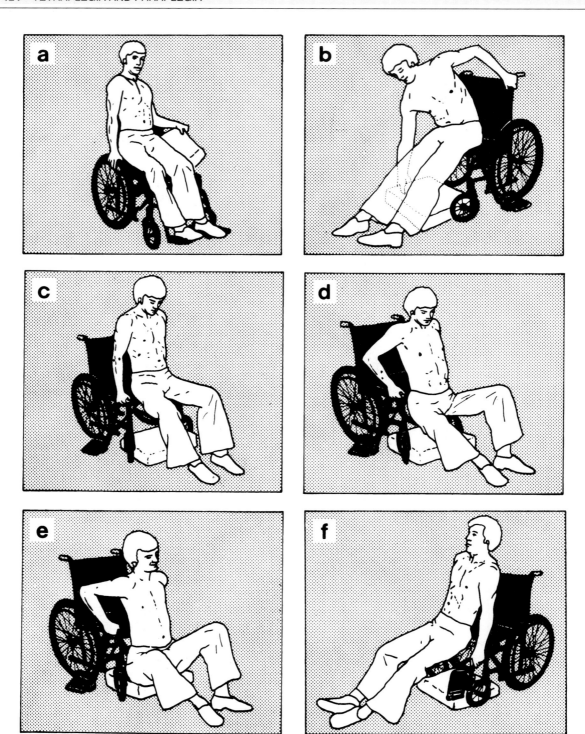

Figure 11.10   a–e: Transfer to the floor. f–i: Transfer back into the chair. Patient with a complete lesion below T11.

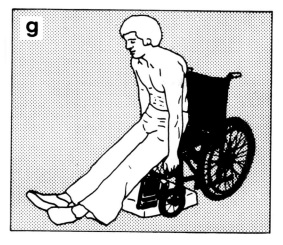

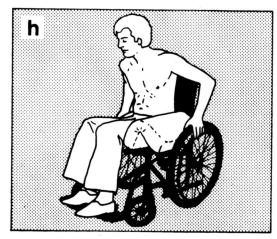

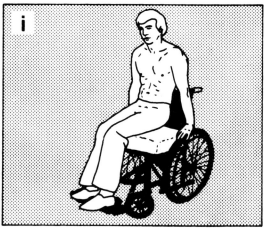

Figure 11.10 cont'd.

2. Wheel the chair forward until it is touching the bed.
3. Keeping the head and trunk flexed, lift forward in the chair. Small children who cannot lift on the armrests may lift by pushing down on the cushion (Fig. 11.11a). Repeated lifts may be necessary (Fig. 11.11b).
4. With the left hand on the bed and the right hand on the cushion, lift the buttocks sideways onto the bed (Fig. 11.11c & d). Repeated lifts will be necessary.

TRANSFERS FROM A HIGH PERFORMANCE WHEELCHAIR

Some adjustment in technique is required when transferring from the high performance wheelchair, which may have rigid footplates and a more forward position of the rear wheels than on the standard chair. When transferring sideways to, for example, the toilet or bath, the angle between the chair and the toilet may have to be altered and, with non-detachable footrests,

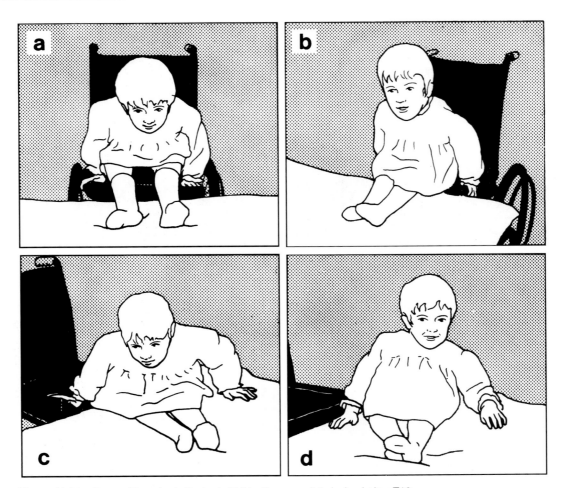

Figure 11.11 Forward transfer to the bed. Child with a complete lesion below T10.

forward transfer to the bed or over the bath end may not be possible.

Transfers to and from the floor are achievable by patients with complete lesions below C7 using the high performance wheelchair.

To transfer to the floor

Action of the patient

1. Bring the hips forward in the chair as described on page 112.
2. Remove the armrests.
3. Lift the feet onto the floor in front of the footplates.
4. Holding the top of the left footrest support

with the left hand, lean forward and to the right until the right hand can take weight on the floor (Fig. 11.12a).
5. Lift towards the right hand, keeping the head and trunk well flexed (Fig. 11.12b) and lower the body onto the floor (Fig. 11.12c).

The high performance wheelchair will move during this manoeuvre, but this should not affect the patient's control of the movement.

To transfer from the floor to the chair

Action of the patient

1. Sit close to the right side of the footplates.

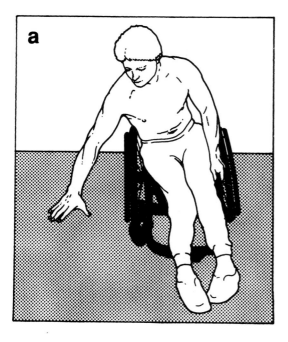

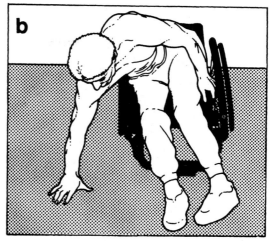

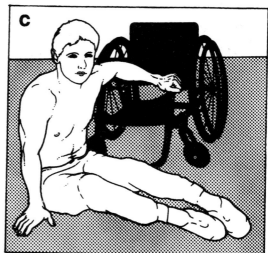

Figure 11.12 a–c: Transfer to the floor from a high performance wheelchair. Patient with a complete lesion below T12.

2. Hold the top of the left footrest support with the left hand and place the right hand on the floor beside the right hip (supported on the knuckles to give extra height if necessary, as in Fig. 11.13a).
3. Flex head and trunk as far as possible.
4. Push on the right hand and pull with the left hand (Fig. 11.13b).
5. Swing the buttocks into the chair. To ensure minimum effort, the lift needs to be performed as quickly as possible commensurate with safety, avoiding

knocking the hips or buttocks on the chair (Fig. 11.13c).
6. As the buttocks reach the chair, hold firmly with the left hand and pull the trunk to the left to regain balance (Fig. 11.13d).

The chair will move during the lift but this should not affect the patient's control of the movement.

The transfer using a hoist is described in Chapter 13.

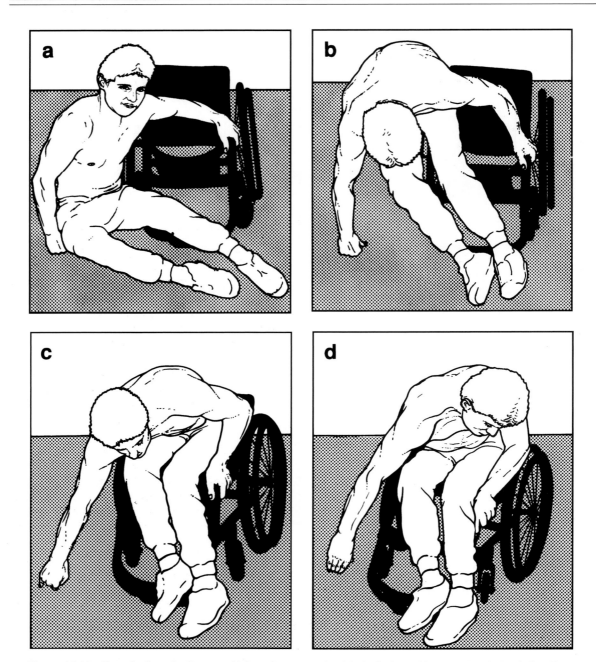

Figure 11.13 Transfer from the floor to a high performance wheelchair. Patient with a complete lesion below T12.

12

Gait training

It is important to put walking into perspective in terms of function in everyday life amongst able-bodied people outside hospital. Although most patients want to learn to walk, the energy cost of walking on crutches is high even for patients with low lesions, and in general only those with lesions at T10 and below, who are not overweight and who demonstrate some athletic ability, are successful and use their walking for functional purposes. Orthoses are expensive. Research has shown that the majority of paraplegic patients use their wheelchairs as their main means of locomotion. Not more than 10% of patients with complete lesions use orthoses for functional activities and a little less than one-third never use them at all (Haln 1970, Hong et al 1990).

As in all rehabilitation, much depends upon the physical proportions, age, sex and previous medical history of the patient, and even more upon his motivation. Further research on predictive factors is required to identify those patients with complete lesions who will become and remain functional walkers.

All patients are encouraged to stand, as the upright posture is believed to have a positive influence on:

- contractures in the lower limbs
- osteoporosis of the long bones with the danger of recurrent fractures
- the circulation
- spasticity
- renal function.

In a study on children with myelomeningocele,

the non-walkers had five times the number of pressure sores and twice the number of fractures than the walking group (Mazur et al 1989).

Most patients with lesions between T1 and T9 are able to walk between parallel bars using a swing-to gait and may progress to walking with crutches or a rollator for exercise only. Some may prefer to use a hip–knee–ankle–foot orthosis and use a four-point gait. Where the terrain is difficult for wheelchair use and motivation is high, some patients with lesions from T6 to T9 may learn swing-through gait on crutches and use it functionally at home, though these are rare exceptions.

Patients with lesions from C5 to C8 use a standing frame (Fig. 12.1) or stand between parallel bars, and those with higher lesions use a tilt table. Standing unassisted between bars aids the retraining of postural sensibility even for those with low cervical lesions, for the patient utilizes all innervated arm and trunk muscles to maintain balance. It is therefore an excellent exercise even for those who will not be able to walk.

Functional gait

The aim is to teach the use of both wheelchair and crutches so that the patient is equipped to use either, as the occasion demands. A widely increased sphere of independence is gained through crutch walking. Independent entrance can be obtained, for example, to buildings with small doorways, hotel accommodation, aircraft and trains. For the active patients, the benefits gained in everyday life far outweigh the patience and effort involved in training.

Concern is sometimes expressed about the effect that weight-bearing has on the shoulder joint. Research to determine the effect of the swing-through crutch walking gait on shoulder degeneration showed that no degenerative changes occurred, and there was an increase in the forearm bone density (Wing & Tedwell 1983). More recent studies have shown that, as most of the activities undertaken by active paralysed people involve the shoulder joints in weight-bearing, in older age problems in the shoulders occur at an earlier age than in the rest of the population (Ch.16).

Appliances

The basic requirements are to fix the knee joints and to hold the feet in dorsiflexion. The over-development of the trunk muscles, together with the creation of a new postural sense, may render any additional bracing unnecessary. Patients with low cervical or high thoracic lesions may walk with a hip–knee–ankle–foot orthosis (HKAFO), which supports the hips and trunk. Research continues to try to improve the function and appearance of these orthoses, the hybrid system of orthosis plus functional electrical stimulation (FES) and FES alone. Important advances have been made, but apart from the KAFO it is difficult to use these orthoses functionally.

Knee–ankle–foot orthosis (KAFO) (calipers)

Knee–ankle–foot orthoses (KAFOs), which allow

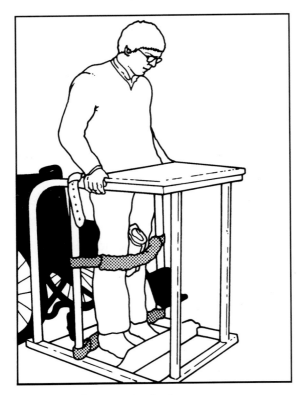

Figure 12.1 Oswestry standing frame.

the legs to bear the weight, are the only essential appliance for many patients. If standing is to minimize the formation of osteoporosis, it is vital that the weight should go through the long bones. Ischial weight-bearing is to be avoided because of the danger of causing pressure sores. A bucket-type thigh corset is used. The knee supports need to be wide. They encircle the knee to prevent lateral movement and give adequate support to the paralysed joint (Fig. 12.2). Round sockets are used in the shoe with backstops. In a small number of cases with extreme plantar-flexion spasticity, toe-raising springs may be needed in addition to the backstops.

These orthoses are made of duralumin as they need to be as light as possible. Where patients are overweight or have severe spasticity, it may be necessary to replace the duralumin with steel. For selected patients, usually those with flaccid lesions or who have minimum spasticity, ortholon cosmetic calipers may be prescribed. The lower section is moulded around the calf and heel and under the foot to just below the metatarso-phalangeal joints, and the upper section is moulded around the back of the thigh. They are cosmetically more acceptable, but care must be taken to ensure that they do not cause pressure sores, particularly around the ankle.

Caution. These orthoses are unsuitable for patients with severe spasticity or oedema of the feet and lower legs.

KAFOs are available which have adjustable locked ankle joints (Scott 1971). The correct angle to gain maximum stability is found with the patient standing in the balanced position between the parallel bars, with hips hyperextended and feet dorsiflexed beyond 90° (see p. 134). The ankle joint is locked with the patient standing in this position. The shoe is flat to take a steel plate and is permanently fixed to the orthosis, which is made of steel and is heavier than if made from duralumin. Greater stability is provided and they may be particularly useful for patients with lesions between T6 and T9 (Duffus & Wood 1983).

Modular KAFOs and plaster of Paris leg splints

Modular KAFOs can be kept in stock to fit on a temporary basis until the made-to-measure orthosis is available. In the absence of modular calipers, posterior shells of plaster of Paris are made for each patient and used to stabilize the knees. The shells extend from 5 cm below the ischial tuberosities to 5 cm above the malleoli. It may be necessary to reinforce the plasters with a strip of steel or Kramer wire for patients who are overweight or who have severe spasticity. Temporary toe-raising springs are used with these splints to hold the foot in dorsiflexion. They consist of a webbing band round the leg, with adjustable straps, a short spring and a narrow webbing band under the shoe (Fig. 12.3).

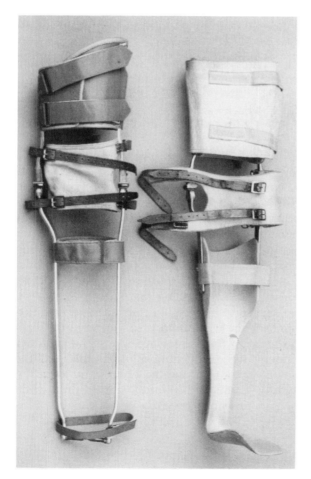

Figure 12.2 Calipers.

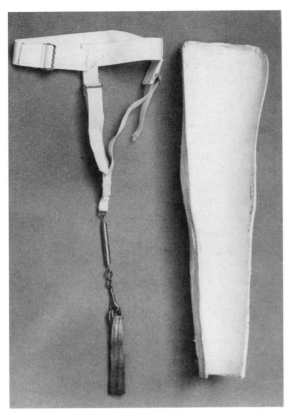

Figure 12.3 Temporary toe-raising spring and plaster of Paris splint.

Shoes

Shoes for use with any type of orthosis should provide good support for the feet and be made of soft leather without toe caps. To prevent pressure sores, all the inside seams, particularly around the heel, must be smooth. Leather soles stitched to the uppers provide the most suitable support for the sockets, back stops, or T straps if necessary. To accommodate for slight oedema and avoid damage when putting them on, the shoe fitting should be at least half a size larger than the size previously worn.

STANDING A PATIENT WITH A KNEE–ANKLE–FOOT ORTHOSIS
Standing between parallel bars

Because of the loss of all postural and equilib-

rium reactions below the level of the lesion, a new postural sense must be developed in the erect position. Compensation by sight for the loss of sensation is essential, and a long mirror is used at the end of the bars and another to the side of the patient. Patients without muscle control at the hips lift their legs by the action of latissimus dorsi and the associated action of trapezius and shoulder girdle muscles. Postural sense in standing is developed largely through the action of these 'bridge' muscles. Occasionally, vasomotor disturbances occur on standing the higher lesions. If necessary, an abdominal binder can be worn temporarily to assist in preventing pooling of the blood in the splanchnic vessels. Fainting is more likely to occur when the patient is tall and thin (Figoni 1984).

Position of the wheelchair

The chair is positioned with the supporting crossbar of the bars behind the front wheels, if possible. This will prevent the chair from slipping backwards.

Height of the bars

For the efficient use of latissimus dorsi and triceps, the bars must be at the correct height. With the hand on the bar and the shoulders relaxed, the elbow must be slightly flexed. This usually brings the wrist approximately level with the greater trochanter, but this depends upon individual physical proportions. For the initial stand, the height of the bars is determined by guesswork. After seeing the patient on his feet, the therapist must make the necessary adjustments. It is a common error to have the bars too high. In this case, elevation of the shoulder renders depression almost impossible and the patient cannot lift the leg effectively. With the bars too low, stability can be gained only when the patient leans forward with his weight on his hands.

To stand a patient

Action of the therapist. Stand facing the patient,

with the feet either side of the patient's legs, ready to grip with the knees to prevent the feet from sliding forward. Step-standing may be preferred, as in Figure 12.4a. Hold the patient under the buttocks and pull the hips forward as the patient lifts.

Action of the patient

1. Sitting well back in the chair, lean forward and place the hands at the end of the bars with the elbows vertically above the wrists (Fig. 12.4a). This position allows the patient to stand by pushing down on the bars. The tendency to reach along the bars and pull up must be avoided.
2. Push down on the hands and stretch upwards, not forward (Fig. 12.4b).
3. As the weight comes over the feet, hyperextend the hips and at the same time extend the head and retract the shoulders.
4. Move the hands a short distance forward along the bars (Fig. 12.4c). If the patient is tall or overweight, a second therapist may be needed to push the feet back as the patient lifts. This will reduce the effort required by the patient.

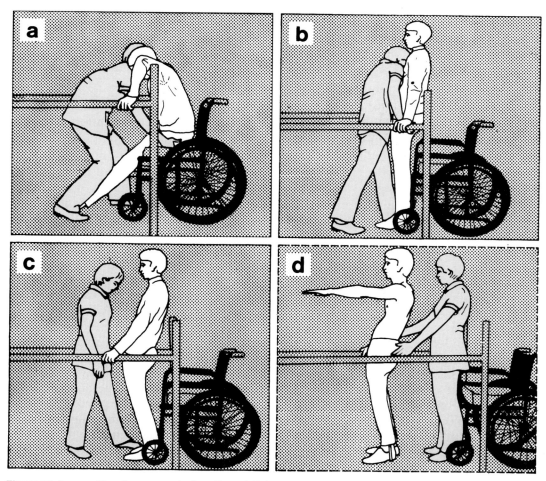

Figure 12.4   a–c: Standing a paraplegic patient. d: Balance exercise in the bars. Patient with a complete lesion below T5.

To get behind the patient and establish the balanced position

Action of the therapist

Keeping the hips in extension with the left hand, and the upper trunk extended with the right arm, move behind the patient by passing under his right arm. At the same time, slide the arms around the patient's trunk to maintain his position (Fig. 12.5).

Brace one hip against the patient's sacrum to maintain hyperextension of his hips. Prevent forward or lateral movement of the trunk with the right hand on the upper thorax and the left hand on the pelvis (Fig. 12.4d). Watching in the mirrors, help the patient to find his point of balance and encourage him to hold it without support.

When this has been achieved, resisted exercises can be given to improve balance and coordination.

Suitable patients with lesions at C6/7 should be able to stand in this way, but will need the assistance of a second therapist to push the buttocks and hips forward and the shoulders back.

If a young and active patient with a lesion at C7 or C8 is anxious to walk, swing-to gait can be taught as for the paraplegic patient.

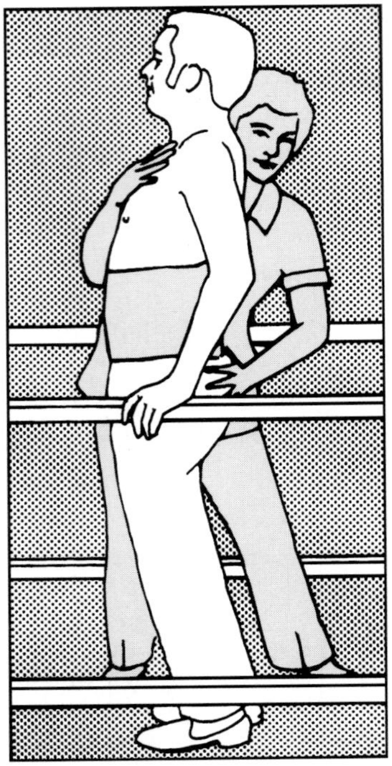

Figure 12.5 Moving behind the patient (note abdominal belt).

Posture correction

The standing posture is corrected so that:

1. weight goes through the heels
2. legs are inclined only a few degrees forward of 90° at the ankle
3. hips are slightly extended so that the line of gravity lies behind the hip joints, through the knee joints and slightly in front of the ankle joints to prevent the 'jack-knife' fall forward
4. spine is as upright as possible. Some adjustment must be made in the upper thoracic spine to compensate for the hyperextended hips. Overcorrection must be avoided
5. bars are held with the hands approximately level with the toes
6. shoulders are relaxed.

The posture of the patient with useful abdominal muscles should be almost erect except for the slight hyperextension necessary at the hip joints. As the level of the lesion rises, a greater degree of compensation will be necessary at the hip joints. In all cases, overcorrection should be avoided. If the patient is allowed to lean forward with the weight over the toes and with the spine and shoulders extended, he will be unable to lift the weight off his feet. A second mirror placed at the side of the patient may assist him to correct his posture by showing the anteroposterior deviations from the vertical.

There is a fine point between over- and undercorrection. This position provides the basic balance point from which all gait training proceeds.

Duration of the stand

Depending upon the height of the lesion the patient may remain on his feet for only 2 minutes or up to 5 or 10 minutes on the first day. A gradual increase in the duration of the stand is most important in order to allow the circulation to adapt with the minimum ill effect on the patient.

Initially it is more beneficial to stand two or three times for a few moments only than to stand once for a longer period. The constant change in posture stimulates the vascular system and promotes a more rapid establishment of vaso-motor adjustment.

To sit down

The therapist, holding the patient under the buttocks and controlling his legs with her knees and feet, allows him to sit down gradually.

Action of the patient

With the feet approximately a foot's length from the chair:

1. Hyperextend the hips and place the hands in their original position on the bars.
2. Take the weight on the arms.
3. Flex the head and trunk, and lower the weight gently until the buttocks reach the chair.

Caution. Care must be taken to ensure that the patient does not knock his hips against the sides of the chair, or drop his weight suddenly onto the buttocks. Bruising, both superficial and in the deeper tissues, can easily occur.

When resting in the chair, with splints or calipers on the legs, the heels must be supported on a stool; otherwise the weight of the leg is taken on the upper end of the femur. If preferred, calipers can be unlocked at the knee joints.

Exercises in standing

As control is gained over the upper thorax, the therapist can place both hands around the hips to support only the pelvis. The hands are placed along the iliac crest, with the fingers over the anterior superior iliac spine. With the hands in this position, the therapist can pull the pelvis back with her fingers (Fig. 12.6a), push it forward with the heel of her hand (Fig. 12.6b), give pressure downwards (Fig. 12.6c) or lift upwards. In this way, the therapist has complete control of the patient and can assist or resist movement in any direction.

Balance exercises

Watching his position in the mirror, the patient is taught to:

- hold, move out of and regain the correct posture
- maintain balance whilst lifting one hand off the bar (Fig. 12.4d). Progression is made by moving the arm in all directions, and later by repeating this with the eyes closed
- move both hands forwards and backwards along the bars.

Exercises for strength and control

Before commencing gait training, the patient must learn to tilt his pelvis by using latissimus dorsi, and to become aware of the degree of control he can achieve with this compensatory mechanism.

Pelvic side tilting

To 'hitch' the left leg, place the left hand on the bar only slightly in front of the left hip, and the right hand about half a foot length further forward. Keeping the elbow straight, press firmly down on the left hand and depress the shoulder.

The leg must be lifted upwards and not forwards.

To lift both feet off the ground and control the pelvis

Place both hands on the bars slightly in front of the hip joints. Push down on the bars, with the elbows straight, and depress the shoulders. To gain control of the pelvis, the patient should practise holding himself at both full and partial lift, rotating the trunk and tilting the pelvis with the feet lifted off the ground.

Resisted trunk exercises

For greater efficiency in balance, strength and control, resisted trunk exercises in the standing and 'lifting' positions and resisted 'hitching' are also given.

Passive stretch in standing

Where strong spasm in the hip flexors and abdominal muscles prevents the patient from assuming the erect posture, a passive stretch can be given. The therapist gives firm pressure forwards with her hip against the patient's sacrum, and with her hands pulls backwards over the front of the shoulder joints.

If the position is maintained for a few moments the spasticity usually relaxes and the patient is able to maintain his balance.

Cautions

1. Stretching must always be performed with extreme care. Unskilled passive stretching has resulted in fracture of the neck of the femur. The top of the caliper becomes the fulcrum and the strain is transferred to the femoral neck.
2. Until the spasm relaxes, the patient may experience some difficulty in breathing. The spasticity is initially increased by the stretch, and the tightness of the abdominal muscles may prevent adequate movement of the diaphragm.
3. The therapist must make sure that she has no hard objects in her pocket which could cause pressure.

Standing frames

Where walking is impractical, a standing frame may be used (Fig. 12.1). Some standing frames have additional supports at each side so that a strap can be used to control the trunk of the tetraplegic patient, if required.

GAIT

There are three types of gait used:

- swing-to gait
- four-point gait
- swing-through gait.

Controlled walking is achieved only through perseverance, perfect timing, rhythm and coordination. The patient is taught always:

1. to move the hands first
2. to walk slowly and place his feet accurately
3. to take the weight through the feet and so ensure that the hands can relax between each step
4. to lift the body upwards and not to drag the legs forwards.

An accurate technique must be achieved in bars if crutch walking is to be successful.

Where it is anticipated that the patient will become an accomplished walker, it is usual to commence training with the four-point gait. It is easier to learn to use the latissimus dorsi muscles at first separately and then together than vice versa.

GAIT TRAINING IN THE BARS

Swing-to gait

This is the universal gait because it is both the simplest and the safest. All patients with lesions above T10 are normally taught this gait first.

The therapist

The therapist stands behind the patient with her hands over the iliac crests. Assistance is given to lift, to control the tilt of the pelvis and to transfer weight as necessary.

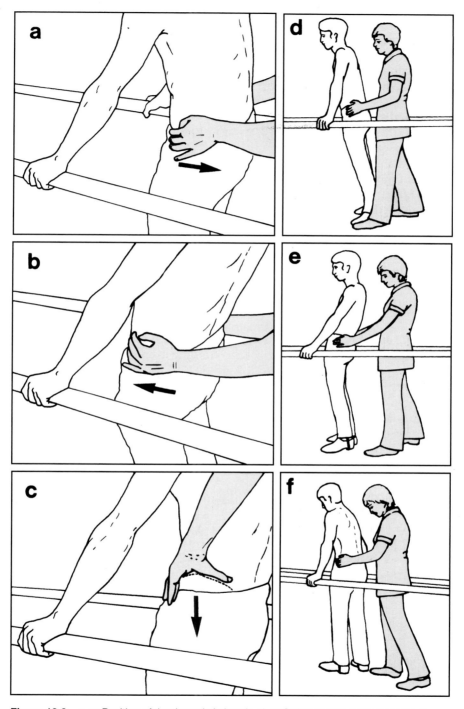

Figure 12.6   a–c: Position of the therapist's hands. d, e: Swing-to gait. f: Four-point gait.

Action of the patient

1. Balance in the hyperextended position.
2. Move the hands, either separately or together, forward along the bars approximately half a foot length in front of the toes.
3. Lean forward, with the head and shoulders over the hands (Fig. 12.6d), and lift the legs, which will swing forward to follow the position of the head and shoulders. The step is short and the feet must drop just behind the level of the hands (Fig. 12.6e). To achieve this, the lift must be released quickly, otherwise the feet will travel too far and land between or in front of the hands. When on crutches, it is unstable and therefore dangerous to have the feet and hands in line. It must therefore be avoided in the bars. The swing-to gait is a 'staccato' gait with no follow through: 'lift and drop'.

The patient should also be taught to swing backwards along the bars.

To turn in the bars. The turn is achieved in two movements by turning through 90° each time. To turn to the right:

1. Place the left hand forward about a foot length along the bars and the right hand either level with or a little behind the trunk.
2. Lift and twist the shoulders and upper trunk to the right. The feet land facing the bar to the right (Fig. 12.7a).
3. Balance in this position and move the left hand across to the right bar (Fig. 12.7b).
4. Twisting the upper trunk to the right, place the right hand on the opposite bar.
5. Lift the feet round to a central position between the bars (Fig. 12.7c).

Four-point gait

This gait is the slowest and most difficult of all and is only achieved on crutches by accomplished walkers. It facilitates turning and manoeuvring in confined spaces. It also provides an excellent training exercise in strength, balance and control.

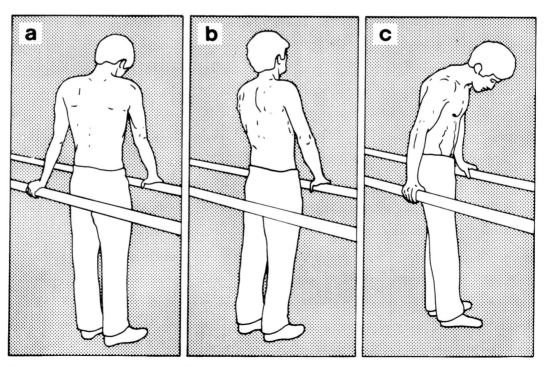

Figure 12.7   Turning in the bars. Patient with a complete lesion below T11.

The therapist

The therapist holds the pelvis in the usual way. Both by instruction and by correction with her hands, the therapist emphasizes each move, ensuring that the patient achieves it correctly. Only when the patient consistently makes a single movement correctly does the therapist stop correcting that component. The patient needs to see and 'feel' the correct posture at each move, and therefore constant repetition is necessary.

Action of the patient

To take a step forward with the left leg

1. Place the right hand forward about half a foot length along the bar and the left one just in front of the hip joint.
2. Take the weight on the right leg, so that the hip is over the right foot and the knee and ankle in a vertical line.
3. With the left shoulder slightly protracted, push on the left hand and depress the shoulder (Fig. 12.6f). The effort is to 'lift' the leg upwards.
4. As the left leg is lifted, it swings forward to follow the shoulder. The 'lift' is released when a large enough step has been made. (Small steps should be taken initially, but the foot must always land in front of the hand.)
5. Take the weight over the left leg.
6. Move the left hand forward along the bar in preparation for moving the right leg. Pelvic rotation must be avoided.

The following are possible reasons for an inadequate lift:

- some weight remains on the moving leg
- the hands are too far forward
- the weight may be over the toes and not back over the heels, in which case the trunk may be hyperextended and the legs consequently inclined too far forward
- insufficient depression of the shoulder girdle on the side of the moving leg
- the bars are too high or too low
- the lift is not held for sufficient time to allow the leg to swing forward.

To take a step backward with the left leg

1. Place the left hand slightly behind the hip joint.
2. Lift the leg and at the same time lean forward on that side.
3. Bend the elbow and 'flip' the leg backwards.

Swing-through gait

This gait requires skilled balance, but it is the fastest and most useful.

The therapist

The therapist gives assistance where necessary with her hands controlling the pelvis until the patient can accurately and slowly perform the movements. The forward thrust of the pelvis to push the weight over the feet usually needs to be emphasized.

Action of the patient

1. Place the hands forward along the bars as for the swing-to gait.
2. Lean forward and take the weight on the hands.
3. Push down on the bars, depress the shoulder girdle and lift both legs. The lift must be sustained until the legs have swung forward to land the same distance in front of the hands as they were originally behind. Considerably more effort is required than for the swing-to gait.
4. As the weight is lifted and the legs swing forward, hyperextend the hips, extend the head and retract the shoulders.
5. To move the trunk forward over the feet, push on the hands, extending the elbows and adducting the shoulders. When the weight is firmly on the feet, move the hands along the bars for the next step.

GAIT TRAINING ON CRUTCHES

Progression is made to crutch walking only when the technique between the bars is good. The height of the elbow crutches is checked as for the bars.

The change from walking in bars to crutch walking is considerable, and all patients are initially unstable and fearful. A high degree of balance skill is essential and this is only achieved with perseverance and much practice.

Balance exercises

Balance on crutches is trained in the same way as when balancing in the bars (Fig. 12.8a). Resisted work is also given to enable the patient to gain adequate control over the trunk and pelvis.

Walking on crutches

Swing-to and four-point gaits are taught first and progression is made to swing-through (Fig. 12.8b & c). Until the new postural sense is established training is again carried out in front of a mirror.

Progression in the four-point gait may be made by using one bar and one crutch if preferred. Otherwise, progression is directly onto two crutches, as there is less tendency to trunk and pelvic rotation.

The technique for each gait is the same as already described for walking in bars. Much greater skill is required and several weeks of practice will be needed to acquire the necessary balance and coordination.

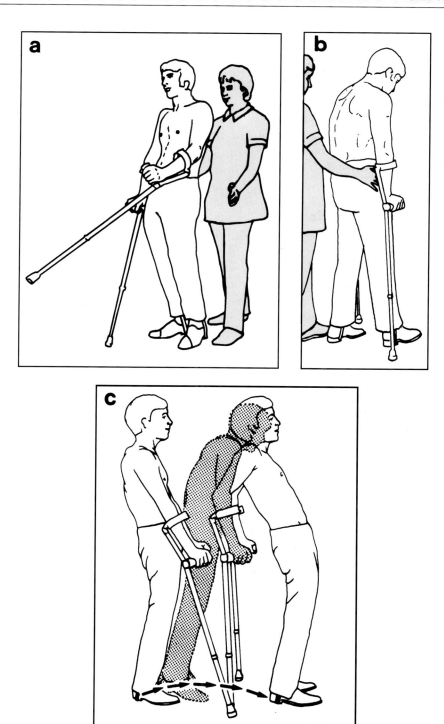

Figure 12.8 a: Balance exercise on crutches. Patient with a complete lesion below T5. b: Four-point gait. c: Swing-through gait. Patient with a complete lesion below T12.

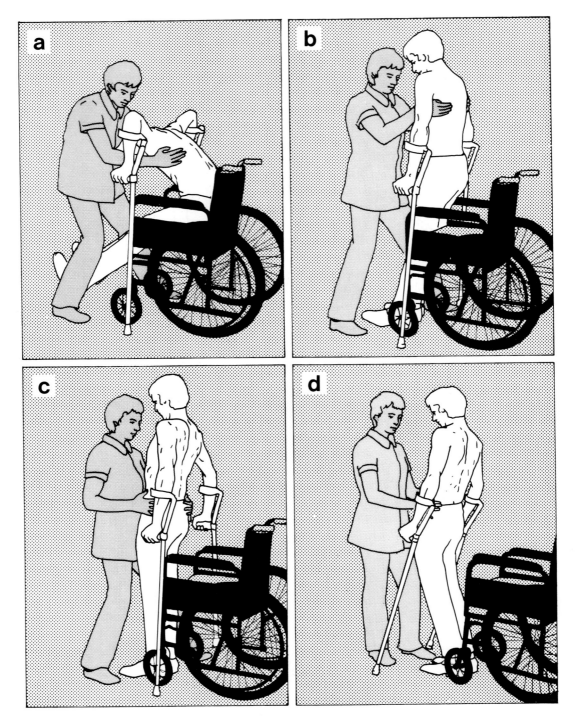

Figure 12.9   Chair to crutches – forwards technique. Patient with a complete lesion below T6.

To transfer from chair to crutches

An unaided exit from a chair is essential if crutch walking is to be functional. There are three techniques used to get into and out of the chair with crutches:

- forwards technique
- sideways technique
- backwards technique.

All three methods are taught where possible, and the patient chooses that which he finds easiest.

Forwards technique

Severe abdominal and/or flexor spasticity which prohibits the necessary hyperextension at the hips, or excessive height, may prevent a patient accomplishing this technique. When the patient is well over average height with the extra length primarily in the legs, the elbows are higher than the shoulders with the crutches in position for the lift. Latissimus dorsi and triceps are thus at a mechanical disadvantage and a balanced lift is impossible.

The therapist

The therapist stands in front of the patient astride the legs and ready to give support with her hands around the scapula region (Fig. 12.9).

Action of the patient

1. Check the position of the chair and swing away the footplates. During early training, when the weight distribution may be incorrect, a feeling of stability is given if the chair is backed against a wall.
2. Sit well back in the chair (Fig. 12.10a).
3. Place the crutches midway between the front and rear wheels, level with each other and equidistant from the sides of the chair (Fig. 12.10b). To avoid rotation during the lift, the position of the crutches must be accurate.
4. Lean forward over the crutches and balance.
5. Lift on the crutches, adducting and extending the shoulders.
6. The feet are lifted backwards, and as the weight goes onto them, hyperextend the hips and retract the shoulders (Fig. 12.10c).
7. When balanced, move the crutches forward and assume the correct standing position (Fig. 12.10d).

To sit down, reverse the procedure, as in Figures 12.10d–a. If the physical proportions of the patient are suitable, an alternative method is shown in Figure 12.10e. The short patient reaches back with his hands, releases the crutch handles and grasps the armrests. Such patients may be able to stand up in the same way. To prevent trauma, which could result in haemorrhage and bursa formation, sitting down should be done slowly without bumping on the chair.

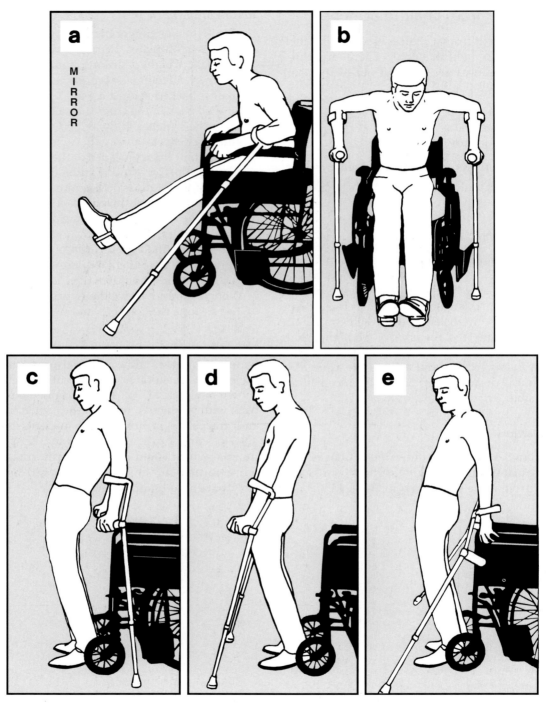

Figure 12.10 a–d: Chair to crutches – forwards technique. Patient with a complete lesion below T9. e: Short patient sitting down.

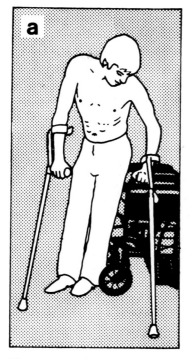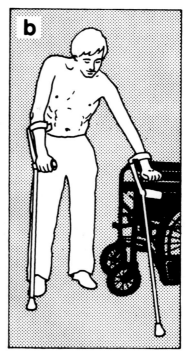

Figure 12.11   Chair to crutches – sideways technique.

Sideways technique

Some patients of below average height are able to get out of the chair using one crutch and an armrest:

1. Put the left arm through the forearm support, position the left crutch and grasp the armrest.
2. Turn through 45° towards the left armrest.
3. Place the right crutch in front and to the left of the midline of the chair.
4. Lift on both arms (Fig. 12.11a & b).
5. With the weight on the feet, balance on the right crutch and grasp the left crutch handle.

Reverse the procedure to sit down.

Backwards technique

The therapist stands in front of the patient ready to control the pelvis or legs as necessary. The following actions are for the patient turning to the left:

1. Cross the right leg over the left (Fig. 12.12a).

2. Lift the buttocks to the right side of the chair (Fig. 12.12b).
3. Turn the trunk to the left, moving the left hand to the right armrest and the right hand to the left armrest (Fig. 12.12c).
4. Push on both armrests to stand (Fig. 12.12d) facing the chair.
5. Hitch the feet to the left (Fig. 12.12e).
6. Put each hand through the crutch forearm rest and return to holding the armrest (Fig. 12.12f).
7. Grasp the handgrips in turn.
8. Walk backwards away from the chair (Fig. 12.12g).

Reverse the procedure to sit down.

Stairs

Climbing stairs is normally functional for patients with good abdominal muscles. Some young and active patients with lesions between T6 and T10, with or without a spinal brace, may also become efficient and independent.

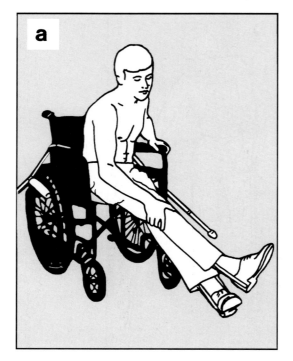

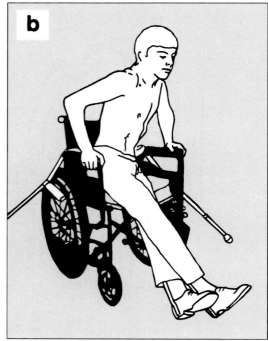

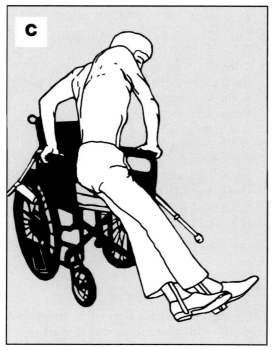

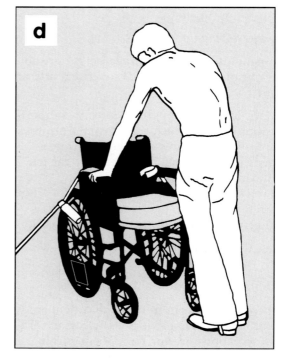

Figure 12.12 a–g: Chair to crutches – backwards technique. Patient with a complete lesion below T12.

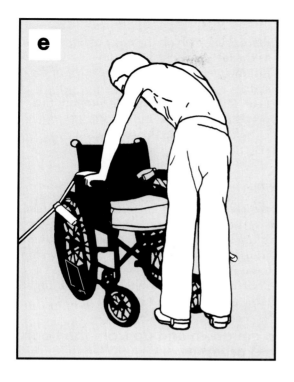

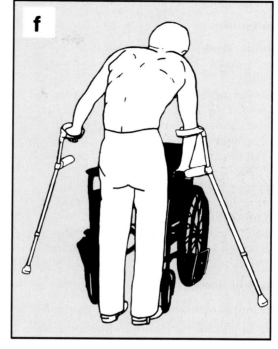

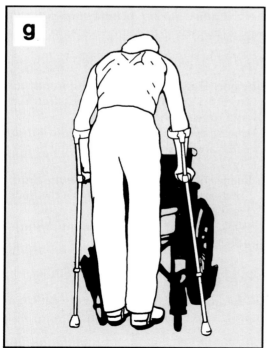

Figure 12.12 cont'd.

Patients can climb the stairs either forwards or backwards. The forwards technique is usually taught first because it has the advantage that the patient can see where he is going. Most agile patients with good abdominal muscles will learn both methods and make their own choice. Where there is severe abdominal and/or hip flexor spasticity, the degree of hyperextension easily obtainable at the hip joints may be too limited for the forwards technique.

Two rails are used initially, progression being made to one rail and one crutch. Finally, the second crutch must be carried, usually in the crutch hand, as illustrated in Figure 12.13.

The therapist

The therapist always stands behind the patient. She holds the trouser band with one hand and grasps the patient round the waist with the other. After the initial attempts, both hands can be placed around the pelvis in the usual position and assistance given, as necessary, until the technique is mastered.

Forwards technique using one rail and one crutch

To walk upstairs

1. Standing close to the rail, grasp it approximately half a foot length in front of the toes.
2. Place the right crutch on the stair above, level with the hand on the rail (Fig. 12.13a). The hands must be level to avoid trunk rotation when lifting. The tendency to grasp the rail too far forward and 'pull' must be avoided.
3. Lean over the hands and lift as high as possible, keeping the trunk and pelvis in the horizontal plane (Fig. 12.13b).
4. As soon as the feet land on the stair above, hyperextend the hips to find the balance point (Fig. 12.13c).

To walk downstairs

1. Standing close to the rail and keeping the body in the horizontal plane, place the right crutch close to the edge of the same stair.
2. Place the left hand down the rail on a level with the crutch (Fig. 12.13d).
3. Lift and swing the feet down to the stair below (Fig. 12.13e).
4. Hyperextend the hips and retract the shoulders as soon as the feet touch the ground (Fig. 12.13f).

Very short patients may need to put the crutch on the stair below the feet and lift down to the crutch.

Backwards technique using one rail and one crutch

To walk upstairs

1. Balance in hyperextension whilst placing the left hand higher up the rail and the crutch on the stair above, keeping the hands level (Fig. 12.13f).
2. Lift backwards (Fig. 12.13e).
3. Regain the balance (Fig. 12.13d).

To walk downstairs

1. Place the crutch on the edge of the same stair as the feet, with the hands level (Fig. 12.13c).
2. Lift the feet backwards to the edge of the stair.
3. Lean forward on the hands, lift and 'flick' the pelvis backwards (Fig. 12.13b).
4. Drop the feet onto the stair below (Fig. 12.13a).

Kerbs

Kerbs are negotiated by putting the crutches on the kerb first and then taking a swing-through step onto the pavement. The same technique is used to descend a kerb. A long shallow step can be mounted in the same way.

Patients are not taught to ascend flights of narrow steps on two crutches.

To get down and up from the floor onto crutches

Crutches to floor

The therapist stands behind the patient and controls the pelvis, feet and legs, as necessary:

1. From the standing position on the mat (Fig. 12.14a), 'walk' the crutches forward one by one (Fig. 12.14b) until the hips and trunk are sufficiently flexed for the outstretched hand to reach the floor.
2. Balance on the right crutch, release the left crutch and put the left hand on the floor (Fig. 12.14c).
3. Balance on the left hand, release the right crutch and put the right hand on the floor (Fig. 12.14d).
4. 'Walk' forward on the hands until lying prone (Fig. 12.14e).

Floor to crutches

The therapist may need to assist the patient to get the weight over his feet initially:

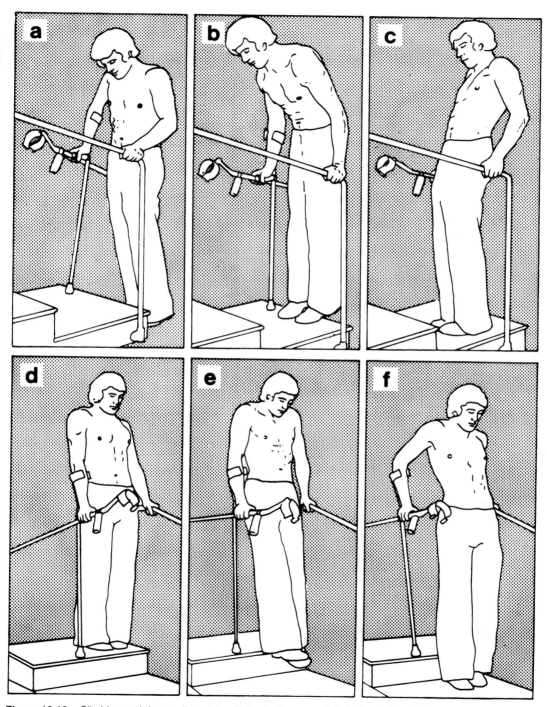

Figure 12.13 Climbing and descending stairs. Patient with a complete lesion below T11.

1. Lying prone, make sure the ankles and toes are dorsiflexed so that the feet are vertical (Fig. 12.14f).
2. Position the crutches, tips forward, well in front of the body and put both forearms through the forearm supports.
3. Press up on the hands, and at the same time use the abdominal muscles to pull the pelvis towards the hands and so prevent the legs being pushed backwards.
4. Maintaining the action of the abdominal muscles, 'walk' the hands towards the feet, trailing the crutches (Fig. 12.14g) until the weight is over the feet (Fig. 12.14h).
5. Balance on the left hand, grasp the right crutch handle and place the crutch on the floor (Fig. 12.14i).
6. Balance on the right crutch and take hold of the left crutch in a similar manner. Balance on both crutches (Fig. 12.14j).
7. 'Walk' the crutches towards the feet until standing erect (Fig. 12.14k).

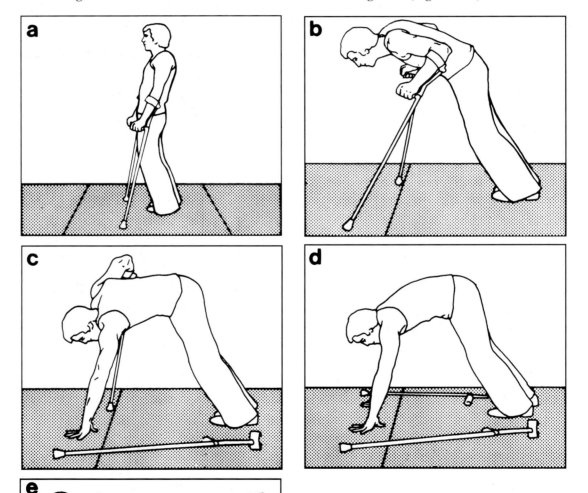

Figure 12.14   a–e: Crutches to floor.

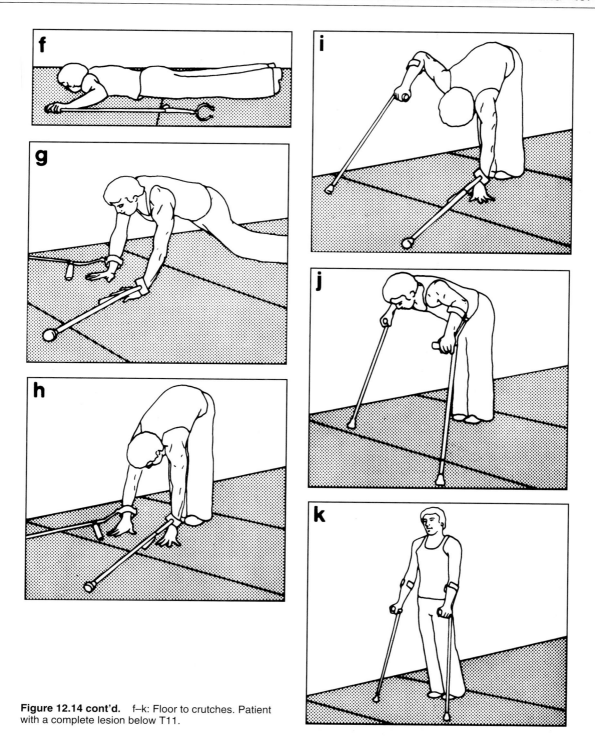

Figure 12.14 cont'd.   f–k: Floor to crutches. Patient with a complete lesion below T11.

To get out of a car onto crutches

1. Turn to face the open door and lift the legs out of the car.
2. Lock the knee joints.
3. With the window open, use the window ledge and the back of the seat, or the seat and a crutch, to lift into standing.
4. Balance with the hips hyperextended and take hold of each crutch in turn.

Final functional activities on crutches

The patient is taught to walk on slopes and over uneven ground such as grass and shale. He must also learn to open and close a door, to sit in and rise from an easy chair, and to sit down at and rise from a table by pushing down on the table with one hand and using the crutch in the other.

GAIT USING HIP–KNEE–ANKLE–FOOT ORTHOSES (HKAFOS)

Over the past few years some of the mechanical problems of the early reciprocating *walking* orthoses (this is a generic term for all the following orthoses) have been eliminated and their popularity has increased. These orthoses enable patients with lesions from C6/7 (with triceps) to T12 to walk with more stability and greater freedom than with KAFOs because they offer support to the trunk, pelvis and hips as well as to the knees and feet.

Work in the late 1960s produced HKAFOs which linked the hips together to allow reciprocal movement of both hips. In the UK, Scrutton (1971) used Bowden cables in an HKAFO for children with spina bifida and Motlock in Canada developed a mechanism based on the use of gears. A refinement on the original design by Scrutton produced the reciprocating gait orthosis at the Louisiana State University (Scott 1971).

At the present time, four main types of reciprocating *walking* orthoses are available internationally.

The *ORLAU* (Orthotic Research and Locomotor Assessment Unit) or *Parawalker* (Hip Guidance Orthosis) was produced in Oswestry, UK, initially for children with spina bifida but more recently for adults with spinal cord lesions (Butler & Major 1971, Stallard 1986). The Parawalker is a rigid structure with good lateral stiffness, which prevents adduction of either hip. The control of adduction is important as the swing leg has less ground clearance if the stance leg adducts (Stallard & Major 1995). The hip joints are free to move between 18° of flexion and 6° of extension when locked for walking. The swing phase is achieved by a pendulum action using gravity and a low-friction orthotic hip joint. The shoes fit onto metal footplates with rocker soles, which adds to the rigidity of the brace but prevents the orthosis being worn under everyday clothing (Fig. 12.15). When the gluteal muscles were stimulated to support hip extension and abduction in an FES hybrid walking project, energy consumption was reduced (Nene & Patrick 1990).

The *Reciprocating Gait Orthosis* (RGO) uses two Bowden cables to link the two sides of the brace (Douglas et al 1983). The front cable assists flexion of the hip and the rear one maintains extension of the brace, effectively acting as the absent hip extensor. This orthosis is more flexible

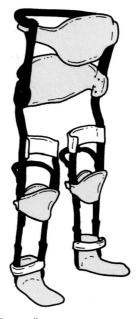

Figure 12.15 Parawalker.

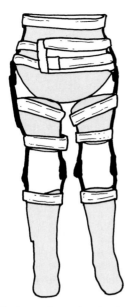

Figure 12.16   Reciprocating gait orthosis.

and lighter than the Parawalker. The foot support is plastic and fits inside the shoe, allowing the orthosis to be worn under normal clothing (Fig. 12.16).

Although patients can don and doff the orthosis, it is difficult to stand up or sit down in it without assistance.

Modifications to the RGO were made by Hugh Steeper Ltd to produce the *Advanced Reciprocating Gait Orthosis* (ARGO). The piston mechanism of this orthosis assists the action of standing and sitting by enabling the knees to extend and flex. The two Bowden cables are reduced to one which is encased in a tube, in an effort to prevent the cables breaking and to improve cosmesis.

Motlock suggested a modification to the RGO which is known as the *Isocentric Reciprocating Gait Orthosis* (IRGO). As the cables in the RGO are the least dependable part of the orthosis and are cosmetically unacceptable, they are replaced by a centrally pivoting bar attached around a pelvic jacket (Motlock 1992). Whereas hip extension in the RGO is adjusted by tightening the Bowden cables, in the IRGO it is achieved by turning the screw threads inside a barrel at each hip joint.

Walkabout. This orthosis was designed in Australia. It is available in the UK and elsewhere, although it is not as extensively used as the Parawalker and RGO in the UK, where it is mainly prescribed for patients with low thoracic lesions.

Plastic shells support the upper and lower legs and pass under the soles of the feet, and the knee joints are hinged. In an attempt to avoid the problems which arise at the hip joints, the KAFOs in this orthosis are joined at the top inside edge by a small bar. This contains the mechanism which allows the swing leg to move forward when the weight on it is released. There are no hip joints, but a flexible thoracic band attached to the calipers by loops can provide some trunk support if required. The Walkabout is more easily concealed beneath normal clothing than either the Parawalker or the RGO.

Similarities and differences in HKAFOs

Most braces have a weight tolerance limit. The recommended weight for the Parawalker is 75 kg. Above 76.4 kg, the Bowden cables tend to snap on the RGO, and over 80.9 kg it becomes a physical struggle for the user to walk.

In the two main types of orthoses, Parawalker and RGO, the aim is similar although the orthoses are different in design and appearance. The body is braced from mid-trunk to the feet with knees and ankles immobilized in both orthoses. Flexion and extension are allowed at the hips but adduction is prevented when the leg is lifted off the ground. Both braces work to bring about flexion of the swing leg after weight transference (Whittle et al 1991).

The Parawalker was designed to be used with crutches and the RGO with a specially designed rollator with the restrictive front bar removed to allow for a more normal stride length. In practice, patients using either orthosis can walk with crutches or rollator.

After 4 months' use, Whittle et al (1991) found no significant difference between the Parawalker and the RGO in the general gait parameters of cadence, stride length and velocity, and effort expenditure was similar. Banta et al (1991) and

Bowker et al (1992) found energy cost less with the Parawalker. Whittle & Cochrane (1989) found that the effort expended through the crutches was less with the Parawalker. The RGO was lighter and therefore easier to transport and its cosmesis was preferred (Whittle & Cochrane 1989). The functional results did not differ between subjects or centres as greatly as expected in a multicentre trial of the Parawalker, RGO and ARGO orthoses in Italy (Lotta et al 1994). The main difference in outcome seemed to depend on the device adopted. For example, patients in the Parawalker cannot climb stairs, but the orthosis never needed repairs, it took the shortest time to don and doff and less time for the patients to learn to use it. Using the IRGO as opposed to the ARGO, energy cost was slightly less and mean velocity slightly greater, although neither was statistically significant (Winchester 1993).

Assessment

If the patient is to be successful in using a reciprocating *walking* orthosis, it is essential that an accurate assessment is undertaken before it is prescribed. More important perhaps than the usual physical factors, such as spasticity or flexion contracture which might mitigate against continued use of the orthosis, is the patient's perception of its functional use and his expectations of the degree of independence it might allow (Sykes et al 1995). Walking with any of these orthoses has many limitations. The gait is slow and the patient can only cover short distances with great physical effort (Whittle et al 1991). Disappointment can only be avoided if the patient appreciates that walking with one of these orthoses is a useful form of exercise. It is not an alternative to wheelchair locomotion (Stallard et al 1989).

As well as the physical and psychological assessment, the home and work situation must also be discussed. Stallard et al (1989) suggest that all the following factors should be considered:

- independence – as well as walking in the orthosis, the patient should be able to don and doff it and be able to get into and out of the wheelchair

- energy cost
- cosmesis
- reliability of the orthosis
- cost.

The problem is to identify those patients who will continue to use the orthoses so that optimal benefit can be achieved with minimal wastage (Sykes et al 1995). The usual practice in spinal cord injury units in the UK is to reassess the patient who shows an interest in using a reciprocating *walking* orthosis approximately 1 year after discharge from the initial period of rehabilitation. The orthosis most suited to the needs of the individual patient can then be selected.

Team

An experienced team consisting of an orthotist, doctor, physiotherapist and orthotic technician must be involved in the assessment, prescription and construction of the orthosis. A tailored fit is crucial and the team approach is essential if the patient is to succeed. When the patient starts to use the orthosis and is learning to walk, the team continues to monitor progress and adjust the fit as necessary.

Training

Before learning to use a reciprocating *walking* orthosis, the patient completes a training programme to increase muscle strength, aerobic power and cardiovascular efficiency.

Gait

To achieve reciprocating gait, three actions must occur:

- the swing leg has to clear the ground
- the swing leg has to move from extension to flexion
- the trunk has to move forward over the stance leg, i.e. the hip has to extend.

Parawalker

The patient transfers to the plinth and the Parawalker is placed in the wheelchair. The patient lifts into it and fastens the straps. The chair is positioned in the bars as described earlier.

Action of the patient
1. Lock the knee joints.
2. With the heels on the ground, lie back in the chair and lock the hip joints. (If low in the chair, lift up until the body is at an approximate angle of 45°.)
3. Hold onto the bars and pull up into standing.

Two therapists usually assist the patient to stand for the first time, one on each side of the bars. As the patient has been at home for at least a year and has undertaken a strengthening programme before being fitted with the orthosis, his arms should be strong and little effort should be required of the therapists.

To walk moving the right leg first
1. Push *sideways* with right hand using latissimus dorsi to transfer weight to left leg.
2. The right leg swings forward.
3. Take the weight on the right leg and continue to push with right hand to extend right hip. Repeat on left side.

Crutch walking is commenced in 2 or 3 days.

To stand up with crutches
1. Lock the knee and hip joints in the wheelchair.
2. Place the tip of the crutches alongside the back of the rear wheels on each side of the chair.
3. Push into standing.
4. Edge crutches forward, one at a time to the balance position with the crutches in front.

Walk as described above.
To sit down reverse the procedure.

RGO

The chair is positioned between the bars as already described.

To stand up
1. Engage the clips at the hip joints.
2. Push down on the bars and stand up.
3. Extend the hips to complete the locking action at the hips.

To sit down. Disengage the clips and lower gently into the chair.

The Bowden cables can be tightened to adjust the degree of extension at the hips or, if the hip flexors are tight, the degree of flexion. One of the most vital adjustments to the brace is the control of extension of the trunk to enable the patient to maintain his balance. The two upper straps at the front and back of the brace can be adjusted to control the position of the trunk within the brace. Extension is controlled by slackening the Velcro fastening on the back strap and then tightening the front strap. The upper body weight is moved backwards over the heels, achieving the balance position and correct posture for a patient with spinal cord injury. If the back strap is too tight, the patient is pushed forward off balance.

IRGO

The pre-selection function of the hip joints of the IRGO enables the patient to stand up and sit down safely.

To stand up
1. In sitting, place the clips at the hip joints (called 'pre-selection' hip joints) in the 'up' position.
2. Push down on the bars and stand up.
3. Forcibly extend the hips; the joints will lock automatically in their pre-selected setting.

To sit down
1. Place the clips at the hip joints in the pre-selected 'down' position.
2. Forcibly extend the hips; the hip joints will unlock.
3. Lower gently into the chair.

To walk moving the right leg
1. Transfer weight onto the left leg.
2. Using latissimus dorsi, lift the right (swing) leg by pushing down on the right hand.
3. The right leg swings forward.
4. Transfer weight onto the right leg.
5. Continue to push with the right arm to extend the right hip.

This movement into full extension on the supporting leg is called the 'tuck phase'.

Repeat to move the left leg.

The patient learns to walk in parallel bars and progresses to rollator or crutches.

To create a relatively normal stride using the rollator, the patient pushes the rollator forward between each step. Crutch walking is described on page 139.

Follow-up studies on the number of patients who continue to use these orthoses when the training period is over are remarkably similar. Sixty-four per cent continued to use the Parawalker (Moore & Stallard 1991) and 62% continued to use the RGO (Ellis 1995).

The effort of walking is the main reason why most patients do not continue to walk after discharge from hospital (Coghlan et al 1980). Using the IRGO as opposed to the ARGO, the energy cost was slightly less and the mean velocity slightly greater, although neither was statistically significant (Winchester 1993).

Although construction problems still exist and the energy required to walk in these orthoses is high, they enable patients with high lesions, including those with low cervical lesions, to stand and walk, and as long as patients are interested progress will continue to be made.

GAIT USING FUNCTIONAL ELECTRICAL STIMULATION (FES) STANDING SYSTEMS

For the past 30 years, experiments have been undertaken to enable patients to walk using electrical stimulation of the relevant muscles. Surface, nerve cuff and deep muscle electrodes have been used. FES is applied to the intact lower motor neurone pathways and is therefore only suitable for upper motor neurone paralysis, as with stimulation of the phrenic nerve (Ch. 5). Initially, FES is used to improve the condition and bulk of the paralysed muscles. When the state of the muscles has improved, electronic implants can be used to activate muscles in functional sequence. Interestingly, 50 years ago Sir Ludwig Guttmann showed that muscle bulk

could be improved in rabbits (Guttmann & Guttman 1942) and later in humans using galvanic stimulation (Guttmann & Guttman 1944).

Surface stimulation

Root stimulation gives access to the whole motor output, whilst surface stimulation reaches only part of it. Usually the gluteal and hamstring muscles are stimulated for standing, and quadriceps and the flexor withdrawal response for walking. To stimulate more muscles is impractical as it is too time-consuming. Surface stimulation is wasteful of current and requires assiduous attention to skin care, and the stimulation varies with movement of the limbs (Rushton et al 1995).

As surface stimulation methods are essentially limited to experimental work and for assessment, the electrode system must be implanted to obtain consistent and selective results.

Implanted electrodes

Three types of implanted electrodes are used:

• Percutaneous wires are inserted through the skin and focused on a motor point. Any number of wires may be used. Formal surgery is not required and the wires are inserted easily by a practised operator. This procedure has a high risk of electrode failure and a high incidence of infection. Cosmesis is unacceptable (Barr et al 1995).

• The nerve cuff electrode is placed around peripheral nerves in a formal surgical procedure.

• The epimysial electrode (disc type of electrode) is placed near the motor point of large muscles. Less dissection is required than for the cuff type but multichannel lower limb systems still require extensive surgery and the cabling also has to be implanted in the limb. As cable connectors tend to fracture, further surgery is often required.

A *Sacral Anterior Root Stimulator Implant* (SARSI) has been widely used to restore bladder control in male and female patients and erectile function in male patients (Brindley & Rushton 1990). A *Lumbar Anterior Root Stimulator Implant* (LARSI) has been used to stimulate lumbar and sacral roots (L2–S2) to restore lower limb function in two patients. Only one is documented to date (Barr et al 1995). These systems are now commercially available, as are some surface and upper limb motor locomotor systems.

Stringent criteria are necessary for the selection of patients for any FES system, which will include psychological as well as physical assessments. For example, joints must have full range of movement and be free of osteoporosis and the patient must be physically fit, as energy consumption is high. Patients gain the usual benefits from standing and walking with these systems, and Jaeger et al (1990) found psychological benefits also, in that the patients' self-esteem and confidence appeared to increase. To use a surface system long term is impractical, but surface stimulation as a non-invasive means of assessment and training is necessary as prerequisite to an implant system (Barr et al 1995). Both systems are useful and in many ways complementary (Rushton 1996).

FES does not restore functional gait. It is a form of exercise and remains experimental. Whatever the technique used, walking speed is slow and, together with energy consumption, is a limiting factor. Major technical problems continue to be encountered, for example in the selection and control of stimulation, failure of equipment and muscle fatigue.

To replace the intricate mechanism of normal gait is an enormous task. It is not surprising that progress is slow. Research continues in many centres worldwide.

In a study to examine the safety of FES, Ashley et al (1993) found evidence to suggest that there was a danger of autonomic dysreflexia during treatment in patients with lesions above the splanchnic outflow, i.e. above T6. Extra caution should therefore be employed with these patients.

GAIT USING HYBRID SYSTEMS – RGO WITH FES

The difficulties of mimicking the voluntary activity of walking by computer-controlled electrical stimulation, and its potential use to restore function, are well documented by Hunter Peckham (1987). With such a large number of sophisticated component parts, computer-controlled gait is open to malfunction and this has given rise to the use of functional electrical stimulation with an orthosis, producing an integrated or hybrid system.

Interest has developed since 1984 when, in the US, the Louisiana State University reciprocating gait orthosis was combined with FES to quadriceps and the gluteal muscles (Petrofsky et al 1985). The reciprocating gait orthosis supported the patient as only a few of the muscles used in walking were stimulated and greater use of the trunk and arms was required to maintain balance. In addition, if the electrical system failed, the patient was still supported.

Research continues in many countries, but a functional system has not yet been developed. In most studies, the quadriceps and hamstring muscles are stimulated but the user still has to lift his body weight with his arms to swing the stride leg forward. The energy cost of paraplegic walking is intrinsically high (Nene et al 1996).

Few patients continue to use the systems after the training programmes are completed. Hip and knee adjustments are required, the electrical connections are fragile and break easily, and other problems occur. This means that the patient needs to be frequently in contact with the rehabilitation team and this is not always practical because of distance.

Researchers are looking at different approaches, e.g. the stimulation of additional muscles to assist hip flexion (Phillips 1989) or the stimulation of the ipsilateral gluteal muscle to improve hip extension of the stance leg (Yang et al 1996). In the Netherlands, a research group is developing a more complicated orthosis with multichannels (Hermans et al 1994). Others are developing a lockable/unlockable knee joint which allows the knee to be unlocked during the swing phase of the gait cycle and relocked for stability in the stance phase (Melia 1997).

Patients will only use a system if it allows them to walk without too much effort and perform other functions when wearing it. Energy consumption, transportability and the gait pattern all need improving if patients are to continue to use these systems (Nene et al 1996).

13

Ultra-high lesions

Injuries to the upper cervical spine (C1–C3) paralyse the diaphragm as well as the other muscles of respiration and prove fatal at the scene of the accident unless the condition is recognized and artificial respiration given immediately.

Due to the knowledge and expertise of the emergency services in the UK, many patients with fractures at this level now reach hospital. The most common injury is at C2 when the cranial nerves are intact and there is partial supply to the accessory nerve but the diaphragm is paralysed and the patient will need ventilation.

Where the injury occurs at C4, the patient usually manages to reach hospital on a partially functioning diaphragm. Most lesions then ascend a segment when a ventilator becomes necessary. The lesion descends in the majority of cases and the patient finally manages to breathe unaided. The major muscles remaining innervated in the patient with a lesion at C4 are the upper portion of the trapezius and sternomastoid supplied by the accessory nerve, and platysma supplied by the facial nerve.

Not only are these patients totally paralysed apart from the head, but if ventilated they have no means of communication and therefore no way of expressing emotions and physical needs. A rudimentary system of communication needs to be established with the patient as soon as possible (Chawla 1993). Eye movements or blinking can be used to indicate 'yes' and 'no'. Later a scanning system can be used, such as selecting alphabet letters, items or words from a chart. The speech and language therapist needs to be involved from the day of admission. All staff need to remember that the patient has no means of initiating conversation.

Verbal independence. Even with so little ability to communicate, the patient's wishes should be taken into account. An early priority is to assist the patient to begin to take control of himself and his environment; for example, as soon as possible, the patient is encouraged to know where his belongings are to be found in the locker and when he needs replenishments.

The ability to describe all aspects of the care he needs is vital for the patient with an ultra-high cervical lesion.

During his rehabilitation the patient must learn, for example:

- the settings for the ventilator
- suction and hyperinflationary techniques
- correct positioning in bed and in the wheelchair
- turning procedures
- bladder and bowel care
- the management of all equipment
- how to avoid pressures sores
- how to recognize indicators of impending problems.

Not only must he master the details of the care taught to him by the various professionals, he must also show that, in turn, he can teach his carers.

Plasticity of the human motor cortex may explain the increase in acuity of sight and hearing which those who treat patients with lesions at C2 observe. Hallett et al (1993) suggested that the relationship between the motor cortex and the muscles supplied may be modified in patients with disability. They used transcranial magnetic stimulation and muscle responses (motor-evoked potentials) to demonstrate the change in cortical mapping which occurs in patients with complete spinal cord lesions. It would appear that cortical representation of intact muscles spreads onto the area previously controlling the now paralysed muscles. Previous studies (Levy et al 1990, Topka et al 1991) support Hallet et al's

findings. However, Brouwer & Hopkins-Russel's (1997) study does not and they suggest: 'there is a need for further investigation to determine the association of pathology and specific rehabilitation intervention strategies with the occurrence or extent of motor cortical expansion'.

Patients with lesions between C1 and C4 have no motor power in the arms, trunk or legs. There is complete loss of sensation, bladder, bowel and sexual function, and vasomotor control. As a result of the paralysis of the vasoconstrictors, there is a marked vasodilatation initially. This causes blockage of the nasal air passages which adds to the difficulties of respiration without a tracheostomy. This phenomenon, known as Guttmann's sign, is often present in patients with lower cervical lesions also (Guttmann 1976d).

When the stage of spinal areflexia is over, spasticity and rigidity of muscle develop, the limbs becoming predominantly spastic in extension.

Physical rehabilitation is limited to training the vasomotor system to enable the patient to lead a wheelchair life and to teaching him control of the power-drive chair and his environment. Special equipment is needed for those patients who return home, and the relatives require expert training.

Physiotherapy during the acute stage

Chest therapy is vital and is described in Chapter 5, including the treatment of a patient on a ventilator.

Treatment will be needed every 2 hours if not every hour for the first 24–48 hours. For patients without a tracheostomy, it is advisable to continue daily postural drainage for several months as a prophylactic measure once the acute stage is over. For patients with a tendency to chest infection, this should be continued throughout life. If a patient with a lesion at this level develops a head cold, he should remain in bed for a day or two to prevent secretions dripping down into the chest when the patient is vertical.

The ventilated patient will need to gain confidence in the physiotherapist and others involved in his care in order to be as relaxed as possible when the respirator is removed for suction or other purposes. Whilst giving the patient encouragement and reassurance, and with his permission, the physiotherapist needs to disconnect the ventilator for very brief periods to acclimatize the patient. If possible, ventilated patients should be taught to breathe using the accessory muscles. Glossopharyngeal breathing is also useful if the staff know how to teach it and if the patient can learn it, but it does prove a difficult task (Pool & Weerden 1973). Later these patients may be assessed for diaphragmatic pacing.

To minimize the effect of the extensor spasticity, the position of the arms is important. From the first day, the correct position is adduction of the shoulder, 45° flexion or mid-position of the elbow, extension of the wrist and flexion of the fingers.

When the fracture is healed, training for the vasomotor system must be taken very slowly. An abdominal binder is often a help for the first few weeks to minimize pooling of the blood in the splanchnic vessels. Some patients may continue to wear them.

PHYSICAL REHABILITATION
The power-drive chair

These patients will require a power-drive chair. The chair will be controlled by pushing a small sensitive lever in the appropriate direction, using the chin, head, mouth or breath. As the power-drive chair is heavy to dismantle and put in a car, the patient will also need a transit chair.

The patient on a ventilator will need to carry on his chair the ventilator unit with back-up system, suction equipment and manual hyper-inflation bag. The non-ventilated patient may need to carry a portable ventilator and the patient with a paced diaphragm will have to fix the pacer to his chair, usually attached to the armrest (Fig. 13.1).

Particular care needs to be taken in choosing a chair and cushion to fit the individual requirements of the user (Chs 6 and 10).

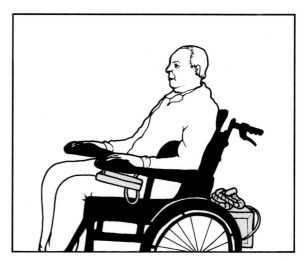

Figure 13.1   A patient with a pacer on the armrest and a ventilator between the rear wheels.

Position of the patient in the wheelchair

The patient has no muscles with which to save himself, and therefore his position in the chair must be carefully checked for safety and stability and to ensure that there are no factors likely to irritate his spasticity.

A semi-reclining backrest assists both stability and respiration, particularly if the patient is ventilated or the diaphragm remains partially paralysed. The arms need to be adequately supported to reduce spasticity and to minimize the strain on the shoulder joints. The forearms and hands can be positioned on a wheelchair tray, cushion on the lap or specific support made for some models of wheelchair (Fig. 13.2).

Physiotherapy

Once the patient is up, treatment is directed towards:

*   hypertrophy of the innervated muscles
*   control of the power-drive chair
*   reducing spasticity
*   educating the patient and relatives / carers in all relevant aspects of care
*   maintaining balance in the chair, for the patient with a lesion at C4.

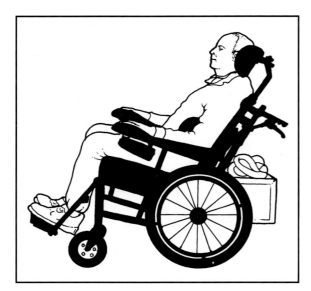

Figure 13.2   Position in the wheelchair of a patient with a lesion at C2.

Patient with a lesion at C2. The patient will not be able to move within his wheelchair. The main priority is to mobilize and strengthen the neck muscles to enable the patient to look around, take his head off the head rest, use a computer, drive the power-drive wheelchair and control his environment by electronic means.

Hypertrophy of the few remaining muscles can be achieved with surprising results.

Free movement and manual resistance are used to mobilize and strengthen. As the neck gets stronger, the head rest is removed for short periods. Passive movements to the arms are continued and, if necessary, to the legs also.

Patient with a lesion at C4. In addition to the above, balance exercises in the chair are carried out in front of the mirror to help the patient (1) become aware of his position in space, and (2) use his head and shoulders to maintain his equilibrium, especially when moving over uneven ground.

1. The therapist sits the patient away from the back of the chair and if necessary reclines the backrest to a greater angle to give more room for the exercise. The therapist finds the balance point and the patient tries to hold the position by moving his head and using trapezius.

2. The patient sits back in the chair, leaning against the backrest and facing the mirror. By flexing the head quickly and then lifting it quickly, the patient can learn to 'bounce' his shoulders away from the backrest. Having bounced the upper trunk away from the chair, the patient side-flexes his head, and his upper trunk moves a few inches to one side. Once learnt, this manoeuvre is invaluable as it aids stability when the chair is being moved. This may require a great deal of practice but repays the effort involved.

Reduction of spasticity

Spasticity may be reduced by passive movements, by reflex-inhibiting postures on the plinth or bed, by careful positioning in bed at night and by standing. Drugs may be given to control severe spasticity.

Standing. A tilt table is used to stand patients with ultra-high lesions as they have insufficient motor power to assist in maintaining their own standing position. A tilting bed may be used at home.

The patient stands for only 2 or 3 minutes on the first day. This is increased to two periods of the same duration on the second day. Subsequently, the time is increased a few minutes only per day until the patient can stand for about 20 minutes.

In time, some patients, even those with lesions at C2, can stand and want to stand for long periods, i.e. 2 hours or more, as they say they enjoy it.

It is helpful for the patient to stand daily whilst training the vasomotor response, but afterwards the patient stands two or three times a week. If possible, a relative is taught the technique so that the patient can continue to stand at home.

Abilities

The patient with a lesion at C2 can learn to operate a computer using the voice, chin, head, mouth or another muscle with a suitably adapted interface.

The patient with a lesion at C4 can learn to use various mouth sticks to operate a computer, type, turn pages, paint and play certain games. A platform can be fitted at a convenient height so that the patient can pick out and replace the mouth sticks required.

Several environmental control systems are available which enable the completely paralysed patient to operate a selection of appliances in his environment. This is done by means of a switch, activated by the lightest touch, for example, of the chin, head or breath, or by the voice. The patient can, for example, control lights, doors, power points, curtains, entertainment systems and use a telephone.

Patients with these high lesions may need to employ carers, and if so, will need to be able to advertise, interview, train and arrange for payment for them.

HANDLING THE PATIENT

To relieve pressure

This is discussed in Chapter 6.

To turn the patient

1. Cross one ankle over the other in the direction of the turn.
2. Turn the shoulders by putting one arm, e.g. the right, across the chest to hang down on the left side and pull the left shoulder back.
3. The therapist thrusts her arms underneath the buttocks until she can grip the anterior superior iliac spine, if possible. The arms are kept close together – the heavier the patient, the closer the arms need to be.
4. Turn the buttocks and at the same time pull them back into the middle of the bed. The 'bounce' of the mattress can be utilized to flip the patient over.

When a turn onto the side is not necessary but pressure over the sacrum and buttocks needs to be relieved, steps 3 and 4 alone can be used to turn the buttocks through 30°. A pillow should be used to support the buttocks.

To transfer a patient with a lesion at C2 from bed to chair using a hoist

Before moving the patient, ensure that the ventilator is appropriately positioned.

1. Sit the patient up and put the sling behind him as low down as possible.
2. Lie the patient down.
3. Lift one leg at a time, to bring the sling under the thighs. Or,
   a. roll the sling lengthwise
   b. roll the patient onto one side
   c. place the sling as far as possible under the back
   d. roll onto the other side and pull the sling through.
4. Attach the sling to the hoist (Fig. 13.3a), which may be free-standing or on a permanent rail in the patient's own home for example.
5. Use the hoist to lift, move and lower the patient into the chair (Fig. 13.3b & c).
6. Lift the thigh to remove the sling on each side.
7. Lean the patient forward and remove the sling from behind his back.
8. Lift buttocks back in the chair (Fig. 13.3d) and correct his sitting position.

Reverse the procedure to move from chair to bed.

Occasions will occur when the patient needs to be transferred but the hoist is not available, e.g. when travelling. In this case, manual lifts will be required; these are described in Chapter 11.

HANDLING THE WHEELCHAIR

To push up a kerb

1. Tip the chair onto its rear wheels by pressing down on the chair handles and one of the tipping levers.
2. Push the chair on the rear wheels until the front wheels are over the kerb.
3. Lower the chair onto the front wheels and push the rear wheels up the kerb.

To push down a kerb

Tilt the chair onto its rear wheels and push down the kerb on the rear wheels only. If the patient

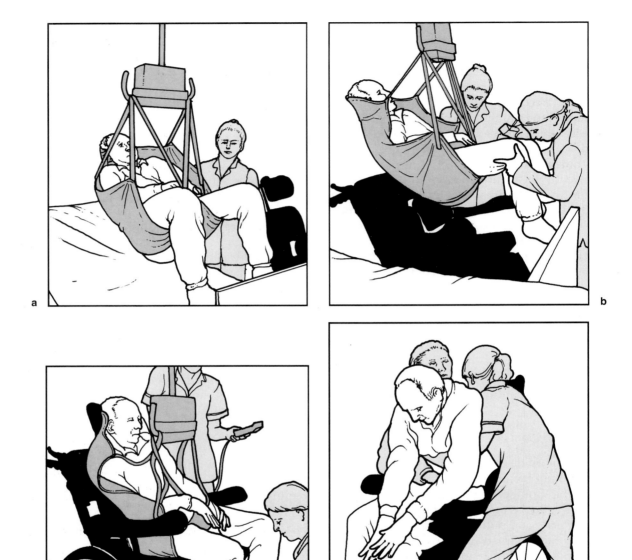

Figure 13.3 Transfer using a hoist.

is large and heavy, or excessively nervous, turn the chair around and allow the rear wheels to descend first.

To put the chair in the boot of the car

Take out the cushion, remove the wheels if applicable, fold the chair and remove the foot-plates if necessary. Check that the brakes are on. With the side of the chair facing the operator, hold onto the crossbars or the wheels. Tip the chair up onto the thighs and pivot it into the boot. Lightweight wheelchairs are more easily handled.

If the wheels are not removable, they are usually placed to the back of the boot. Deep boots entail lifting the chair the depth of the boot before it can be taken out. Therefore, unless two chairs need to be carried, a boot in which the floor is level with the door is more convenient.

PERMANENT CARE

It is a tribute to the medical social workers, to the social services and particularly to the relatives that so many of the patients with ultra-high lesions return to their own homes. Some patients have large families where the strain of caring for the disabled person is spread between several members. In other cases, there is only one relative available. Some depend on maximum social support, while others accept only a little help.

Patients with additional problems may need permanent hospital care. Others may have no suitable relative young and fit enough to cope with the full-time care needed. Some of these patients may be able to pay for the necessary assistance, while others will need to go into long-term care in homes with heavy nursing wards. Many questions are still to be answered regarding long-term planning for people with high spinal cord lesions (Mathson-Prince 1997).

The person who is to care for the patient with a very high lesion at home needs special training which should start as soon as possible. If willing and able, carers are encouraged to assist the staff in suctioning techniques from an early stage. There are many tasks for them to learn and the carer should spend a minimum of a week at the hospital before the patient is discharged. The carer will need to learn how to handle the patient and the wheelchair, how to dress the patient and attend to the bladder and bowels. It is also important for the carer to see what the patient can do for himself and how best to help him achieve even minimum independence.

The staff need to assist the patient and carer to find the most appropriate way of dealing with all the tasks so that in time they will occupy a less prominent role in home life. The presence of a ventilator-dependent person in the home obviously has a profound effect on family life.

The most important factors in successful adaption appear to be the level of communication with the family and the degree of commitment between all family members (Glass 1993).

Equipment

Beds

An electronically manipulated bed and/or special mattress is usually required for home use. These aids do not negate the necessity to turn the patient but either lengthen the period between turns or facilitate the turn itself. Beds are available which raise the patient from supine to the sitting position and there are also beds that turn the patient. Some relatives may prefer to turn the patient manually. In some cases and with suitable adaptions, the patient may be able to operate the bed himself, thus achieving a small measure of independence.

These patients, with or without a pacer, will require ventilators, suction equipment with all disposable supplies, a manual chair and a power chair at home.

Hoists

The hammock sling supports the head and is completely safe for patients with high cervical lesions. As the support for the lower body is under the thighs, not under the buttocks, it can easily be removed during the day so that the patient does not have to sit on it

Hoists are available to get in and out of the car but are often cumbersome and bulky to use.

The patient with a C2 lesion will need to travel in a car in his wheelchair. Mechanisms are available which enable the patient in a wheelchair to be lifted either into the area of the passenger's seat or into the rear of a hatchback car or van.

Safety procedures for patients with a lesion at C2 are vital. When at home, someone who knows how to suction the patient and who can cope with any other possible problem should always be able to see, and be seen by, the patient. All equipment needs to be taken with the patient when he travels by car and someone should travel with the patient in addition to the driver.

Robotics technology

Studies on the use of robotics technology in the development of manipulative aids for personal care and control of the environment continue. Further work in this interesting field is required in order to simplify the devices and make them effective but less expensive, and to establish the rehabilitation potential and acceptability to the user of this approach.

14

The incomplete spinal lesion

Susan Edwards

INTRODUCTION

The term 'incomplete lesion' encompasses all patients with some sparing of neural activity below the level of the lesion.

The number of patients with incomplete lesions as opposed to complete lesions is increasing. Bedbrook (1985) attributed this to the widespread use of seat belts and improved early care of the spinal injured patient. According to a recent study carried out in America looking at demographic and treatment trends between 1973 and 1986, of the total number of patients with spinal cord injury, there was an increase in the number of incomplete lesions from 43.6 to 51.4%. This percentage increase was most notable in those with sensory sparing (De Vivo et al 1992).

Although data relating to spinal cord demographics and treatment outcome is usually reported in the spinal cord injury literature, it is important to recognize that many patients with spinal cord lesions are never admitted to a spinal injuries unit. Non-traumatic incomplete spinal cord lesions account for at least 1.2% of all neurology out-patient consultations (Stevenson et al 1996).

The functional outcome for patients with complete lesions, e.g. a C6 or T12, is more predictable than for those with incomplete lesions. As with all lesions, the pre-morbid status of the patient is of paramount importance in influencing outcome. Patients with incomplete lesions include not only those who sustain their injury as a result of trauma, but also those with more diverse pathologies, many of which are progressive. Prognosis for these patients is ill-defined.

Patients with incomplete spinal cord damage as a result of pathological causes include those with:

- vascular accidents or disease
- tumours
- cervical myelopathy
- inflammatory disease.

CLASSIFICATIONS

No two lesions will be identical. The pathology will always be different because of the complex nature of the spinal cord. However, certain types of lesions are referred to as syndromes. These include:

- central cord syndrome
- anterior cord syndrome
- Brown–Séquard syndrome.

Central cord syndrome

The central cord syndrome (CCS) was initially described by Schneider et al (1954). It is the most common type of incomplete spinal cord injury (Shaw 1995).

The American Spinal Injury Association (ASIA) define this syndrome as: 'a lesion, occurring almost exclusively in the cervical region, that produces sacral sparing and greater weakness in the upper limbs than in the lower limbs' (ASIA 1994).

The acute CCS is commonly stated to arise from an injury which affects primarily the central part of the spinal cord and is frequently haemorrhagic (Morse 1982, Maroon et al 1991). However, Quencer et al (1992) found no evidence of haemorrhage into the substance of the cord and concluded that CCS was not primarily a grey matter lesion but that the neurological disability, at least in part, was due to damage to the white matter tracts. They suggested that the most common mechanism of injury may be direct compression of the cord in an already narrowed spinal canal. This would explain the predominance of axonal injury in the white matter of the lateral columns.

Roth et al (1990), in a study of 81 traumatic CCS patients, found that more than 90% of patients had neurological recovery of both upper and lower limbs, neurological recovery being defined as an increase in strength of one muscle grade. This recovery generally occurred in the order of lower limbs, bladder function, upper limbs and finally the hands. The extent of recovery is greatest in younger patients, who have a better prognosis for recovery in activities of daily living and in becoming functional walkers (Penrod et al 1990, Roth et al 1990).

It is possible that arteriosclerosis may compromise blood supply to the cord in older subjects and that the initial damage may be more severe due to cervical spondylosis (Scher 1995). Progressive neurological deterioration, characterized by spasticity, has been identified in older patients with CCS, whereby patients who were initially functionally ambulant became wheelchair-dependent (Maroon et al 1991).

Cause

This type of lesion usually affects older people with cervical spondylosis who sustain hyperextension injuries in falls or in motor vehicle accidents. Older men, over the age of 40, with predisposing narrow cervical canals and osteoarthritis of the cervical spine have also been identified to be at risk of CCS following body surfing accidents (Scher 1995).

However, CCS may occur in people of any age and be associated with other aetiologies, injury mechanisms or predisposing factors (Fig. 14.1) (Roth et al 1990). In older age groups, fracture of the cervical spine is less common than in younger subjects (Penrod et al 1990), and in the absence of a fracture, this lesion may be difficult to diagnose. Computerized tomography or magnetic resonance imaging will provide confirmation and additional information.

Clinical picture (Fig. 14.2)

The general clinical picture is of:

- disproportionately more motor impairment of the upper than lower extremities

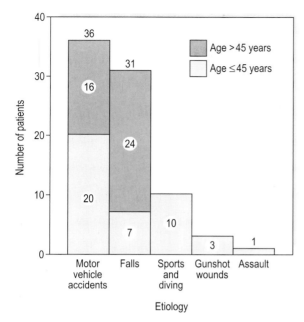

Figure 14.1 Aetiology distribution of central cord syndrome patients (Roth 1990).

- bladder dysfunction, often with urinary retention
- varying degrees of sensory loss.

Spasticity, shoulder pain, hand oedema and dysaesthetic pain are noted complications (Roth et al 1990, Maroon et al 1991).

Motor deficit. At the level of the lesion, there will be damage to the anterior horn cells resulting in a flaccid paralysis of those muscles supplied from this level (Scher 1995). For example, a lesion occurring at the C5 level will give rise to flaccidity, most notably of deltoid and biceps. The gradual wasting of these muscles gives rise to the fairly typical picture of the central cord lesion.

Hand dysfunction is an outstanding feature of cervical myelopathies (Nakajima & Hirayama 1995) but this is variable in CCS. The hands may be relatively uninvolved, but without the background of proximal stability, selective upper limb function cannot be achieved.

In other cases, the hands may be paralysed. The predominant loss of muscle function in distal

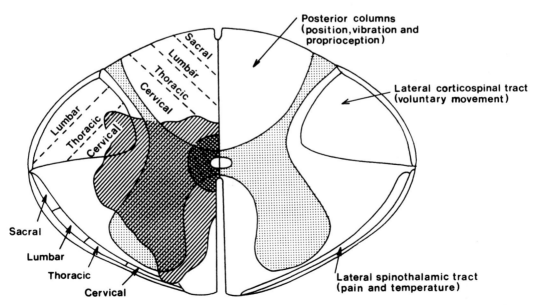

Figure 14.2 Cross-section of cervical spinal cord. Hatched areas represent a zone of central haemorrhage (■) and surrounding oedema (▨). The impingement on pathways, especially central cervical fibres, in part subserving upper extremity function, is readily apparent. (After Morse 1982.)

muscles may be explained by axonal damage. Disruption of axons, particularly in the lateral columns in the region occupied by the cortico-spinal tracts, reflects their importance for hand and finger function (Quencer et al 1992).

Paralysis of the hands may lead to the development of stiff and painful joints or cervical hand syndrome (pages 25, 218) and swelling may occur compounded by the effect of gravity.

The development of contractures and/or painful joints of the upper limbs will remain a very real danger throughout all stages of rehabilitation. Roth et al (1990) found that the number of patients with shoulder pain and dysaesthetic pain increased over time to be greater at discharge than during rehabilitation.

Many patients with CCS will achieve an inde-pendent gait with or without the use of walking aids. In a sense, these patients differ from virtu-ally all other patients with neurological dis-ability, in that use of the arms in gait re-education is recommended. All too often, these patients walk independently before they have significant recovery of the upper limbs. The importance of the use of the arms while learning how to walk again cannot be overemphasized. Once the patient is able to walk independently, there may be little if any opportunity for the arms to be involved in function (Fig. 14.3).

Depending on the severity of the lesion, the patient will demonstrate some degree of motor deficit in the trunk and lower limbs which is invariably characterized by the presence of spasticity.

Sensory deficit. This is extremely variable, ranging from severe sensory loss to virtually no impairment.

The disability of these patients is often under-estimated. Those who are ambulant may appear less disabled, and yet, without the use of their upper limbs they are invariably more impaired than the chairbound paraplegic.

Anterior spinal cord syndrome

Cause

Traumatic. This syndrome may result from a forced flexion, compression injury which may

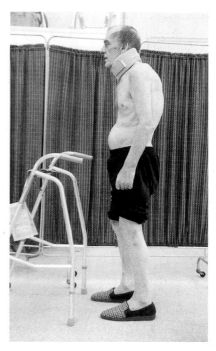

Figure 14.3 Standing posture of patient with central cord syndrome.

occur in diving or road traffic accidents (Foo et al 1981).

Non-traumatic. The anterior cord syndrome may result from infarction secondary to anterior spinal artery thrombosis, spinal cord angioma or rupture of aortic aneurysm. Significant neuro-logical recovery following spinal cord infarct is unusual unless there is improvement within the first 24 hours (Geldermacher & Nager 1989; cited in Stevenson et al 1996).

Clinical picture

This syndrome results from damage to the anterior part of the spinal cord. The clinical signs and symptoms are those of:

- motor loss
- loss of pain and temperature sensation
- preservation of tactile and joint position sense.

The severity of impairment will depend upon the extent and exact site of the damage.

Patients presenting with motor loss and sensory sparing are classified as Frankel B, or B on the ASIA impairment scale. However, these scales make no distinction between the types of sensory sparing, e.g. tactile, joint position sense and pain and temperature.

A clear distinction has been made between the different types of sensory sparing. Those with preserved pin prick have been shown to have an excellent prognosis to regain a functional gait. Crozier et al (1991) found that 66% of Frankel B patients with preservation of pin perception recovered to become functional walkers, whereas only 14% with light touch were able to walk (*n* = 33).

Vibration sense, tactile and joint position sense are served by the dorsal columns, whereas pain and temperature sensation is dependent upon the spinothalamic tracts. Preservation of pin prick indicates some integrity of the spinothalamic tracts in the anterolateral aspect of the spinal cord and therefore the possibility of some sparing of the adjacent corticospinal tracts (Foo et al 1981).

Body awareness enables patients with anterior cord lesions to respond more quickly to the rehabilitation process, often achieving their treatment goals in a shorter time. However, management of these patients is the same as that for Frankel A patients. Continuous pain has been identified as a key feature following spinal cord infarction (Pelser & van Gijn 1993).

Sensory sparing clearly indicates that the lesion is incomplete, but a significant difference in outcome to those with incomplete lesions is only possible where there is some motor recovery.

Brown–Séquard syndrome

This syndrome results from a transverse hemisection of the spinal cord, whereby half of the spinal cord is damaged laterally (Sullivan 1989).

Cause

Lateral damage to one side of the cord may be caused by penetration injuries such as stab wounds but may also result from other aetiologies and injury mechanisms such as road traffic accidents and rugby football injuries. Fracture-dislocation of a unilateral articular process and acute ruptured intervertebral disc have also been reported to give rise to this syndrome (Sullivan 1989).

Although knife injuries may result in the classical picture of Brown–Séquard syndrome, they are relatively uncommon. In over 1600 cases of spinal cord injury in America, only 1.1% were due to penetrating injuries other than gunshot wounds (Waters et al 1995). However, in South Africa, of 1600 patients admitted to a spinal injuries unit, a quarter were the result of stab wounds. Of these, 50% had Brown–Séquard syndrome (Peacock et al 1977).

Clinical picture

Motor deficit. Motor loss occurs on the same side as the lesion due to destruction of the pyramidal tracts.

The lower motor lesion, resulting from damage to the anterior horn cells at the level of the lesion, will be particularly significant at the cervical or lumbar enlargements.

Sensory deficit. Destruction of the posterior column results in loss of position sense, vibration and tactile discrimination below the level of the lesion on the affected side.

Destruction of the lateral spinothalamic tract causes loss of sensation of pain and temperature *on the side opposite to the lesion*. As the fibres entering this tract do not cross for several segments, the upper level of this sensory loss is likely to be a few segments below the level of the lesion. Fibres entering the cord at the level of the lesion may be involved before they cross, causing a narrow zone of similar pain and temperature loss *on the same side*.

Typical cases of Brown–Séquard syndrome are rare. Many patients with incomplete lesions will present with some asymmetry whilst not fulfilling the exact criteria of this syndrome. Patients with a total severance of the lateral half of their spinal cord will have little if any recovery, whereas those with contusions or contracoup injuries are likely to show significant functional improvement.

The majority of these patients will walk independently, with a reciprocal gait, as only one leg has lost or reduced motor power. An orthosis and/or walking aids may be required.

Even among the three syndromes described above, there is considerable variability in the severity of neurological damage and thus in the functional outcome. Incomplete spinal cord damage resulting from other pathologies, such as tumours, inflammatory disease, cervical myelopathy and vascular disease, is often more diverse and the outcome even more unpredictable.

Psychological factors

Obviously, with both complete and incomplete lesions, the psychological factors resulting from such a devastating injury have to be taken into account throughout all stages of rehabilitation.

The patient with an incomplete lesion may have a particular problem in coming to terms with his disability. Being incomplete, prognosis is ill-defined, and it is particularly difficult, even for those with a substantial functional recovery, to accept less than 100% normality (Sullivan 1989).

If surrounded by patients with complete lesions, it is easy to consider the patient with an incomplete lesion fortunate because he has some sparing. Although this is true, even those patients making a good recovery may still be unable to return to their normal lifestyle.

Understanding the patient's psychological response to his condition is crucial for effective rehabilitation. The physiotherapist, because of her close contact with the patient, may be the one chosen as 'confidante' by both the patient and his relatives. It is important that she allows him to express his fears and/or frustrations while offering constructive advice. Where more professional counselling is thought to be required, the patient and/or relatives should be encouraged to talk to a clinical psychologist.

TREATMENT
General comments

The therapeutic management of a patient with an incomplete lesion differs significantly from that of a patient with a complete lesion. Therapists working in spinal injury units develop great skill in maximizing the potential of patients with complete lesions and may be tempted to treat the patient with an incomplete lesion along similar lines.

Clearly, it is essential for all persons involved in the rehabilitation of the patient with an incomplete spinal cord injury to assess the disability of each patient as it relates to that individual and not to compare him with other patients, especially those with complete lesions.

Young (1994) stated that: 'spinal cord injury has been relegated to rehabilitation with the primary goal of maximizing remaining functions rather than restoring lost functions. This pessimistic attitude is not warranted.' Although his comments relate to the use of methylprednisolone within the first 8 hours post-injury, this statement may equally apply to the therapeutic management of incomplete spinal cord injured patients.

It has been suggested that patients with incomplete spinal cord lesions, particularly those caused by slowly progressive pathologies, are best managed in a neurological rehabilitation unit as opposed to a spinal injury unit (Stevenson et al 1996). Given that over 50% of all spinal injured patients have incomplete lesions, this statement is of enormous significance to the future management of this client group.

However, the patient with an incomplete spinal cord lesion may have severe disruption of bladder and bowel function, which requires the specific expertise of a spinal injury unit. Greater liaison and transference of skills should be made between therapists and other staff working in spinal injury units and neurological rehabilitation centres.

Patients with incomplete spinal cord lesions demonstrate many diverse disabilities depending on the level and extent of the pathology. It is important that both the patient and therapist have realistic expectations in terms of functional outcome and that appropriate short-term goals are selected to demonstrate progress. Accurate initial and ongoing assessment is essential to set and monitor these mutually agreed goals with appropriate, objective outcome measures to determine the efficacy of treatment.

Normal movement is the ultimate goal of rehabilitation, but all too often this is not achievable for patients with extensive neurological damage. Compensatory strategies may be necessary in order for the patient to attain his optimal level of function. The therapeutic skill lies in determining that compensation which is necessary and even essential for function and that which is unnecessary and potentially detrimental to the patient.

Analysis of movement and implications for treatment following incomplete spinal cord damage

Many authors describe the analysis of normal movement as the basis for the development of treatment techniques for patients with neurological damage (Bobath 1990, Shumway-Cook & Woollacott 1995, Carr et al 1995, Edwards 1996). However, the emphasis differs with regard to treatment approaches. For example, Bobath (1990) advocates the control of abnormal reflex activity and the underlying tone to improve coordination of movement, whereas Carr et al (1995) direct movement training towards improving performance of everyday actions, thereby enabling the patient to learn control of muscle activity and develop strength and endurance during functional motor performance.

Over recent years, the emphasis of the Bobath approach has changed significantly in that the musculoskeletal consequences of neurological damage are now recognized to be of equal importance to the tonal problems. Unfortunately, although this more holistic approach is now widely taught on Bobath adult hemiplegia courses in the UK, there is no current literature to describe this change of emphasis.

Normal movement is dependent upon an intact CNS which can receive, integrate and respond to stimuli. The complexity of this processing is illustrated by Harris-Warwick & Sparks (1995), where they refer to 'motor plans being implemented through networks that determine the order, timing and strength of movement around each joint, which is translated into a choreography of motoneurone activity that drives the individual muscles at the right moment and with the right force'. Spinal cord damage will affect this processing, the extent to which it is damaged being determined by the site and severity of the lesion.

The key features of normal movement are:

- normal postural tone
- reciprocal innervation
- sensory motor feedback and feedforward
- postural and balance reactions
- normal biomechanical properties of muscle.

Normal postural tone

Normal postural tone is dependent upon an intact CNS, which enables an individual to maintain an upright posture and adapt to a varying and often changing base of support, and which allows selective movement for function. (The base of support is the area within the boundaries of each point of contact with the supporting surface; Edwards 1996).

Neurologists assess muscle tone as the resistance to stretch in a state of voluntary relaxation (Davidoff 1992), which clearly has implications for both the neurological component of the movement disorder, e.g. spasticity, and the biomechanical changes to muscle.

Following spinal cord damage, postural tone may be impaired as a result of spasticity and/or weakness. The management of patients with incomplete spinal cord lesions will be determined to a large extent by the alterations in postural tone. Positioning in bed, particularly during the early stages, passive/active movements, facilitation of transfers, posture in the wheelchair and standing will all be influenced by the underlying tone. Equally, the manner in which these activities are carried out will in turn influence the prevailing postural tone.

Facilitation of active movement on a background of impaired tone, particularly low tone, is often more difficult when the patient is fully supported. Bed rest is often essential in the immediate aftermath of traumatic spinal cord injury, and therefore alternative positioning is not possible. However, as soon as the medical condition allows, positioning against gravity with appropriate support is recommended to stimulate a more active response (Edwards 1996).

Reciprocal innervation

Reciprocal innervation is the graded interaction of agonists, antagonists and synergists during the maintenance of a posture or the performance of a movement (Bobath 1990).

Reciprocal innervation is best illustrated in the postural adjustments which occur prior to and during movement. Horak et al (1984) examined the activation times for trunk and leg movement while lifting the arm. Activity in these postural muscles preceded the arm displacement, presumably to provide stability for the ensuing movement. The sequencing of these postural adjustments was found to be more variable during slower movements. As less stabilization is required during slower movement, the preparatory muscle activity is not programmed as rigidly as with more rapid movement.

These early changes in postural muscles were significantly decreased if the subject was supported at the shoulder or even touched a rail with a single finger (Cordo & Nashner 1982).

These two factors, the speed at which the movement is performed and the support provided during movement, are of particular significance for patients with neurological damage such as may result from spinal cord injury.

Many patients will be unable to move as quickly as normal subjects, and changes in the postural adjustments may be related to the speed of the movement as much as the pathology.

The order and timing of postural adjustments will be influenced when providing assistance for a patient to stand and walk. Clearly it is important to facilitate a more normal posture or movement, but it may be of equal value to allow the patient to correct his own posture. If the therapist constantly supports the patient, the postural adjustments will always be dependent upon this support.

Normal sensorimotor feedback system

Postures and movements are guided by a mixture of motor programmes and sensory feedback because calculations made ahead of time in the CNS are always corrected after central and peripheral reports about reality (Brooks 1986).

Rothwell (1994) describes the production of voluntary movement as being sequential in terms of the idea or reason to move, the motor plan which is constantly updated to fit the requirements of the muscles involved in the movement and the execution of the movement. This interaction between central and peripheral systems may be considered a cyclical event whereby movement skills are constantly reinforced and refined by repetition.

If the patient is unable to move due to significant paralysis, he will be unable to reinforce his movement skills. Hallett et al (1993) demonstrated the change in cortical mapping of a patient with a complete cervical spinal cord lesion using transcranial magnetic stimulation. The cortical representation of deltoid expanded to encroach on the territory previously subserving the paralysed muscles innervated below the neurological level of the lesion.

Patients who develop spasticity may create new motor programmes that are dictated by the stereotyped activity. Movements attempted on a background of increased tone will involve effort and produce an abnormal sensory input to the CNS.

The aim of physiotherapy is to modify this stereotypical response by facilitation of more normal movement patterns. Prolonged use of a limited repertoire of movement patterns such as occurs with spasticity creates a dominant abnormal response which becomes increasingly difficult to reverse. Once established, re-education of more purposeful movement can sometimes only be achieved with outside intervention such as localized injections of botulinum toxin to weaken the dominant spastic muscles (p. 193).

The direct effect of sensory loss is more difficult to quantify. Patients who have full muscle power but who have no appreciation of movement can be as disabled as those without motor control. Clearly any specific sensory loss will have implications for the initiation, guidance and control of movement.

Posture and balance reactions

Postural control, which provides stability and orientation, requires:

- the integration of sensory information to assess the position and motion of the body in space
- the ability to generate forces for controlling body position (Shumway-Cook & Woollacott 1995).

Automatic reactions occur in response to alteration of body alignment to maintain the centre of gravity within the base of support. Different types of responses are described: equilibrium, righting and protective reactions (Bobath 1990) or alternatively the ankle, hip and stepping strategies (Shumway-Cook & Woollacott 1995).

Equilibrium reactions. The equilibrium reactions are synonymous with the postural adjustments which occur throughout the body and are effective only on a background of normal postural tone. Postural adjustments occur during any movement, and any alteration in the position of the body's centre of gravity requires modification of tone throughout the body musculature.

For example, during quiet stance, the muscles of the feet and lower limbs are constantly making minute adjustments to maintain the body's centre of gravity over the base of support. Shumway-Cook & Woollacott (1995) refer to this response as the ankle strategy, in that the body is maintained or restored to a position of stability through body movement centred primarily about the ankle joints.

Equilibrium reactions or the ankle strategy are used more commonly in situations where the demands placed on postural control are small. This means of maintaining balance is dependent upon normal range of movement and strength around the ankle joint.

Righting reactions. These reactions are activated when the more discreet postural adjustments or equilibrium reactions prove to be inadequate. The arms become increasingly involved the greater the balance displacement.

Shumway-Cook & Woollacott (1995) refer to this response as the hip strategy, which is used to restore balance in response to larger, faster movements. The hip strategy is most apparent when the support surface is compliant, or smaller than the feet, such as when standing on a balance beam. Olympic gymnasts may be able to maintain control with an ankle strategy when performing on a balance bar, but this is certainly not the case with the amateur where hip and arm movements become increasingly pronounced as they strive to stay upright.

For patients with incomplete spinal cord lesions, the hip strategy will be called into play if there is inadequate control at the ankles, which may result from weakness, muscle imbalance or spasticity. A typical example of this is in patients with a positive support reaction whereby the foot is unable to adapt to and accept the base of the support. The patient is unable to transfer weight over the full surface of the foot and the ankle remains in a degree of plantarflexion. The compensatory response is flexion at the hip to maintain the body weight over the base of support (Bobath 1990).

Righting reactions also refer to the alignment of body segments, the head, trunk and limbs, with each other and with the environment (Bobath 1990). They are observed in virtually all sequences of movement, such as rolling, sitting up and lying down, and are dependent upon the interaction between flexion and extension which allows for rotation. Any traumatic injury to the spine will interfere with these responses in that there is invariably a reduced range of movement following any acute injury.

Righting reactions are often grossly impaired following immobilization of the cervical spine with halo pelvic traction. It has been observed in clinical practice that even those patients who have full neurological function have severe difficulties in effecting correct body alignment following prolonged immobilization in this type of support. Although a valuable means of stabilization, it would appear that the rigidity of the device virtually negates muscle activity between the points of contact. It is therefore not unusual to see an anterior tilt of the pelvis and poking chin, with little if any neck and trunk rotation, on removal of the support.

Protective reactions. Protective reactions or the stepping strategy are called into play when the equilibrium and righting reactions fail to maintain the centre of gravity within the base of support. The initial movement is often a step in the direction to which balance is displaced, but the parachute response, putting the arms out to protect the face, may have to be utilized as a last line of defence.

Patients with impaired movement control are often apprehensive, realizing that their response to sudden and unexpected perturbations may be inadequate to maintain balance. Movements are consequently slower and the background postural tone higher, particularly when standing and walking, in anticipation of potential falls.

Biomechanical properties of muscle

The different types of skeletal muscle are referred to as slow oxidative (SO), fast glycolytic (FG) and fast oxidative glycolytic (FOG). Their characteristics are summarized in Table 14.1 (Rothwell 1994).

The SO muscles are those which participate in long-lasting but relatively weak contractions, such as in the control of posture, whereas the FG muscles generate large forces but are readily fatigued. The recruitment order of a motor unit is dependent upon the size of its motor neurone (Henneman et al 1956; cited in Rothwell 1994) and is in the order of SO, FOG, FG. From a functional perspective, the SO muscles provide postural control to allow for the FG to perform the more selective movements.

Table 14.1 The characteristics of different types of skeletal muscles (from Rothwell 1994, Table 3.1, with permission)

Fibre type	I SO	IIA FOG	IIB FG
Motor unit type	Slow (S)	Fast fatigue resistant (FR)	Fast fatiguable (FF)
Fibre diameter	Small	Medium–small	Large

Muscles alter their characteristics in response to function, that is to say it is the activity of the muscle which determines the muscle type (Dietz 1992). Following spinal cord injury, the disturbance of spinal cord circuitry leads to disordered muscular activation patterns which will alter the muscle characteristics.

Damage to anterior horn cells at the level of the lesion gives rise to flaccid paralysis or weakness of the affected muscle groups as a result of disuse. This is well illustrated in patients with central cord syndrome at the level of C5 where the shoulder muscles are often significantly wasted. The postural, anti-gravity muscles (SO) are more profoundly affected by this disuse, exhibiting rapid and extensive atrophy in response to the deprivation of normal activity patterns (Goldspink & Williams 1990, Given et al 1995).

Spasticity, which is often a complication for patients with incomplete spinal cord lesions, will impose different activity patterns on muscle due to the stereotyped movements. The more spastic muscles, as a result of the overactivity, undergo a transformation from FG to SO (Dattola et al 1993). As they become more SO, they will be recruited more readily, thereby exacerbating the spastic response.

The length and stiffness of the muscle are key determinants for normal functional use. The length-associated changes of muscle will affect patients with paralysis and/or spasticity in that, in both instances, full-range active movement is impaired and normal motor function is not possible (Ada & Canning 1990, Goldspink & Williams 1990, Edwards 1996).

Imposed length changes have been shown to alter the mechanical properties and structure of muscle. Immobilization in a shortened position produces short, stiff muscles with fewer sarcomeres and an increase in connective tissue. These length changes and sarcomere loss are accelerated when the muscle shortening is induced by electrical stimulation or tetanus toxin. It is suggested that these results provide a model for the rapid length changes seen in spastic muscle (Herbert 1988).

The main remit of the physiotherapist is to maintain the range of movement in all affected muscle groups. This is of particular significance for patients with incomplete spinal cord lesions in that the majority of patients will have some degree of neurological recovery. As recovery occurs in a specific muscle, if the antagonist muscle has become shortened, it will be more difficult, if not impossible, to maximize this recovery.

An understanding of these features of normal movement is essential for the development of treatment techniques for the patient with incomplete spinal cord injury. Of all patients with neurological damage, the patient with an incomplete spinal cord injury often presents with the most diverse functional problems, which will depend upon the site and extent of the lesion.

In order to develop appropriate treatment strategies, it is important to distinguish between the primary deficit and the secondary compensation. Analysis of positions and movement sequences in normal subjects is useful to draw comparison with the postural and movement deficits which may result from incomplete spinal cord damage. In this way, the distinction between the primary cause and secondary compensation can be more readily made.

Analysis of specific positions

Although few individuals demonstrate identical characteristics when assuming any one position,

certain features are remarkably similar. A detailed description of the normal characteristics of supine-lying, prone-lying, side-lying, sitting and standing is to be found in Edwards (1996).

Table 14.2 provides a summary of the identified features when assuming each of these positions. This table is by no means conclusive. Its purpose is to allow comparisons to be drawn between normal subjects and patients with movement disorders. Analysis of these positions in this way provides a structure for the assessment of patients with physical disability and for the selection of the most appropriate position in which to treat the patient. For example, patients with flaccidity should be stimulated by treatment in positions requiring anti-gravity activity. Those with spasticity should be mobilized in an appropriate position to inhibit the spasticity in order to prepare them to accept the base of support.

Key points of control

Key points of control are described as areas of the body from which movement can be most effectively controlled and from where movement may be centralized. The proximal key points are the trunk, shoulder girdles and pelvis, and the distal key points are the hands and feet (Bobath 1990).

Trunk mobilization is recognized as an important treatment modality and in the majority

Table 14.2 Characteristics of supported positions and positions requiring anti-gravity activity

	Supported positions			Positions requiring anti-gravitiy activity	
	Prone	Supine	Supported sitting	Sitting	Standing
Head	To side	Midline	Midline	Midline	Midline
Shoulders	Forwards of CKP	Backwards of CKP	Forwards of CKP	Forwards of CKP	Forwards of CKP
Pelvis	Forwards of CKP (anterior tilt)	Backwards of CKP (posterior tilt)	Forwards of CKP (posterior tilt)	Backwards of CKP (anterior tilt)	Backwards of CKP (posterior tilt)
Upper limbs	Flexion, adduction, medial rotation	Extension, abduction, lateral rotation	Flexion, adduction, medial rotation	Flexion, adduction, medial rotation	Flexion, adduction, medial rotation
Lower limbs	Adduction, medial rotation	Extension, abduction, lateral rotation	Flexion, adduction, medial rotation	Flexion, abduction, lateral rotation	Extension, abduction, lateral rotation
Overall influence	Flexion	Extension	Flexion	Flexion	Extension

WB = weight-bearing; NWB = non-weight-bearing; CKP = central key point.

of cases is a prerequisite for the facilitation of movement of the limbs (Davies 1990, Edwards 1996). If the trunk is unable to make the required postural adjustments to movement of the limbs, then these distal movements will inevitably be abnormal.

Posture and movement within the trunk may be effectively controlled by manual guidance from a central point between the xiphisternum and the T8 vertebra. This is called the central key point. The relationship of the central key point with the proximal key points provides a basis for the analysis of abnormal patterns of posture and movement. In the normal subject, although asymmetrical postures may be adopted, the relationship between the central key point, the head and the proximal key points is generally symmetrical. Although asymmetry may be seen, as in cross legged sitting, it is in no way comparable to that of a patient with neurological dysfunction (Fig. 14.4).

As a basis for the analysis of neurological damage and the resultant impaired movement, it is helpful to assess the patient in terms of the midline deviation. This may be considered in three planes of movement:

- the sagittal plane
- the coronal plane
- the horizontal plane.

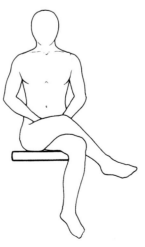

Figure 14.4 Cross-legged sitting.

The relationship of the key points to the midline will vary in different positions depending upon the ability of the individual to:

- support himself in anti-gravity situations
- accept the base of support in supported positions.

A key point from which to influence movement is determined by the ability of the individual to respond to facilitation of movement. Facilitation from a distal key point, e.g. the hand, can only be safely used if there is adequate postural control within the trunk. If the patient is unable to make the required adjustments, the shoulder may be traumatized.

This analysis demonstrates that there can be no stereotyped picture of what is 'normal'. Individuals have different levels of postural tone in accepting the base of support and reacting to the effects of gravity. Similarly, movements from one position to another will show similarities but may vary quite considerably whilst still being accepted as being within a normal range.

Pathophysiology

The movement deficit of patients with incomplete spinal cord lesions may originate from:

- impairment of supraspinal control through damage to descending tracts (Dimitrijevic et al 1983)
- disturbance of spinal cord circuitry which leads to disordered muscular activation patterns and abnormal reflex activity (Fung et al 1990)
- weakness due to anterior horn cell damage at the level of the lesion or as a consequence of spasticity
- change in the mechanical properties of muscle (Given et al 1995)
- muscle imbalance, as a result of either spasticity or unopposed muscle action.

Disability following incomplete spinal cord injury therefore arises primarily as a result of spasticity and/or weakness, through both neural and mechanical mechanisms.

Spasticity

Spasticity is a common consequence of spinal cord injury and is often more severe in patients with incomplete lesions, particularly those classified as Frankel B and C (Maynard et al 1990, Heckman 1994).

The classical definition of spasticity is that it is 'a motor disorder characterised by a velocity-dependent increase in tonic stretch reflexes with exaggerated tendon jerks resulting from hyper-excitability of the stretch reflex as one component of the upper motoneurone syndrome' (Lance 1980). While this may be an accurate definition of the 'neural component' or positive feature of spasticity (Carr et al 1995), it is of little relevance to the patient. What have been described as the negative or associated features of spasticity – decreased dexterity, fatigability, paresis or weakness, impairment of coordinated movement and changes in posture (Katz & Rymer 1989, Brown 1994) – are the symptoms which are more disabling for the patient. Factors which are thought to contribute to the increased mechanical resistance to movement include reduced tendon compliance and physiological and histochemical changes in muscle fibres (Dietz 1992).

There are two major balancing descending systems which control tone in humans. These are the inhibitory dorsal reticulospinal tract and the facilitatory medial reticulospinal and vestibulospinal tracts. Damage to the dorsal reticulospinal tract leaves the action of the facilitatory pathways unopposed and leads to extensor spasticity, whereas damage to the vestibulospinal and medial reticulospinal tracts may contribute to the release of flexor spasticity. Damage to the corticospinal tract leads to paresis as opposed to spasticity (Brown 1994).

A characteristic feature of spasticity is impaired reciprocal inhibition (Boorman et al 1996), frequently termed reciprocal innervation by physiotherapists (Edwards 1996). This is associated with an increase in the degree of antagonist muscle contraction seen during alternating muscle actions. It has been suggested that muscle relaxation is accomplished, not simply by inhibition of the active motoneurone pool, but also by active, possibly presynaptic, processes which speed 'de-recruitment' of the motoneurones. These active processes are impaired in patients with incomplete spinal cord lesions with spasticity (Boorman et al 1996). Dietz et al (1995) proposed that reduced modulation of EMG patterns observed during locomotion – a longer lasting tonic gastrocnemius EMG activity and coactivation of antagonist leg muscles – may be due to impaired function of polysynaptic spinal reflexes.

Acquired spasticity may be considered as a dynamic phenomenon and reflects the age, site and size of the lesion responsible for its genesis. The reorganization of neural pathways following spinal cord injury occurs as a result of the sprouting of new neuronal connections and through unmasking of existing but functionally inactive pathways. Whereas sprouting occurs over time, unmasking is evident within hours (Topka et al 1991).

In the uninjured spinal cord, the efficiency of synaptic function and the pattern of synaptic connections within the neural circuitry responsible for learning have been shown to be activity-dependent. This dispels the concept that the spinal cord is relatively non-plastic and serves simply to relay supraspinal commands. There is evidence supporting both activity-dependent and injury-induced plasticity after spinal cord trauma (Muir & Steeves 1997).

One hypothesis for physiotherapy in the treatment of patients with incomplete spinal cord injury may be that of channelling regenerating axons to appropriate target neurones through facilitating movement to maximize function.

Pathological activity associated with spasticity

The positive support reaction. This term is used by physiotherapists to describe a pathological extensor response in the lower limb evoked by a stimulus of pressure on the ball of the foot (Bobath 1990, Edwards 1996).

This reaction, which is considered to be of distal origin, prevents transference of weight over the full surface of the foot. The patient, with extensor spasticity of the lower limb and plantarflexion and inversion of the foot, is unable to accommodate to the supporting surface. This extensor response prevents hip extension during stance phase of gait, the patient having to flex forward at the hip to maintain balance.

Although the knee is held in extension, this position is not maintained with normal quadriceps activity and it is not uncommon to observe wasting of this muscle group. The knee becomes hyperextended due to the inability to attain normal alignment of the pelvis over the foot, impaired reciprocal innervation between agonists and antagonists, and shortening of gastrocnemius (Edwards 1996).

Patients with a positive support reaction are in danger of developing contractures of all muscle groups held in a shortened position. Those most notably affected are:

- soleus and gastrocnemius
- tibialis posterior
- intrinsic foot musculature and plantar fascia
- iliopsoas
- rectus femoris
- hip adductors.

The clinical picture of the positive support reaction is most apparent during gait. The extensor spasticity prevents release of the knee and the patient has to hitch the leg forward during the swing phase of gait. It may also affect the patient's ability to stand up or sit down, the extensor spasticity preventing mobility at the knee.

Inhibition of this pathological response must incorporate desensitization by mobilization of the foot itself. Physiotherapists are often advised to avoid contact with the ball of the foot. However, in this instance, mobilization of the foot, the posterior crural muscle group and the Achilles tendon is recommended to desensitize against both the intrinsic and extrinsic stimuli (Lynch & Grisogono 1991, Edwards 1996). This distal intervention should be used in conjunction with facilitation of more normal alignment of the pelvis over the weight-bearing foot.

The flexor withdrawal response. This response occurs as a protective mechanism in normal subjects and may be observed as an individual withdraws the hand from a hot stove, or the foot when stepping on a nail. It is determined by the direction of the noxious stimulus and therefore may not necessarily be into flexion (Rothwell 1994). Patients with incomplete spinal cord lesions may demonstrate this response, but in a more stereotyped and consistent pattern and in response to a fairly innocuous stimulus such as removal of the bedclothes. As the term implies, the flexor withdrawal is associated with flexor spasticity.

The withdrawal response in the lower limbs is that of flexion and lateral rotation at the hip, flexion at the knee and dorsiflexion or plantarflexion at the ankle. The foot may be everted or inverted, often being everted with dorsiflexion or inverted with plantarflexion at the ankle.

Noxious stimulus on a background of abnormal tone may give rise to this response. For example, a pressure sore, pain or an ingrowing toenail may cause an increase in spasticity with flexion of the limb. It is essential to determine if there is an external cause and to treat this prior to undertaking more radical intervention to manage the spasticity. The short-term influence of such a stimulus may be readily reversible, but prolonged exposure may have more residual effects such as the development of contractures (Edwards 1996).

The clinical picture of the flexor withdrawal response is most apparent during the swing phase of gait where there is exaggerated flexor activity. Weight-bearing through the affected limb(s) was previously recommended but this should be carried out with caution. Attempts to stand the patient on a leg which is contracted into flexion will further aggravate the situation, not least by imposing an additional painful stimulus (Edwards 1996).

The crossed extensor reflex. The crossed extensor reflex as described by Magnus (1926; cited in Bobath 1985) is a spinal reflex involving a flexion reflex of one limb and the simultaneous increase of extensor tone in the supporting limb.

Although this reflex may be referred to in patients with incomplete spinal cord damage, it is rarely seen in its 'pure' form. More often than not the clinical picture is one of increased extensor activity bilaterally in the lower limbs (Bajd et al 1989). The extensor tone may interfere with general function, such as dressing, transferring and turning in bed, but its influence is most apparent during gait (see p. 186).

Paralysis/weakness

Weakness may result from damage to the anterior horn cells producing peripheral denervation or as a consequence of damage to the corticospinal tract.

With a complete spinal cord lesion, there is total ablation of the anterior horn cells at the level of the lesion and therefore no 'final common pathway' to the muscle. This produces a flaccid paralysis of muscles innervated from that level of the spinal cord.

In incomplete lesions, the extent of this destruction will be variable depending on the site and severity of the lesion. The lesion may affect virtually all efferent and afferent neurones at a certain level but not causing complete interruption of their function. Alternatively, there may be lesions where there are distinct parts of the spinal cord which are completely damaged but others that are preserved intact (Bajd et al 1989).

In many instances, the strength of the muscle will be reduced, but some control may remain, producing weakness as opposed to a complete paralysis. EMG investigations have revealed that the active units could be divided into those under normal control, spontaneous active units which could not be activated by the subject and units which could only be slowly and weakly activated (Stein et al 1990).

Muscle fibre and connective tissue changes associated with use and disuse are described in detail by Goldspink & Williams (1990) and have been discussed earlier (p. 174).

The acute lesion in bed

One of the main aims of physiotherapy is to minimize the effects of spasticity and to prevent length-associated changes in muscle to enable more appropriate function.

Changes in cortical representation of body parts due to loss of function have been shown to occur within minutes (Hallet et al 1993) and

therefore early treatment is essential to minimize these adverse effects.

The spinal cord damage gives rise to the presenting signs and symptoms with regard to spasticity, but it is how the patient copes with this pathological movement that will determine the outcome in terms of muscle, neural and soft tissue changes.

Although this section relates to the early management of these patients, it is of relevance throughout all stages of rehabilitation.

Positioning

In the early stages of traumatic spinal cord injury, the positioning of the patient is determined by the management of the fracture site. The position

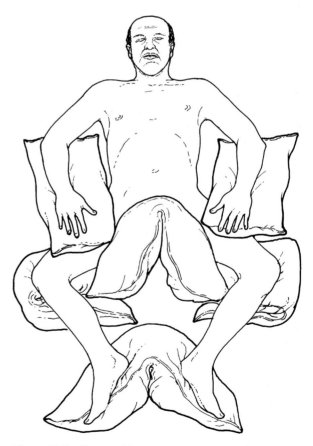

Figure 14.5 Frog position.

of the incomplete lesion is, therefore, the same as that for the complete lesion.

Where severe spasticity is a complicating factor, it may be necessary to avoid the supine position and to use pillows and sandbags to support the fracture site and keep the patient in side-lying. If the extensor aspect of the patient's body is in contact with the bed, as is the case even when on his 'side' on the Egerton–Stoke Mandeville electric turning bed, a stimulus is provided for him to push against which may exacerbate his spasticity and may therefore be contraindicated.

The 'frog position', where the hips are abducted, laterally rotated and flexed to approximately 40°, can be used to break up severe extensor spasticity (Fig. 14.5). Patients positioned in this way to control extensor tone should be closely monitored for any increase in flexor tone, as it is possible to reverse the pattern of spasticity completely.

Alternate positioning of the arms is also recommended in certain spinal injury units. The crucifix position and positioning of the arms in lateral rotation (Fig. 14.6a & b) should be used with caution as they are at the extreme end of range. Any shortening of, for example, the pectoral muscles or medial rotators of the shoulder may place undue stress on an already vulnerable joint. The neural structures may also become shortened and specific tension tests are recommended to maintain or restore adaptive lengthening of the nervous system (Davies 1994).

Clearly the aim is to prevent this shortening occurring in the first place, but even with the most rigorous intervention with regard to positioning and movement in the early stages, it is very difficult to replicate the full repertoire of normal movement. Any normal subject, lying in the crucifix position will appreciate the discomfort felt over a relatively short period of time.

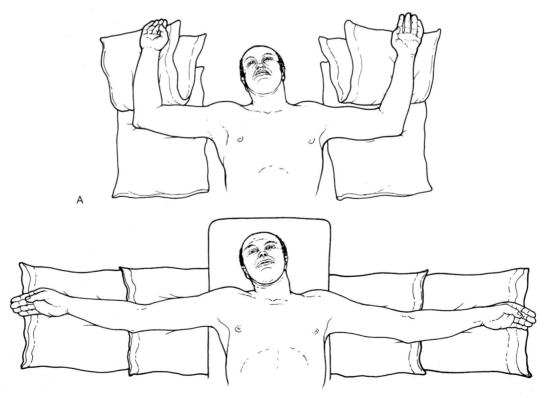

Figure 14.6 Positioning of arms. A: The arms in lateral rotation. B: Crucifix.

Passive/active movement

Assisted movements should be carried out with the patient's full awareness and participation. Regenerating axons in the adult CNS are capable of forming synapses with both appropriate and inappropriate target neurones. Facilitation of appropriate patterns of activity will assist in establishing functional connections between regenerating supraspinal axons and spinal neurones (Muir & Steeves 1997).

Motor learning is an active process and can only occur as a result of relatively permanent changes in the capability for skilled movement (Schmidt 1991). Passive movement, while of value in maintaining muscle and joint range, does little to effect functional change unless there is some participation on the part of the patient. As such, the term 'passive' is inappropriate in that the patient should always be involved in the activity. In the early stages following spinal cord injury, no active movement may be possible. However, given that there is often significant anatomical continuity across the injury site, even in patients with minimal function below the lesion (Dimitrijevic et al 1983), it is imperative to ensure that the patient is aware of, and contributes to, the desired movement.

The physiotherapist must appreciate changes in tone and, by her handling, modify this tone before taking the limb through normal joint range. If movements are performed in this way, with close communication between patient and therapist, there will be less danger of trauma and of the joints becoming painful and contracted.

Effort during movement should be avoided where spasticity is present. The physiotherapist gives sufficient guidance and assistance to the patient to reduce to a minimum the effort required to perform the movement. This is particularly important where spasticity may jeopardize stability at the fracture site. Some patients may be particularly sensitive to any stimulus, even removal of the bedclothes prior to doing the movements, and with cervical lesions it may be necessary for another person to support the shoulders to eliminate excessive movement around the fracture site.

In the majority of patients, extensor spasticity is the dominant pattern in the lower limbs (Bajd et al 1989) and this spastic posturing may also be in evidence in the arms and trunk of a patient with a high cervical lesion. A combination of both flexor and extensor spasticity frequently occurs and movement initially may be from one total pattern to the other.

In those cases where there is severe extensor spasticity, it may be necessary initially to move the limbs into the total flexor pattern in order to have any effect on the predominant extension. After breaking up the total extensor synergy, it is important to work recovering muscles out of any stereotyped pattern. For example, with the leg flexed, the patient is encouraged to use any active hip flexion with adduction and medial rotation, and when moving into extension this should incorporate abduction and lateral rotation, always maintaining control to avoid an extensor thrust.

Partial preservation of brain influences contribute to the central excitatory state of segmental reflexes and spasticity, and as control of movement improves, there is often a notable reduction in the level of spasticity (Maynard et al 1990).

Compensatory movements

Teaching compensatory movement patterns may be considered to be inappropriate in the early stages, but this is dependent upon the functional outcome. For example, with a complete C6 lesion, in the absence of triceps, extension of the elbow can only be accomplished by means of lateral rotation at the shoulder with distal support at the hand. Although the resultant movement is compensatory, it in no way precludes recovery of triceps. Clinical experience suggests that the reverse is true, in that with extension of the elbow and using this movement in functional activities, activity in triceps is stimulated.

It has been shown that the cortical representation of extensor carpi radialis varies according to the function. Some parts of its cortical representation are concerned with this muscle as a 'prime mover', e.g. when used in the tenodysis grip, while others are concerned with its role as a stabilizer of the wrist during movements of the hand (Turton et al 1993). The early use of the tenodysis grip is therefore more difficult to substantiate. Patients with no finger movement but with wrist extension will readily use a tenodysis grip to maximize function. However, if finger movements then recover at a later date, it is often difficult for the patient to cease to rely on this grip, thereby impeding functional use of the fingers.

Compensatory movement must therefore be viewed on merit in the light of the presenting signs and symptoms and the expected prognosis, always assuming a positive outcome.

The shoulder

Patients with cervical cord damage, particularly those with central cord lesions, will invariably have abnormal movement at the shoulder due to the imbalance of muscle activity (Roth et al 1990). The shoulder joint is the most mobile joint of the body, sacrificing stability for this mobility. With paralysis or weakness of the muscles around the shoulder, functional activities are severely compromised.

It is essential to understand the components of normal activity at the shoulder in order to prevent trauma and possible contracture through inappropriate handling and movement. The shoulder joint cannot be viewed in isolation. Movements of the shoulder joint are dependent upon the integrity and responsiveness of the shoulder girdle, trunk, pelvis and lower limbs. For example, full elevation of the arms is dependent upon adequate extension within the thoracic spine (Crawford & Jull 1993).

The normal shoulder mechanism is dependent upon the structure and relationship of seven articulations (Fig. 14.7). The scapula lies in a slightly laterally rotated position, there being a ratio of approximately 2:3 in the distance between the medial edge of the spine of the scapula and the vertebral column, and the inferior angle and the vertebral column (Fig. 14.8a).

The glenoid fossa faces anteriorly, laterally and superiorly in its articulation with the head of

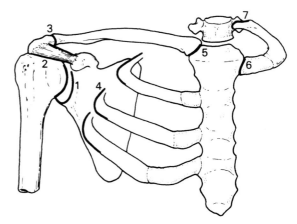

Figure 14.7 Composite drawing of the shoulder girdle. 1, glenohumoral; 2, suprahumeral; 3, acromioclavicular; 4, scapulocostal; 5, sternoclavicular; 6, costosternal; 7, costovertebral. (From Cailliet 1987.)

the humerus. This relationship between the head of the humerus and the glenoid fossa provides a degree of stability described as the locking mechanism of the shoulder (Basmajian 1978).

Functional movement of the upper limb requires coordination of movement between the glenohumeral (shoulder) joint and the scapula on a background of dynamic co-contraction and stability in the trunk. This interaction is dependent upon normal muscle activity. In patients with cervical cord damage, this muscle activity will be impaired.

The patient with flaccidity/low tone, on assessment in the sitting position, demonstrates the following:

- The scapula adopts a more vertical position (Fig. 14.8b), the inferior angle lying the same distance from the vertebral column as the spine of the scapula. Winging of the scapula is apparent.
- The glenoid fossa lies vertically in its articulation with the head of humerus, thereby creating a position of abduction at the glenohumeral joint. This nullifies the locking mechanism, and the support of the arm now depends primarily on the capsule and the coracohumeral ligament. Subluxation frequently occurs.
- The upper fibres of trapezius become hyperactive in an attempt to counteract the weight of the upper limb.

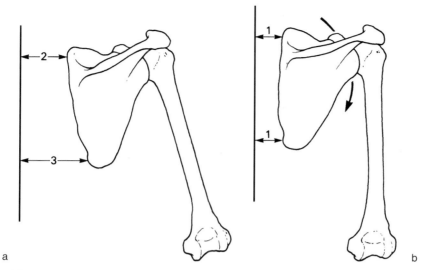

Figure 14.8 Relationship of the shoulder girdle and vertebral column. a: Normal relationship. b: Abnormal relationship.

The patient with spasticity/high tone, presents with similar malalignment, but the situation is exacerbated by the increased tone:

• The scapula will be pulled medially towards the vertebral column under the influence of spasticity of the rhomboids. In extreme cases, the position of the inferior angle of the scapula will be closer to the vertebral column than that of the medial aspect of the spine of the scapula. Winging of the scapula is often pronounced.
• The degree of abduction at the glenohumeral joint may be increased.
• Spasticity of the medial rotators of the upper limb will cause further malalignment of the glenohumeral joint, producing a spastic, anterior subluxation.
• In some cases, the medial rotators of the upper limb may become shortened.

Movements of the arm away from the body will, in this situation, create a hypermobile scapula. The inferior angle will rotate laterally around the chest wall and there will be little or no isolated movement at the glenohumeral joint.

Because of the variability in injuries sustained, it is not possible to describe in detail the particular problems that any one patient with cervical cord damage will have. However, it is important to recognize that although contractures are more likely to occur in the presence of spasticity (Yarkony & Sahgal 1987), profound disability has been reported as a result of reduced joint mobility in patients with Guillain–Barre syndrome, a peripheral CNS disorder (Soryal et al 1992).

This analysis describes a basic concept of normal movement, to enable the therapist to identify the patient's individual problem(s) and select appropriate treatment techniques. In every case, treatment must attempt to restore a more correct alignment of the upper limb, shoulder girdle and trunk. Movements of the upper limb, be they passive or active, must be performed with a full understanding of the normal shoulder mechanism and an accurate analysis of the patient's problem.

The pelvis and gait

Extensive work has been carried out in the field of gait analysis taking into consideration:

• kinematics – monitoring the gait pattern

- electromyography – monitoring muscle activity
- kinetics – monitoring forces that produce change/motion
- efficiency of gait – measuring energy expenditure, speed and endurance.

An understanding of these aspects of normal gait is invaluable when assessing patients with incomplete spinal cord damage. This detailed analysis using highly sophisticated equipment allows the primary errors in walking to be distinguished from compensatory changes, which is essential in planning effective treatment (Sutherland 1992).

The different problems that may arise as a result of incomplete spinal cord damage are too numerous and diverse to enable a standardized treatment approach. However, there are certain aspects of gait which must be considered with observational analysis and in planning treatment:

- the quality of postural tone, both the neural and mechanical components
- the speed and efficiency of gait
- the midline orientation of the central key point and the proximal key points of the shoulder girdles and the pelvis in terms of the sagittal, coronal and transverse planes
- the ability of the feet to accept the base of support.

In addition, each patient must have a full neurological assessment to determine the motor and sensory deficit. Special attention must be paid to aspects such as skeletal deformity or surgical intervention in the form of vertebral fusion or the insertion of, for example, a Harrington rod.

Normal walking is dependent upon a continual interchange between mobility and stability, which requires free passive mobility and appropriate muscle action (Perry 1992). Box 14.1 provides a summary of normal muscle activity and function during gait. This box illustrates the complexity of gait. The muscles identified do not have one single action but may work concentrically, eccentrically or isometrically at different stages of the gait cycle.

This is of particular relevance when considering the use of muscle or nerve blocks. For example, the role of the plantarflexors during gait is to contribute to knee stability, provide ankle stability, restrain the forward movement of the tibia on the talus during stance phase, and minimize the vertical oscillation of the whole-body centre of mass (Sutherland et al 1980). Therefore, whilst muscle or nerve blocks will reduce undesirable hyperactivity such as may occur with spasticity, they may also lead to knee and ankle instability and increased energy expenditure.

Normal gait has four major attributes which are frequently lost in abnormal gait. These are:

- stability in stance
- sufficient foot clearance during swing
- appropriate swing-phase prepositioning of the foot
- an adequate step length (Gage 1992).

For example, with predominant extensor spasticity, both legs are used for weight-bearing and the extensor spasticity prevails, preventing adequate flexion of the moving leg.

The most obvious features are:

- extensor spasticity of the lower limbs with adduction and medial rotation at the hips and plantarflexion and inversion at the ankle and foot
- a posterior tilt of the pelvis
- the compensation of the trunk and upper limbs, which is dependent upon whether or not the arms are used for support or balance.

The compensatory mechanisms often used to overcome this pathological activity include the following:

- The patient rises higher on his toes, throwing his trunk backwards to propel the moving leg forward with a minimum of flexion at the hips and knees. The patient walks with a 'scissor gait' with gross overactivity of the upper limbs to preserve balance.
- With the increased extensor activity in the trunk, the tilt of the pelvis may be altered, the resulting anterior tilt reversing the pattern of spasticity in the legs to one of flexion.

Box 14.1 A summary of normal muscle activity and function during gait (after adaptation by Gage 1991, after Perry 1989, with permission from MacKeith Press)

Terminal swing
Muscle function. Ends swing and prepares limb for stance.

- Hip flexors – these muscles are usually not active at this time
- Hamstrings – eccentric action decelerates the forward swing of the thigh and leg
- Quadriceps – concentric action to extend knee for stance
- Tibialis anterior – ankle dorsiflexion supports the ankle at neutral to prevent foot drop

Initial contact
Muscle function. Acts to allow smooth progression and stabilizes joints while simultaneously decelerating the body's inertia.

- Gluteus maximus – controls flexor moment produced by ground reaction forces (GRFs)
- Hamstrings – inhibit knee hyperextension and assist in controlling flexion moment at hip
- Tibialis anterior – initiates the heel rocker

Loading response
Muscle function. Acts to allow smooth progression and stabilizes joints while simultaneously decelerating the body's inertia.

- Hamstrings – concentric action unlocks the knee
- Tibialis anterior – decelerates foot fall by eccentric contraction and pulls the tibia anterior to the body's weight line which results in knee flexion
- Quadriceps – eccentric contraction to decelerate knee flexion and absorb shock of floor contact
- Gluteus maximus – concentric action to extend hip and accelerate trunk over femur. Its action through the iliotibial band contributes to knee extension
- Adductor magnus – concentric action to advance and internally rotate pelvis on stance limb
- Gluteus medius – eccentric action to abduct hip and stabilize pelvis to minimize contralateral pelvic drop

Midstance
Muscle function. Acts to allow smooth progression over a stationary foot while controlling position of the GRF referable to hip and knee.

- Soleus – eccentric action to decelerate ankle dorsiflexion over the planted foot during the period of the second rocker

- Quadriceps – stabilizes flexed knee. Action ceases when GRF vector passes in front of knee
- Gluteus maximus – ceases action when GRF becomes posterior to hip

Terminal stance
Muscle function. Acts to provide acceleration and adequate step length.

- Soleus – intensity of action increases to limit dorsiflexion. Also acts as invertor of subtalar joint to provide stability
- Gastrocnemius – concentric action to stop forward motion of tibia and begin plantarflexion of ankle
- Tibialis posterior – stabilizes the foot against eversion forces
- Peroneals – stabilize the foot against inversion forces
- Long toe flexors – stabilizes metatarsophalangeal (MTP) joints to augment forefoot support

Pre-swing
Muscle function. Muscle control ends stance and prepares limb for swing.

- Gastrocnemius – may unlock the knee so that it may resume flexion
- Adductor longus – concentric action advances the thigh
- Rectus femoris – eccentric action at knee to decelerate the inertia of the shank. Concentric action at hip to augment hip flexion

Initial swing
Muscle function. Provides ability to vary cadence and maintain foot clearance.

- Hip flexor group (iliacus, adductor longus, sartorius, gracilis) – concentric action to advance thigh and works in conjunction with shank inertia to create knee flexion
- Biceps femoris (short head) – augments knee flexion during slow gait when inertial forces are inadequate
- Tibialis anterior – concentric action to dorsiflex foot
- Long toe extensors – concentric action with tibialis anterior to dorsiflex foot

Mid-swing
Muscle function. Little muscle action necessary because inertial forces are propelling the limb.

- Tibialis anterior – concentric action to prevent foot drop

• Use of crutches or a frame may result in overuse and fixation into flexion of the upper limbs and trunk.

The positive support reaction is invariably present. Treatment must therefore combine desensitization of the feet with appropriate re-education and facilitation of more normal standing balance and gait. Treatment will be determined by the compensatory mechanism used by the patient. It is important to realize that in many patients it is possible to completely reverse the pattern of spasticity. There is inadequate normal extensor activity in the supporting limb, and facilitation of flexion of the moving limb may produce a reciprocal inhibitory effect in the supporting limb, causing the patient to collapse.

It must be appreciated that some patients depend upon their extensor spasticity to allow them to walk. While it is important to inhibit this spasticity in order to facilitate more normal extensor activity, overinhibition may prevent the patient maintaining himself upright against gravity. There is a very fine line between a functional gait, albeit abnormal, and the wheelchair-bound patient.

The essential requirement for normal walking is a comprehensive feedback system affording balance, stability and selective movement. This can only exist on a background of normal postural tone and full range of movement of muscles and joints. Although the lower limbs provide the dynamic movement component of gait, postural stability within the trunk and contralateral arm swing are equally important.

The importance of the pelvis in providing dynamic stability throughout the gait cycle cannot be overemphasized. It provides the integration of all phases of the gait cycle, allowing for movement at the swing phase and stability during the weight-bearing stance phase, with reciprocal interchange of action. For example, flexor spasticity of the lower limbs is associated with an anterior pelvic tilt with compensatory hyperextension of the lumbar spine and overuse of the upper limbs for balance. Treatment in this instance would initially be in standing, to encourage normal extensor activity in the legs

(Brown 1994) while mobilizing the pelvis to prevent the often unnecessary degree of compensation (Edwards 1996).

Basic principles of treatment which should be observed in all cases include:

• Standing balanced with the body in correct alignment and with the weight taken throughout the entire surface of the feet.
• Standing without using the arms. If this is impossible the patient is encouraged to use his arms for balance only, rather than for weight-bearing. If the patient learns to push down with the hands in front, the weight is brought forward over the ball of the foot. This will tend to elicit the positive support reaction in those patients with spasticity and predisposes to flexor contractures of the hips.
• Pelvic control. Pelvic alignment and stability are essential to ensure dynamic control of the lower limbs. Weakness or paralysis of the hip abductors and extensors, producing instability at the pelvis, may well give rise to hyperextension of the knee. Treatment must be directed at improving control at the pelvis rather than correction of the more apparent problem at the knee (Edwards 1996).
• Weight transference in both the sagittal and coronal planes with appropriate release of the non-weight-bearing leg.
• Selective movement of the lower limb without excessive use of the trunk.

A means of enabling the patient to walk when he may otherwise have insufficient hip and/or knee control is by the therapist using a stool on wheels. The therapist sits on the stool in front of the patient with the patient's hands on her shoulder(s) (Fig. 14.9). This enables the therapist to have sufficient control at each phase of gait and to facilitate a more normal gait pattern.

The use of splints or othoses must be carefully assessed. In normal gait, foot clearance is only 0.87 cm in midswing, leaving very little room for error (Gage 1992). Weakness of the dorsiflexors or excessive tone or shortening of plantarflexors will compromise a normal gait pattern and lead to compensatory mechanisms such as a high stepping gait or 'hip hitching'. The therapist must deter-

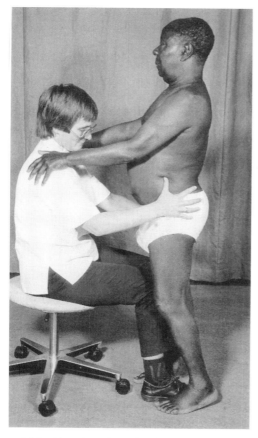

Figure 14.9 Use of stool on wheels.

mine the benefits or otherwise of AFOs, or indeed KAFOs, depending on the degree of paralysis, abnormal tone and changes in muscle length.

Functional electrical stimulation (FES) has been reported to be effective in the treatment of incomplete spinal cord injured patients (Biss & Fox 1988, Granat et al 1993, Stein et al 1993) and has been recommended as an orthotic approach in the management of patients with incomplete spinal cord injury (Bajd et al 1989). Stimulation of the common peroneal nerve stimulates the flexor withdrawal response, thereby aiding the swing-through phase of gait (Granat et al 1993). It has been suggested that FES may be of assistance in the prevention of pressure sores, contractures, muscle atrophy and bone demineralization (Bajd et al 1989).

More recent advances in gait training for these

patients include the use of a treadmill with the body weight supported (Fung et al 1990, Dobkin 1994, Dietz et al 1995, Muir & Steeves 1997). It is suggested that by supporting the body weight with treadmill training, the activation of spasticity and some of the functional consequences of disordered motor control may be reduced (Dobkin 1994). The spinal cord has the capacity not only to generate a locomotor pattern, but also to 'learn' (Dietz et al 1995). This method of enhancing lower limb movement may prove useful in guiding and strengthening functional synapses of regenerating axons to maximize their contribution towards restoring function (Muir & Steeves 1997).

Walking aids

Where possible, the aid should be used to assist balance rather than as a means of support.

Crutches, a rollator or the patient's own wheelchair are preferred to a frame, as they enable the patient to obtain a greater degree of hip and trunk extension and in consequence a more normal walking pattern. With the frame in the forward position, prior to the patient taking a step, flexion and retraction occur at the hips, thereby increasing the danger of hyperextension of the knees.

If either one or two sticks are required, they should be slightly higher than is usually prescribed (to the height of the greater trocanter). This prevents the patient using them for excessive support and initiating walking by means of trunk flexion and trunk side-flexion.

Orthoses and splints

The choice of orthosis will depend upon the degree of paralysis and the severity of spasticity. Not only the rehabilitation staff, but also the patient must be involved in this choice. Unless the patient believes that the orthosis will benefit him, and is prepared to use it, there is no value in supplying one.

There has been considerable improvement in the orthoses available, with particular emphasis on their cosmetic appearance. The lightweight, moulded orthoses are often appropriate for patients with flaccid paralysis and may also be used for some patients with spasticity (Edwards & Charlton 1996).

To assess the benefit of a below-knee orthosis, a bandage can be used to maintain the foot in dorsiflexion. Where spasticity is present, the bandage must hold the foot in eversion as well as dorsiflexion to inhibit the spastic invertors (Fig. 14.10). Not only does this allow the physio-

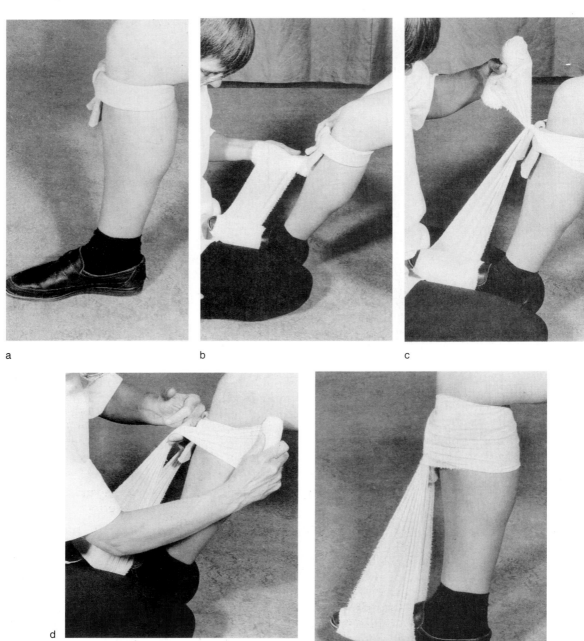

a

b

c

d

Figure 14.10 Application of bandage to hold the foot in dorsiflexion and eversion. Note the small band of foam (a) to protect the skin from the pressure of the bandage.

e

therapist to assess the patient's gait with the appropriate correction, but it also indicates if the patient is likely to develop proximal spasticity in response to the corrective device on his foot. The main disadvantage of this bandage is that it may restrict the blood flow to the lower leg and can therefore only be used for short periods of time.

Splinting materials may also be used as an adjunct to treatment and/or as a means of evaluating the effect of a more permanent orthosis. A combination of 'Soft-cast' and 'Scotch-cast' splinting materials is increasingly being used in clinical practice to support or maintain range of movement of a limb.

'Soft-cast' is impregnated with a polyurethane resin, which sets on exposure to water or the air (Schuren 1994). Once 'set', this material has a rubberized texture which provides only semi-rigid immobilization. Reinforcement with Scotch-cast enables specific control across a joint as the clinical presentation dictates. *Rubber gloves are essential when working with these materials.*

An example of the use of these materials is illustrated in Figure 14.11. Two layers of stockinette extend from the knee to the end of the toes. An additional piece of stockinette is placed between these two layers to facilitate removal of the splint (Fig. 14.11a). Microfoam padding is placed over the malleoli. A bandage of Soft-cast is applied around the lower leg, with each turn of the bandage covering half of the preceding one (Fig. 14.11b). A slab of Scotch-cast is applied extending from below the head of fibula to the end of the toes. A section is cut out around the heel to encase the ankle joint (Fig. 14.11c & d). A second Soft-cast bandage is then applied, following immersion in water, to secure the Scotch-cast slab in place. A wet crepe bandage is used to ensure lamination of the cast (Fig. 14.11e).

The speed at which the cast hardens is dependent upon whether or not the bandages and back slab are immersed in water and the temperature of the water. Using dry bandages gives more time for moulding whereas soaking in hot water produces a much quicker reaction. A combination of the first Soft-cast bandage and the Scotch-cast slab used dry, with the final Soft-cast soaked in tepid water, appears to be the ideal solution.

The Scotch-cast slab becomes rigid within approximately 10 minutes. At this point the crepe bandage and the piece of stockinette between the other two layers are removed (Fig. 14.11f). This additional piece of stockinette gives a little more room when removing the splint using *blunt-ended scissors* (Fig. 14.11g), which is of particular relevance when cutting round the ankle joint. The section over the toes is cut away and the ends of the splint are trimmed (Fig. 14.11h). Straps and buckles are then attached to enable its reapplication (Fig. 14.11i).

The main benefit of these materials is that the cast allows some flexibility while controlling unwanted movement. If the below-knee cast described above is used to counteract a positive support response, some movement is still possible into dorsiflexion but plantarflexion is prevented. In addition, the fact that the cast is removable enables continued mobilization of the muscles during physiotherapy treatment sessions as opposed to their being inaccessible as is the case in a rigid, non-removable cast.

Patients with incomplete spinal cord injury show varied problems necessitating different orthoses or casts which can range from KAFOs or back slabs to a single below-knee splint. Splints may also be required to maintain range of movement in the upper limb or to provide stability at one joint to facilitate movement at another (see the section on 'botulinum toxin').

Great care is taken with selection and the patient must be assessed at regular intervals following discharge from hospital to ensure that the orthosis remains appropriate to his needs.

Gymnastic ball

Treatment using the gymnastic ball was originally devised by Klein-Vogelbach and was adapted for use in neurological conditions by Hasler (1981).

The ball, which is made of resilient hard plastic, comes in various sizes and may be used with good effect in the treatment of some patients with incomplete spinal cord injuries (Silva & Luginbuhl 1981). The choice of size depends

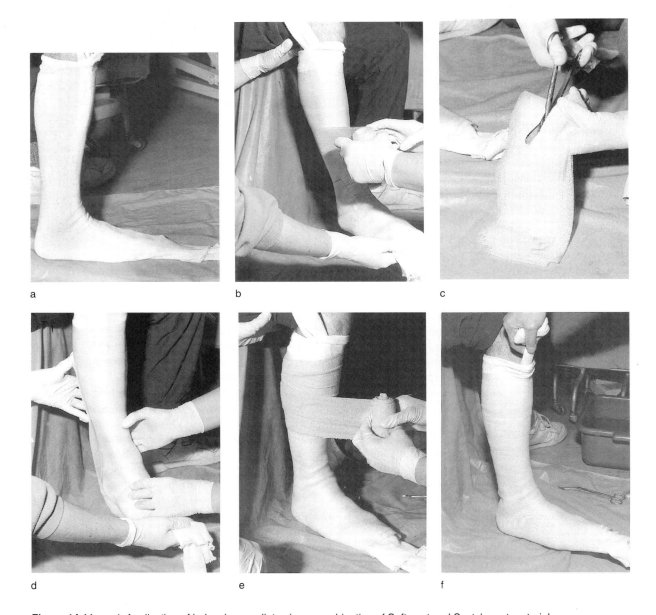

a

b

c

d

e

f

Figure 14.11   a–i: Application of below-knee splint using a combination of Soft-cast and Scotch-cast materials.

upon the reason for which the ball is being used and the physical proportions of the patient.

The ball is useful:

- as a means of inhibition and proximal mobilization where there is excessive spasticity
- in retraining balance reactions and coordination, thereby improving body awareness
- in giving controlled strengthening exercises where weakness of specific muscle groups is apparent.

It is essential that the patient is totally confident and unafraid. If the patient is frightened, not

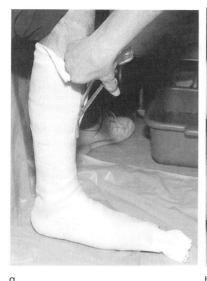
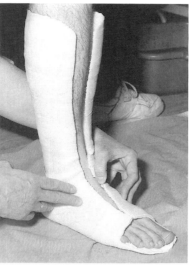
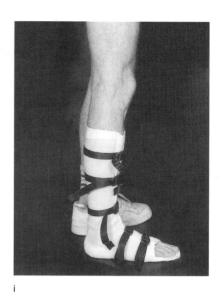

g   h   i

Figure 14.11 cont'd.   Application of below-knee splint using a combination of Soft-cast and Scotch-cast materials.

only will the treatment be ineffective, but it may cause a significant increase in spasticity and therefore prove to be detrimental (Lewis 1989).

More recent advances in the medical management of increased tone

Botulinum toxin for the management of focal spasticity and intrathecal baclofen for the treatment of more global spasticity are increasingly being used in the management of patients with neurological disability.

Botulinum toxin

Botulinum neurotoxin A (BoNT/A) is a potent neurotoxin which produces temporary muscle weakness by presynaptic inhibition of acetylcholine release at the neuromuscular junction (Anderson et al 1992). This weakness does not occur immediately but usually takes between 10 and 14 days, depending on the size of the muscle injected and the dosage. Recovery occurs over a period of approximately 10 to 12 weeks through terminal sprouting.

BoNT/A is widely accepted as an effective treatment for focal dystonias and it is licensed for use in the treatment of blepharospasm, hemifacial spasm and cervical dystonia. Although several papers advocate the use of BoNT/A in the treatment of spasticity, its usefulness is by no means clearly defined (Das & Park 1989, Snow et al 1990).

Where specific, localized muscles are considered to be a major influence in the production and maintenance of the spastic response, BoNT/A may be a useful adjunct to rehabilitation. The main reasons for its use in the treatment of spasticity are to:

• redress problems created by muscle imbalance
• enable improved hygiene
• evaluate the effects of surgery (this is primarily for children with cerebral palsy) (Cosgrove et al 1984).

The purpose of intervention with BoNT/A is to weaken the dominant spastic muscle or muscles to enable clearly identified treatment goals to be accomplished. For example, patients with a positive support reaction are unable to transfer their weight over the full surface of the foot during stance phase of gait due to spasticity of the posterior crural muscle group. The compensatory strategies which may be adopted by the patient in response to this reaction are described above (p. 180). Treatment of the spastic muscles with BoNT/A weakens the calf muscles enabling an improved gait pattern for the duration of the toxin's effect. It is hypothesized that during this period, the improved gait pattern will become established as a more normal motor programme, thereby enabling carryover in the longer term (Scrutton et al 1996). However, the adverse effects that this weakness may have on gait have been discussed (p. 186) and the toxin should be used with caution.

Patients with incomplete spinal cord lesions may also have muscle imbalance which is due to dominant muscle activity precluding recovery of the weaker antagonists. BoNT/A has been used successfully in the treatment of a patient with an incomplete C6 lesion. Recovery of the finger extensors was impeded by the dominance of finger and thumb flexion and reliance on a teno-dysis grip. BoNT/A was administered to flexor digitorum superficialis, flexor pollicis brevis and adductor pollicis. A removable cast was applied, 3 weeks post-injection, to control the position of the wrist in a neutral position. This prevented use of the tenodysis grip. With this splint, the patient was able to use his finger extensors selectively.

The use of BoNT/A in the treatment of spasticity differs to that in the treatment of focal dystonia. Patients with focal dystonia usually attend at 3-monthly intervals for reinjection. For patients with spasticity, the treatment may be only a single event which should always be used in conjunction with physiotherapy. Splinting is often of value to supplement the effects of the toxin. If splinting is to be incorporated as part of the therapy programme, application of the cast should be delayed until the effects of the toxin are apparent, approximately 3 weeks after injection.

It is essential to determine that the cause of the movement impairment is due to spasticity and not to mechanical changes of muscle and soft tissue. BoNT/A weakens muscle and it is therefore of no use whatsoever for patients who no longer demonstrate increased muscle activity, characteristic of spasticity. Assessment with electromyography (EMG) is therefore essential. It is possible to identify the more superficial muscles with surface EMG electrodes, but the more deeply sited muscles require needle EMG to ensure accurate administration of the toxin.

The essential criteria for effective use of what is an expensive treatment are:

- a clearly defined functional goal
- the use of EMG to confirm increased muscle activity as the cause of the movement disorder
- an ongoing physiotherapy programme to re-educate movement for the duration of the toxin's effect.

BoNT/A is suitable only for more focal spasticity, as the dose that can be administered is limited. Patients with more widespread, lower limb spasticity may be more effectively managed with intrathecal baclofen.

Intrathecal baclofen

Baclofen is a gamma-aminobutyric acid (GABA) receptor agonist. GABA is the major inhibitory neurotransmitter of the central nervous system. Baclofen binds to GABA receptors and has a presynaptic effect on the release of excitatory neurotransmitters. It also acts postsynaptically, directly decreasing the firing of motor units (Losseff & Thompson 1995).

Oral baclofen does not readily cross the blood–brain barrier but is equally distributed to the brain and spinal cord. This may lead to centrally mediated effects such as drowsiness, dizziness and confusion without adequate relief of spasticity. Intrathecal administration permits direct access of the drug to the receptor sites in the dorsal horn of the spinal cord, thereby minimizing these central effects (Porter 1997). Doses of less than one-hundredth of those required orally have been shown to be effective in the management of spasticity (Gianino 1993).

Indications for usage. Uncontrolled spasticity may be so severe as to cause pain, interrupt sleep and interfere with function. Although more widely used in the treatment of patients with complete spinal lesions and multiple sclerosis with severe flexor spasticity, intrathecal baclofen is also effective in regulating spasticity in patients with incomplete cord lesions. Severe spasticity may mask underlying active movement and reduction of this hypertonus may enable the patient to utilize this potential function.

In spite of the potential side-effects of oral baclofen, this would always be the method of choice. It is only those patients who are refractory to oral administration, or who have intolerable side-effects, who may be considered suitable for intrathecal baclofen.

The patient must be free of noxious stimuli such as pressure sores, infection or constipation as these may prevent an accurate assessment of the patient (Porter 1997).

Delivery system. The delivery system consists of a pump with a reservoir of baclofen which is connected to the intrathecal space by means of a catheter, the tip of which is sited at the level of the L1 lamina (Penn 1988; cited in Porter 1997). The pump lies subcutaneously in the abdomen. There are two types of pump, one a mechanical device and the other computer-programmable. Although the latter is more expensive, it is more flexible, delivering bolus or continuous infusion at a predetermined rate (Losseff & Thompson 1995). The pump needs to be refilled every 4–12 weeks and the dose adjusted as required (Gianino 1993).

The patient's response to intrathecal administration of baclofen is assessed by means of a temporary intrathecal catheter before proceeding to permanent infusion (Porter 1997). Potential complications of intrathecal baclofen are overdose, which may lead to respiratory arrest, and infection (Losseff & Thompson 1995). Although these complications are very rare, this procedure should be carried out in a specialist centre where there are standardized protocols and patients are regularly monitored.

If the patient has a favourable response to the test dose and is conversant with the implications of long-term intrathecal therapy, he may proceed to surgical implantation. The surgical procedure lasts approximately 2 hours and is performed under general anaesthetic. The exact placement of the pump is discussed with the patient prior to surgery and a subcutaneous pouch is made in the abdomen and the pump placed within it. The catheter is tunnelled from the pump to the lumbar subarachnoid space. The pump reservoir is then filled with baclofen and programmed to deliver the drug at the prescribed rate (Porter 1997).

Depending on the severity and possible functional use of the spasticity, the dose may be a simple continuous cycle or less during the day to enable function and more at night to allow sleep (Gianino 1993).

Intrathecal baclofen may be contraindicated in patients who depend on their spasticity for function. For example, patients who are ambulant, albeit with a grossly spastic gait, may no longer be able to walk following this intervention. The majority of patients in this situation will opt to keep mobile for as long as possible unless the purpose of the intervention is management of pain.

SUMMARY

Patients with incomplete spinal cord lesions demonstrate many different and diverse movement disorders necessitating thorough assessment and individualized treatment programmes. The prognosis is less predictable than for patients with complete lesions and the therapeutic management must reflect the variability of the presenting signs and symptoms.

The analysis of normal movement presented in this chapter provides a basis for a problem-solving approach to treatment. Improved understanding and awareness of movement enable the therapist to identify how a posture or movement differs from the normal and thereby to select appropriate treatment strategies.

For those patients with non-progressive pathology, throughout all stages of rehabilitation, treatment is aimed at improving functional abilities without the use of unnecessary compensation. Patients with progressive pathology, e.g. those with carcinoma, may benefit from the use of early compensation to allow them to return home as soon as possible to give them the maximum time in their familiar environment.

Normal movement is the ultimate goal of rehabilitation, but all too often this is not achievable for patients with extensive neurological damage. There must be a balance between re-education of more normal movement patterns and acceptance, and indeed promotion, of necessary and desirable compensation (Edwards 1996). As previously stated, the therapeutic skill lies in determining that compensation which is necessary, and even essential, for function and that which is unnecessary and potentially detrimental to the patient.

15

Spinal cord injury in children

Ebba Bergström

The incidence of spinal cord injury in children under 13 years is much smaller than in teenagers and adults.

The cause of accidents is similar to the adult population and is always reflective of the surrounding society. In the industrialized world, road traffic accidents are the most common cause of injury (including a larger proportion of pedestrian injuries among children), followed by falls from heights, sporting injuries and assault. In some urban areas, gunshot wounds are reported to equal the number of road accidents (Haffner & Hoffer 1993).

Due to the anatomical characteristics of the immature spine, children are vulnerable to certain traumas. They have a higher frequency of upper cervical cord injuries than teenagers and adults as well as spinal cord injury without radiological abnormalities (SCIWORA) (Osenbach & Menezes 1989, Pang & Pollack 1989), although there may be severe spinal cord damage. It has been suggested that, through its elasticity and cartilaginous properties, the spine of a young child can withstand gross distortion, especially in flexion and rotation, without fracturing bones. The spinal cord cannot stand the same degree of stretch; consequently, traction results in cord damage.

An approximately equal number of spinal cord lesions in children result from non-traumatic causes such as transverse myelitis, vascular accidents and cysts.

The aim of rehabilitation is the same for the child with spinal cord injury as for the adult, namely to:

- maximize potential in order to reach as high a degree of independence as possible
- teach the child and its carer how to prevent complications.

A child's potential depends on age and size as well as on the distribution of the neurological damage. The child's normal intellectual development will have an influence on the timing and progression of rehabilitation. Some skills may have to be postponed until the child is mature enough to tackle them. For example, it is inappropriate to teach a 2-year-old to dress or a 5-year-old to catheterize himself. The size of the child may also mean that some transfer techniques need to be modified.

Continuing growth predisposes the child to many problems, particularly spinal deformity (Lancourt et al 1981, Mayfield et al 1981) and contractures.

All these factors necessitate that rehabilitation is an ongoing process, undertaken at least once a year until the child reaches maturity.

During the acute phase, physiotherapy for the child is the same as for the adult patient. Some modification to therapy is required in certain aspects of rehabilitation, but the major difference in the treatment of children at the National Spinal Injuries Centre (NSIC), Stoke Mandeville Hospital is in the approach to the management and monitoring of the development of the spine through weight-bearing and correct alignment in standing, sitting or lying.

SPINAL DEFORMITY

The prevention of spinal deformity and contractures must be addressed from the beginning of rehabilitation. In order to prevent or minimize these problems, normal growth and development of the skeleton needs to be promoted.

Normal bone growth is influenced by weight-bearing as well as the forces of compression and traction produced in walking and running. For the paralysed child, it is important therefore to stand and walk with the aid of orthoses as

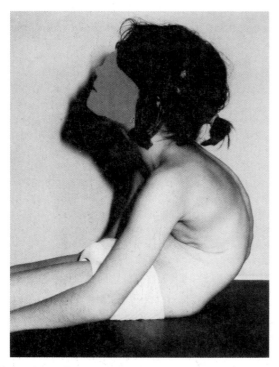

Figure 15.1 Forward flexion. Patient aged 9 years (injured at 2 years) with a complete lesion below T5.

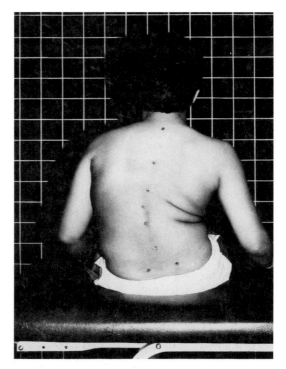

Figure 15.2 Side flexion. Patient aged 11 years (injured at 5 years) with a complete lesion below T6.

frequently and for as long as possible, in order to stimulate normal use of the joints. Similarly the musculoskeletal apparatus will conform to the stresses exerted upon it and, because of continuing growth, the soft tissues will lengthen under constant stretch as well as shorten due to disuse. If full range of movement of joints and muscles is not regularly maintained, contractures will develop. If the skeleton is constantly subjected to abnormal forces during growth, it will gradually shape accordingly and give rise to skeletal abnormalities and spinal deformity. Such forces include:

- gravitational pull when tone is low or absent, causing a collapse of the spine
- unilateral muscle pull, through asymmetrical paralysis or spasticity, habitual asymmetrical posture, sometimes adopted for safety, and contractures.

Deformities of the spinal column commonly seen in children with paraplegia and tetraplegia include:

Collapsing spine

The spine may collapse into forward flexion giving rise to a long 'C' curve which results in weight-bearing on the sacrum and total obliteration of the lumbar lordosis (Fig. 15.1). In most cases, this posture will be followed by external rotation of the femur and, in time, extension contracture of the hip which makes correction of the posture difficult.

The spine may also collapse into side flexion with rotation of the vertebral bodies causing a long C-shaped scoliosis with an oblique pelvis or a lumbar scoliosis with a compensatory curve above it (Fig. 15.2). The collapsing spine is readily correctable with traction (Figs 15.3 and 15.4) but in time develops severe structural change.

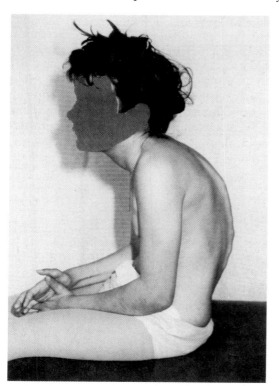

Figure 15.3 Correction of spinal deformity with traction. Patient aged 10 years (injured at 4 years) with a complete lesion below C7.

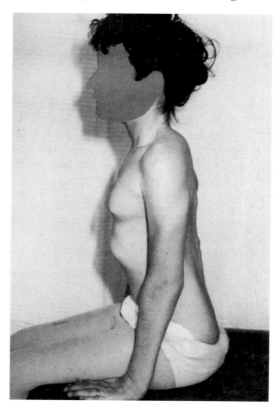

Figure 15.4 As Figure 15.3.

Reversal of the lumbar lordosis and thoracic kyphosis

Flattening of the lumbar lordosis, usually caused by poor sitting posture or extensor spasticity, will lead to compensatory extension of the spine higher up and flattening of the thoracic kyphosis (Fig. 15.5). In severe cases, these curves can be reversed. Flattening of the thoracic kyphosis causes rotation of the vertebral bodies, giving rise to scoliosis.

Hyperlordosis of the lumbar spine

This may be caused by active hip flexor muscles pulling the pelvis forward, or it can be secondary to an accentuated thoracic kyphosis due to a displaced fracture (Fig. 15.6) as well as postural collapse. With few exceptions, this will lead to hip flexion contractures which, if allowed to develop, will make it difficult to stand and to fit the orthosis.

Scoliosis

Unilateral muscle pull due to asymmetrical neurological deficit or spasticity often gives rise to side flexion contractures. It can also mean that the patient has to position himself asymmetrically in order to balance during two-handed activity, which will exacerbate the contracture.

Secondary deformity of the ribcage

All scolioses will give rise to rotation of the spinal column. The rotation will cause a posterior rib hump on the convex side of the scoliosis (see Fig. 15.3). The ribs on the convex side will be more horizontal than normal, whilst those on the concave side will be more vertical (Fig. 15.7).

Any spinal deformity will add to the problems of paraplegia and tetraplegia. It will diminish the chest cavity and further compromise lung function. Uneven pressure will heighten the risk of pressure sores. Poor posture will influence balance and general function. All spinal deformities will alter the position of the neck and may in the future cause musculoskeletal changes and give rise to pain and impaired movement of the neck, shoulders and arms.

Common deformities of other joints also influence the spinal column.

Hip joint

For the acetabulum and the head of the femur to form a stable joint with well-rounded surfaces, the hip joint has to be held and loaded in normal alignment.

Internal rotation and adduction of the femur, whether by the femur on the pelvis or through pelvic obliquity and rotation on the femur, will give little or no surface contact in the joint. Poor development of the joint (Fig. 15.8) and a predisposition to subluxation or dislocation will follow.

Due to contracture of the hip flexor and/or abductor muscles, full extension of the hip joint may only be seen when the leg lies in abduction – it cannot be obtained with the limb in midline. When passive movements are performed, correct alignment of the limb must always be maintained.

Knee joint

Valgus deformity of the knee joint (Fig. 15.9) is caused by either internal rotation of the femur or collapse of the longitudinal arch of the foot when standing, or a combination of the two (Fig. 15.10a). The consequent contracture of the biceps femoris muscle and incorrect alignment of the hip, knee and foot only allow extension of the knee when the hip falls into internal rotation and the knee into the valgus position. The valgus deformity should not be compensated for in the fitting of the orthosis as this will exacerbate the problem.

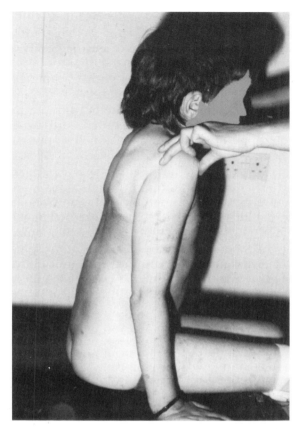

Figure 15.5   Flattening of lumbar lordosos. Patient aged 11 years (injured at 8 years) with a complete lesion below C8.

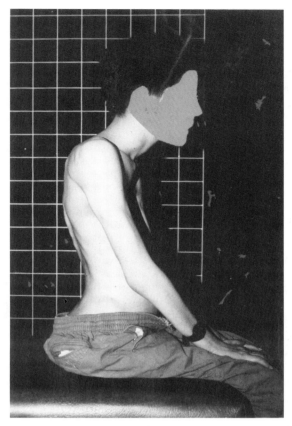

Figure 15.6   Hyperlordosis of the lumbar spine. Patient aged 18 years (injured at 8 years) with a complete lesion below C7.

The caliper should be made as straight as possible (seen in the sagittal plane), allowing the knee to remain in the degree of flexion necessary for the limb to be in correct alignment.

The action of the knee brace should be augmented by passive stretching of the knee into extension, maintaining the limb in midline. Weight-bearing with the knee in the valgus position will result in an altered angle between the tibial condyles and the shaft of the tibia. This may cause torsion of the tibia, pulling the foot into external rotation. This deformity should not be corrected by positioning the foot in neutral as it will increase the valgus deformity of the knee and cause further internal rotation of the hip joint. The foot should be allowed to remain in

external rotation in the caliper. However, the degree of rotation of the tibia varies in normal children so that sometimes the foot is naturally externally rotated. In this case also, where no other deformity is present, the design of the caliper should allow the foot to remain in its natural position.

Foot

Collapse of the medial arch will cause eversion of the foot, and if the foot is allowed to remain in this position, the tendo Achilles will shorten on the lateral side. When passively stretching the tendo Achilles, first the heel must be pulled towards midline and only then should the foot

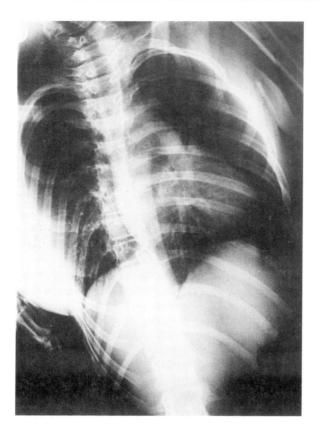

be dorsiflexed. Footwear must be fitted with a medial longitudinal arch support (Fig. 15.10b) and this should reduce the valgus deformity at the knee.

The opinion of clinicians with considerable experience in treating these children is that spinal deformity and contractures are to some degree inevitable consequences of spinal cord injury and, once established, are impossible to reverse. The risk of deformity and its severity are closely related to the age at onset of paralysis (Burke 1974).

A study was undertaken at the National Spinal Injuries Centre (NSIC), Stoke Mandeville Hospital (Bergström 1994) to assess the impact of childhood spinal cord injury (SCI) on spinal deformity and growth in the now adult individual. The 80 subjects taking part in the study came from 189 patients who had an acute onset

Figure 15.7 Postero-anterior X-ray of rib cage. The ribs on the convex side are more horizontal than normal, while those on the concave side are more vertical. The left lung volume is decreased.

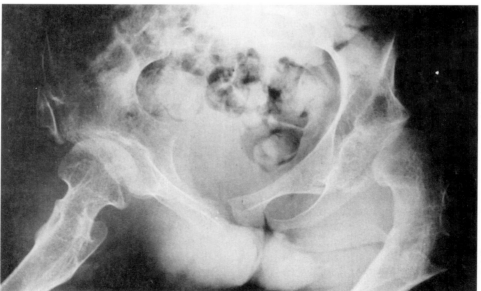

Figure 15.8 Antero-posterior X-ray of pelvis. The left acetabulum is relatively flat and the head of the left femur is grossly abnormal. (The apparent pelvic deformity is mainly projectional).

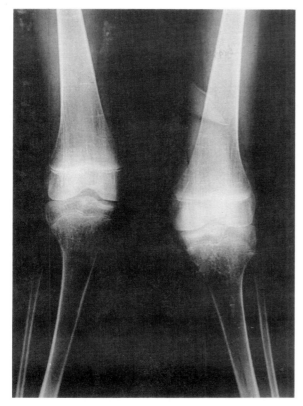

Figure 15.9 Valgus deformity of knee joints.

SCI before their 16th birthday and were treated at the NSIC from within 1 year of onset.

Seventy-six of the subjects had radiographs of their whole thoracic and lumbar spine taken in their habitual upright position (56 seated and 20 standing) in a standardized manner. The statistical analysis was primarily based on two-way subdivisions of the subjects (due to the small sample) as follows:

- level of lesion – tetraplegic/paraplegic
- severity of lesion – complete/incomplete lesion
- age at injury – <11 years, >11 years.

Scoliosis, lordosis and kyphosis were measured from the radiographs according to Cobb (1948). For the purpose of cross-tabulation, these three parameters were divided into three groups:

- scoliosis – mild (<20°), moderate (20–59°), severe (>59°)
- lordosis – hypolordosis (<35°), normal (35–64°), hyperlordosis (>64°)
- kyphosis – hypokyphosis (<25°), normal (25°–49°), hyperkyphosis (>49°).

Of the 76 subjects analyzed, 78% had a scoliosis of more than 10° and 53% had one of moderate to severe magnitude; 42% had a hyperlordosis and 41% a lordosis that was too flat; 45% were hyperkyphotic, while 14% had a thoracic spine that was too flat. Only one subject had a 'normal' spine.

Both level and severity of paralysis as well as age at onset have a strong influence on the magnitude of the scoliosis as illustrated in Table 15.1.

The level of lesion, expressed simply as tetraplegia and paraplegia, has a clear inverse relationship with the degree of scoliosis. The paraplegics have a greater scoliosis than the tetraplegics and also appear in proportionally larger numbers in the increasingly more severe scoliosis group.

The severity of lesion, when only divided two ways into complete and incomplete lesions, shows a positive relationship with the magnitude of scoliosis. The complete lesions have more severe scoliosis than the incomplete lesions. The proportion of complete lesions also increases as the magnitude of the scoliosis increases.

Age at onset is closely related to the occurrence and magnitude of scoliosis. The very young at onset have a more severe scoliosis and are proportionally more numerous in the increasingly more severe scoliosis group.

When analysing the lordosis angle separately for the seated and standing subjects, those seated show a significantly greater lordosis in the paraplegic subsection than in the tetraplegic (50° and 28°, respectively) and also among those with severe (15°) hip flexion contracture compared with those with no or mild (<15°) hip flexion contracture (56° and 27°, respectively) (Table 15.2).

Among the 20 standing subjects, there was a significant difference of lordosis angle when subdivided according to level of lesion only. The lordosis was significantly larger in this group

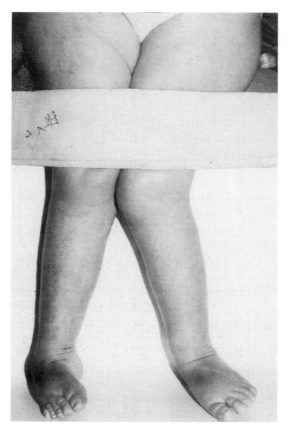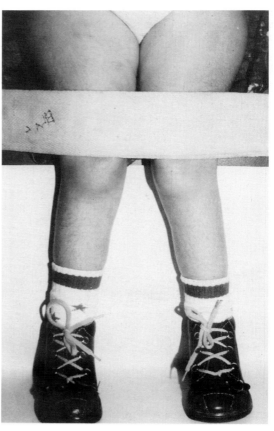

a   b

Figure 15.10   a: Valgus deformity of the left knee with collapse of the medial longitudinal arch of the foot. Patient aged 5 years (injured at 1 year) with a complete lesion below T12/L1. b: Medial longitudinal arch supported.

(mean 71°). The majority (15) had hyperlordosis, and 13 of those had no or mild contracture of the hips (Table 15.3).

These subjects illustrate the connection between hyperlordosis and hip flexion contractures when constantly seated. However, this is not the case for those who predominantly walk.

Measurements of body segments were carried out in accordance with Weiner & Laurie (1969).

In order to eliminate the effect of spinal deformity and contractures on the growth measurements, the humerus and the tibia were compared and analyzed in isolation. The humerus was chosen as the single bone least likely to be affected by the paralysis and the tibia as the bone

most likely to be affected. Table 15.4 shows the mean tibial length to be longer than the mean humeral length among both female and male subjects. In the female subjects, the mean tibial length is shorter in those injured before age 11. The male subjects show a shorter tibia in the paraplegic, incomplete and 'injured before 11 years' groups than their respective counterparts.

In order to examine the effect of a lower motor neurone injury on growth, the humeral/tibial relationship was re-examined in the same manner, separately for those nine subjects with neurological damage at L1 and below (see Table 15.5). The lower motor neurone lesion is thought to have greater retarding influence on growth

Table 15.1   The distribution of scoliosis (Cobb angle) by level of injury, severity of injury, age at onset, duration of injury and range of hip movement in 76 childhood SCI subjects

	Level of injury		Severity of injury		Onset age (years)		Duration (years)		Flexion contracture	
	Tet	Par	Comp	Incomp	<11	>11	<20	>20	<15°	≥15°
Number	26	50	42	34	17	59	38	38	42	32
Mean Cobb angle	17°	33°	36°	18°	38°	24°	22°	33°	21°	37°
Level of significance	**		***		*				**	
Scoliosis										
0–19°	18	18	12	24	4	32	20	16	25	9
20–59°	8	23	23	8	8	23	16	15	15	16
≥60°	0	9	7	2	5	4	2	7	2	7
Level of significance	**		**		*				*	
Missing cases									2	

Tet = tetraplegia; Par = paraplegia; Comp = complete lesion; Incomp = incomplete lesion.
*, $P < 0.05$; **, $P < 0.01$; ***, $P < 0.001$.

Table 15.2   The distribution of lordosis angle in 56 seated childhood SCI subjects by level of injury, severity of injury, age at onset, duration of injury and range of hip movement

	Level of injury		Severity of injury		Onset age (years)		Duration (years)		Flexion contracture	
	Tet	Par	Comp	Incomp	<11	>11	<20	>20	<15°	≥15°
Number	17	39	42	14	14	42	27	29	25	30
Mean lordosis angle	28°	50°	40°	51°	51°	41°	38°	48°	27°	56°
Level of significance	*								**	
Lordosis										
0–34°	12	18	24	6	6	24	15	15	20	10
35–64°	3	6	7	2	2	7	5	4	3	6
≥65°	2	15	11	6	6	11	7	10	2	14
Level of significance									**	
Missing cases									1	

Tet = tetraplegia; Par = paraplegia; Comp = complete lesion; Incomp = incomplete lesion.
*, $P < 0.05$; **, $P < 0.01$; ***, $P < 0.001$.

Table 15.3   The distribution of lordosis angle in 20 standing childhood SCI subjects by level of injury, severity of injury, age at onset, duration of injury and range of hip movement

	Level of injury		Severity of injury		Onset age (years)		Duration (years)		Flexion contracture	
	Tet	Par	Comp	Incomp	<11	>11	<20	>20	<15°	≥15°
Number	9	11	–	20	3	17	11	9	17	2
Mean lordosis angle	62°	78°	–	71°	69°	71°	66°	78°	71°	71°
Level of significance	*									
Lordosis										
0–34°	1	0	–	1	0	1	1	0	1	0
35–64°	2	2	–	4	2	2	3	1	3	1
≥65°	6	9	–	15	1	14	7	8	13	1
Level of significance										
Missing cases									1	

Tet = tetraplegia; Par = paraplegia; Comp = complete lesion; Incomp = incomplete lesion.
*, $P < 0.05$; **, $P < 0.01$; ***, $P < 0.001$.

Table 15.4   Mean humeral length and tibial length for female and male subjects by level and severity of lesion and age at onset

	Female			Male		
	Humerus (mm)	Tibia (mm)	n	Humerus (mm)	Tibia (mm)	n
All	338	350	34	363	366	41
Level of injury						
Tetraplegic	347	369	12	358	379	14
Paraplegic	333	340	22	366	359	27
Severity of injury						
Complete	340	345	17	363	359	25
Incomplete	336	355	17	364	376	16
Onset age						
<11 years	334	354	6	370	357	13
>11 years	339	354	28	360	370	28

Table 15.5   Mean humeral length and tibial length for female and male subjects with neurological damage at and below L1 by severity of lesion and age at onset

	Female			Male		
	Humerus (mm)	Tibia (mm)	n	Humerus (mm)	Tibia (mm)	n
All	333	345	9	338	342	3
Severity of injury						
Complete	342	335	4	360	351	1
Incomplete	327	351	5	327	338	2
Onset age						
<11 years	326	305	1	360	351	1
>11 years	334	349	8	327	338	2

than upper motor neurone lesions, as the upper motor neurone lesion has an intact neural arc. This allows involuntary motor function below the lesion level which ensures better circulation and some muscular stresses on the bones. Both are important factors in stimulating growth. The relationship between the two bones now shows a similar picture for the females and the males. The mean length of the tibia is longer for both sexes, but when subdivided as previously, the complete lesions and those injured before the age of 11 have a shorter mean tibial length than mean humeral length.

These results indicate that SCI does affect the growth of a child, but the many factors potentially influencing growth are confounding one another in this small sample.

TREATMENT

From the beginning, treatment for children with spinal cord injury is aimed at halting, or at least slowing down, the development of the deformity. For maximum effect, this means holding the spine in correct alignment and starting whilst correct alignment is obtainable. Once the spine has started to deform, it may be impossible or extremely difficult to make a cast for a corset in the correct position.

Contractures of the hips and / or asymmetry of the pelvis are deemed to be the main precipitating factors in the malalignment of the spinal column. Therefore, it is of the utmost importance that the hips and pelvis are kept in their anatomical position, avoiding the sitting position

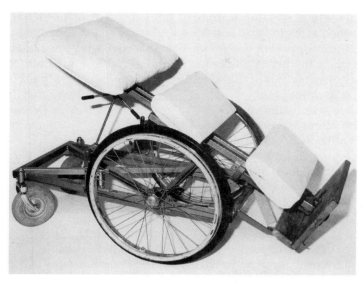

Figure 15.11 Prone trolley.

which encourages poor alignment and resulting deformity. For these reasons, the child is mobilized from bedrest immediately to the upright position by means of an inclined prone trolley (Fig. 15.11). A temporary plasterzote jacket is provided to protect the spine from collapsing. In addition, the child with a cervical injury may wear a collar as prescribed for the adult. The child stands in a semi-inclined position, 30° from the horizontal, and is up for approximately 30 minutes initially, providing there are no orthostatic problems. In this way, the sitting posture is avoided as much as possible, the child gets used to standing as part of a normal day, and its importance is emphasized to him and his parents.

The child will continue to use the prone trolley until the orthosis is completed or temporary back slabs are made to splint the legs. These will be used in conjunction with a suitable standing frame or chariot. Standing and walking will be pursued for as long as possible during the day. It is advisable to allow the child to sit for only 1 hour at a time, although it is recognized that this is a goal that is difficult to achieve and probably will become more so as the child grows and educational and social pressures increase.

Orthoses

As soon as the child can stay up long enough, a cast is made for a body jacket. In order that the child feels well during this procedure, any orthostatic blood pressure problems should have been overcome. He should also be familiar with the people and the procedure so that he can cooperate with maintaining a good position in correct alignment (with a lumbar lordosis) for at least 20 minutes. Knee–ankle–foot orthoses (KAFOs) are made for all children, regardless of the level of the lesion. Children with a very low or incomplete lesion, with no neurological deficit of the trunk, may not need a brace. In these cases also, the development of the spine will need to be closely monitored. The brace will be worn at all times when the child is up (except for swimming and specific exercises) but not in bed. Block leather is used in preference to plastic materials as it is a natural material and, although very firm, is not totally unyielding. It offers more comfort and better protection against pressure points than the lighter and more easily worked modern materials.

The brace should be as near to normal in alignment as possible, with special care taken of the lordosis so that the child remains upright with minimal force applied at the top and bottom of the brace. For maximum support of the spinal column and stabilization of the pelvis, the brace needs to be as long as possible whilst allowing for shoulder depression in order to lift.

The KAFOs are made with extensions above and below the knee to allow for growth. Knee joints will be included as soon as practical, i.e. as soon as the child's leg is long enough to allow the joints to be incorporated in the length of the orthosis. For stability of the knee in the median plane and for some control of rotation of the leg (either from the hip or from the foot), a wrap-around knee extension strap is used (see p. 131). This can be reversed to offer a different directional pull on the leg. In most cases, the KAFOs will be attachable to the brace to achieve stability of the hips and make walking easier (Fig. 15.12). If the brace is to be worn on its own, the hip joints

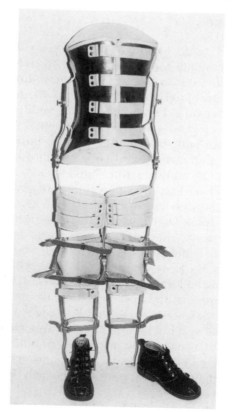

Figure 15.12 Hip–knee–ankle–foot orthosis.

must be part of the KAFOs and not the brace. Alternatively a separate brace for sitting only is provided. Footwear should provide a stable support and include the ankle and an extensive opening to provide easy access to check size and the position of the toes. T-straps may be added to give extra support to the ankle joint in the sagittal plane.

Gait

Plaster of Paris back slabs may be used initially to achieve the upright position while waiting for the completion of the orthosis.

Gait training with crutches or rollator is commenced at the age when the able-bodied child would start to walk, i.e. 12–18 months old. Where possible, all three gaits are taught. When the child is wearing the hip–knee–ankle–foot orthosis (HKAFO), it is only possible to teach swing-to and swing-through gaits (see Ch. 12). He will need to use slightly longer crutches since he cannot flex the trunk when lifting, due to the restriction of the brace. A rollator is preferred to crutches, especially in crowded environments such as school. However, this is a slower method of walking than with crutches, especially when the child is bigger. His height prevents the young child from getting out of the chair onto his crutches using the forwards technique. The child can usually lift himself onto his feet by lifting on both armrests, or using the sideways method.

Other equipment

Although the first choice is to use the HKAFO, as this provides maximal support in the correct position, the practicality of using it all day in school and at home presents problems, and compromise may be necessary.

To enable the child to ambulate throughout the day, it may be necessary to use a swivel walker, chariot or standing frame. The swivel walker (Fig. 15.13) allows the child mobility without using his hands for support, thus freeing them for other activities, and it can be used by a child with a very high lesion. Donning and doffing is easier than with the orthosis, which is appreciated by busy school staff. However, it does not

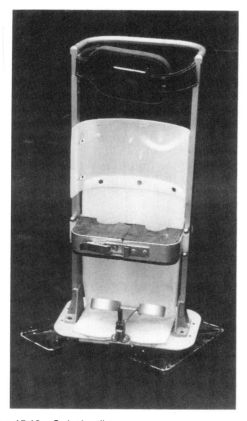

Figure 15.13 Swivel walker.

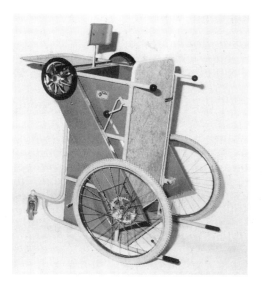

Figure 15.14 Chariot.

provide such a good support for the limbs and walking is slow. The chariot (Fig. 15.14) is a self-propelling device that the child stands in wearing his orthosis. This offers independent mobility for the child with a higher lesion and freedom to use the hands when stationary.

Elbow crutches offer a faster gait with more independence, e.g. climbing stairs, but a walking frame may be needed for safety for most small children, especially at school and in other crowded areas where the risk of being inadvertently knocked over is high.

INVOLVEMENT OF THE SCHOOL

The education of the physically disabled child is of paramount importance. He must be enabled to make the best use of his intellectual resources since so many manual occupations will be inaccessible for him. The Education Act (1981) has introduced in Britain the principles of the integration of children with special educational needs with able-bodied children and the development of facilities to meet the special needs of disabled children. It is desirable that, after spinal cord injury, children should return to mainstream schools and playgroups when their initial period of rehabilitation is concluded. They will then integrate at an early age with able-bodied children and will also have the same chance to achieve the necessary qualifications for higher education. It is encouraging that more schools are welcoming the child back to school after becoming disabled, and are making the necessary alterations to school buildings.

As a large part of the child's day is spent at school, it will be necessary for the school to be involved in the special routines incorporated in the child's care. Special provision for standing may be necessary, such as a standing frame or a high table in the classroom. The child may have to don and doff the orthosis for toileting or rest, and the skills needed have to be passed to the appropriate person(s) at the school. Access to the school will have to be considered as for the home or the workplace for an adult, and any necessary adaptations undertaken.

Wheelchair

The chair should offer the child a good posture and mobility with minimum energy expenditure. Since children do not look like scaled down adults, it is not sufficient to have a scaled down adult chair. A child's wheelchair should be adjustable to allow for growth.

Seat height from the floor needs to be considered. Small children mainly play on the floor and have their environment, such as school and infant school, furnished to their size. In this environment the paralysed child needs a chair that will bring him into contact with his peer group. The adult carer needs push handles that are extended above and behind the backrest, in order not to impede the child's mobility. To give the maximum ergonomic advantage for the carer, the push handles need to be angled away from the backrest. Various sizes of wheels, castors and forks for the castors are available. These allow the seat to be raised to accommodate the growing child. The backrest can be adjusted in height and, on some models, the seat and back canvasses are provided in several sizes.

MODIFICATIONS NECESSARY TO ADULT REHABILITATION PROGRAMME

Postural sensibility

Children aged 3 years and over are given short periods of training, sitting on the plinth in front of the mirror in the usual way. This is augmented for small children by play therapy on the mat. Games and activities involving the use of first one and then both hands are encouraged whilst the unassisted sitting position is maintained. Children under 3 years are usually treated daily on the mat only, but where possible a mirror is used to give the child the necessary visual feedback.

Mat work

The ability of the young child to sit up from lying down is very important, as it releases the mother from going to the child early in the morning to sit him up in his cot to play. Where this activity has not been taught, the mother may continue to lift the child even when he is 5, 6 or 7 years of age.

To sit up from lying down on the mat:

1. Turn the upper trunk and left arm to the right (Fig. 15.15a).
2. Push up onto both elbows (Fig. 15.15b).
3. 'Walk' on the hands to the sitting position (Fig. 15.15c & d).

The child is also taught to turn over, to roll into the prone position and to move himself and his legs around on the mat.

Muscle strength

In order to prevent spinal deformity, particularly if the child is wearing a brace, it is important to hypertrophy the back muscles and latissimus dorsi and to continue these exercises throughout growth.

Dressing and self-care

The child with spinal cord injury is taught to dress and wash at the same age as the able-bodied child. He is also taught as early as possible to look at his own legs for pressure marks, to put pillows between the legs when turning in bed, and to lift and move with care.

Transfers

Some of the techniques of transferring may have to be altered due to the size of the child. The brace will also influence the transfer technique. For example, it gives stability to a collapsing spine and in this case becomes a helpful aid. It is important that the transfers are taught wearing the brace since different postures will alter the biomechanical relationships of the body and thereby necessitate a different technique. (It can be difficult to motivate a child to learn the same task twice, with and without the brace.)

It is easier and safer for the young child to get onto the bed forwards (see Ch. 9).

When transferring onto the toilet, the child will need to keep his feet on the footplates or have them propped on a solid stool of suitable height until the feet reach the floor.

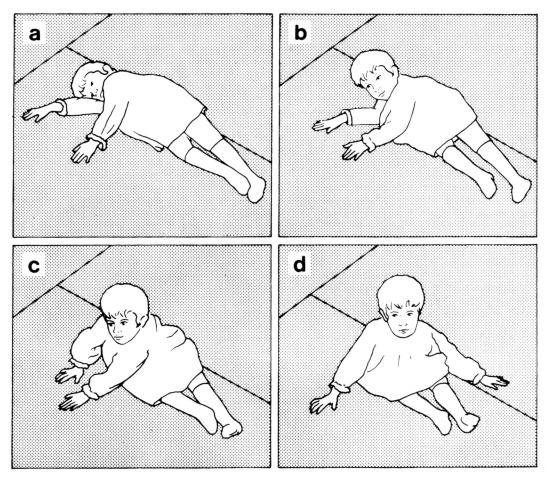

Figure 15.15   Sitting up. Child with a complete lesion below T10.

The lifts involved are usually too great for a child to transfer onto the floor or into the bath without assistance. Stools of varying height can be used as stepping stones for the child to get from his chair to the floor and back. A bath seat may be used in a similar way.

To transfer into a car, a sliding board may be necessary if the gap is too wide for the small child.

INVOLVEMENT OF PARENTS

The responsibility for any child's physical well-being and care falls to the parent, as does the responsibility for the majority of decisions regarding his life. The parents should therefore be involved in all aspects of rehabilitation and great care needs to be taken to make sure that they have a clear understanding of all the special tasks and techniques as well as the reasoning behind them. It is essential that the parents learn in detail the care of the bladder, bowels and skin, and see how the child walks and how to give him any necessary assistance. It is important also for the parents to see what the child can accomplish by himself, e.g. in dressing and transfers, and be taught how important it is that the child should continue his independence when home, even if he is slow at first. The parents must be involved in such a way that they feel confident to try, confident to come back for further advice, and if necessary confident to admit failure and ask for help.

The treatment outlined in this chapter is very demanding for the child, but perhaps more so for the parents. It can be very difficult to allow the child maximum independence when it means very slow progress through the day's tasks. To motivate a child to stand and walk – in the knowledge that he is quicker, gets less tired and can participate in more social activities if he uses a wheelchair – is hard for any parent, and even more so if it causes conflict with the child and threatens to undermine their relationship. Therapists and medical staff must face these realities, take their share of responsibility and assist the parents and child to arrive at a working compromise.

FOLLOW-UP

Due to the child's continued physical and intellectual growth, a regular and frequent follow-up system is necessary, usually taking place every 6–9 months. The most important aspect of the follow-up is to monitor the development of the spine and to check the fit of orthoses and other equipment. This needs to be done as objectively as possible. A simple method in common use is to photograph the children in a standardized manner. With the spinal column and the posterior superior iliac spine marked, posterior and lateral views are taken with the convex side of the spine furthermost when the child is seated unsupported (to see the maximum deformity) and suspended either by lifting himself or by being lifted under the axilla (to see the spontan-eous correction). A skyline (contour) view at the angle of maximum deformity is also taken. When the camera is kept at a constant distance from the child and at a constant height in relation to the seat, some comparison between the pictures can be made and a trend in development can be seen. However, it needs to be augmented with radiographs every 2 years, and yearly if deformity is evident, as this is more revealing than inspection only. This will enable a more realistic assessment of the development of the spinal deformity to be made and intervention of a more vigorous form such as internal fixation to be considered if and when necessary.

As the child matures intellectually, he needs to take on more of his own care and further intensive periods of rehabilitation may be required. The child should be given every opportunity to achieve his potential so that he can gain his maximal social and intellectual as well as physical independence.

Children with spinal cord injury will succumb to the complications of spinal deformity and contractures much more readily than adult patients. All concerned should work to slow down this process so that the child reaches adulthood with as near normal a posture as possible. The spine needs to be kept mobile, not only to prevent deformity and possible consequent damage to internal organs, but also to ensure maximum success should surgical stabilization of the spine be considered when the child gets older.

A longitudinal study on over 200 children is being undertaken at the NSIC to determine whether this treatment regimen is able to curb the inexorable development of spinal deformity in children with spinal cord lesions.

16

Complications

AGEING

Over the last few years, it has been acknowledged that spinal cord injury is not a static unchanging state, and studies have been undertaken on the problems associated with ageing in patients with long-standing spinal cord injury. Survival following spinal cord injury was relatively rare prior to World War II. Medical advances since 1945 have greatly enhanced both the initial and long-term survival of this group of permanently disabled people. Efforts have inevitably concentrated on improving initial care, emergency medical services, rehabilitation and social reintegration through the establishment of spinal cord injury centres.

Morbidity

Mortality, morbidity, health, function and psychosocial outcomes were examined in an extensive study with 834 individuals who had had their spinal cord injury at least 20 years ago (Whiteneck et al 1992). The study was carried out on patients treated at two spinal cord injury centres in the UK. As is to be expected, the decade in which the injury occurred and therefore the initial care given influenced morbidity. The mean survival rate for those injured in the 1940s was 26 years, whilst the rate for those injured in the 1960s was 33 years. Patients with incomplete lesions and those with lower lesions lived longer. The study confirmed that renal failure is no longer the primary cause of death in patients with spinal cord injury and, as deaths from renal failure decreased, the causes of death more closely resembled those of the general population.

Changes in functional ability with age

The 282 survivors were medically examined, revealing significant changes in functional abilities associated with the ageing process. Problems were related to pressure sores, kyphosis or scoliosis, restricted neck flexion, loss of range of movement at the shoulders and hip flexion contractures.

Changes in functional ability were assessed in a further study involving 297 individuals with long term spinal cord injury (Gerhart et al 1993). All had received initial and follow-up care at one of the same two spinal cord injury treatment centres in the UK. All had sustained their injuries between 20 and 47 years ago. Almost one-quarter reported that their need for physical assistance had increased over the years. The majority reported generally good health and rated their quality of life as either good or excellent. Quality of life increased with length of time post-injury, but those who needed more assistance felt their quality of life had declined (Gerhart et al 1993). Ages at which physical decline appeared, late 40s for tetraplegics and early 50s for paraplegics, are considerably younger than would be expected in non-disabled individuals.

Factors identified as contributing to the need for more assistance were fatigue/weakness, specific medical problems, pain and stiffness, weight gain and postural changes. Pain in the shoulder was significantly more frequent in the group which needed more assistance.

Pain in the shoulders

The shoulder is a key weight-bearing joint for individuals who use wheelchairs or ambulation devices (Bagley et al 1987). When a patient transfers, the intra-articular pressure in the shoulder joint rises dramatically and the bones, joints and soft tissues of the upper body are subjected to considerable stress while supporting the body weight (Jansen et al 1994). The same study showed that the level of physical strain is not uniform for patients with the same level of lesion performing the same activities of daily living.

A Wheelchair Users' Shoulder Pain Index (WUSPI) has been developed by therapists in the United States to measure shoulder pain causing limitation of function in individuals who use wheelchairs (Curtis et al 1995). It can be used as a tool for research purposes and for clinicians to document baseline dysfunction. Subjects in this study experienced the most pain when performing functional activities requiring extreme range of shoulder movement or a high level of upper limb strength, or when performing movements with the arm above the head. Activities such as wheeling up an incline or on outdoor surfaces, lifting an object from an overhead shelf, transferring from bath to wheelchair or washing the back caused the most pain. An Australian study (Pentland & Twomey 1994) identified the same tasks as being most painful and also included driving.

Professional support

If problems with posture or in other areas are to be identified early and avoided or delayed, professionals who understand the ageing process and know the patient over a long period need to be involved in their regular check-up. It is possible to address problems related to strength, pain and posture by using adaptive equipment, lightweight or power drive wheelchairs, customized seating systems and specialized cushions (Gerhart et al 1993). Advice should be given to patients about warming up before stressing limbs, checking the environment and avoiding overreaching and sudden unusual stresses, e.g. long-distance pushes or inaccessible toilet transfers.

Changes with age occur in the general population. Individuals with spinal cord injury need to realize the importance of respecting and protecting their upper limbs, to expect that their equipment needs will change and acknowledge that accepting assistance or using equipment does not signify failure (Whiteneck et al 1993b).

Longitudinal studies are required to resolve the many issues involved in the ageing process in patients with permanent disability. 'Do the cumulative stresses from years of wheelchair propulsion, altered ambulation or other adaptive yet repetitive activities hasten the ageing process across the whole population of spinal cord injured people? Or is age itself the factor most closely associated with increased physical dependence?' (Gerhart et al 1993).

Although research has only recently commenced in this field, the indications are that, like non-disabled persons, the lives of many spinal cord injured survivors can continue to be satisfying and rewarding into and beyond what we typically think of as 'old age' (Stover et al 1995).

CONTRACTURES

Contractures introduce delays and difficulties into the patient's programme of rehabilitation. It is the direct responsibility of the therapist and nursing staff to prevent their occurrence.

Causes

The causes of contractures are:

- incorrect positioning in bed or incorrect posture in the wheelchair
- inadequate physiotherapy
- spasticity.

It is difficult to separate these three closely linked factors in relation to the formation of a contracture.

Conservative treatment of established contractures

- Passive movements, including accessory joint play
- Prolonged passive stretching
- Active exercises
- Splinting
- Passive and active exercises in a heated pool
- Ice therapy and ultrasound.

Passive movements

Passive movements are always given at every treatment in addition to any other methods employed. In conjunction with the passive movements, a passive stretch is also given in the position of maximum correction.

Prolonged passive stretching

A prolonged passive stretch can be given for flexion contractures of the hips and knees and adduction contractures of the hips by strapping the limbs in the corrected position. In bed, the corrective position is maintained by using pillows and padded straps. For example, when the knee flexors are contracted, the legs are kept in extension with a strap over the knees. To avoid pressure, pillows are placed (1) under the lower legs to keep the heels off the bed, (2) between the knees to prevent the apposition of skin surfaces, and (3) over the knees, underneath the strap.

Flexion contracture of the hips. The patient lies prone on the plinth. Two or three pillows are placed under the knees and similarly under the trunk, with a gap at the level of the hip joints. To avoid pressure, a pillow is placed between the knees, and the toes must be over the end of the plinth (Fig. 16.1). Correction is obtained by strapping the hips down to the plinth. The strap placed over a pillow on the sacrum is tightened gradually. Care must be taken to arrange the two groups of pillows so that the stretch is given to the hip flexors. If the space between the pillows is too wide, the stretch merely increases the lumbar lordosis. The ankles can also be tied down with a padded strap if there are flexion contractures of the knees. The stretch is normally maintained for 20–30 minutes.

Active exercises

Hold–relax techniques are used to obtain relaxation where the muscle groups are innervated and resisted work is always given to the antagonists.

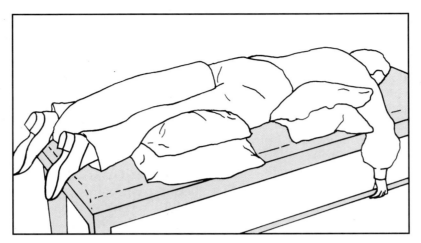

Figure 16.1 Passive stretch for the hip flexor muscles.

Splinting

To avoid excessive pressure, it is advisable to make serial splints and not try to obtain maximum correction initially. The contracture may involve more than one joint. In this case, maximum correction is obtained firstly in the joint principally controlled by the major muscle involved. For example, where the elbow, wrist and fingers are flexed, biceps is the major muscle and maximum correction is given at the elbow joint. Air-filled plastic splints are commercially available and can be useful in some cases.

Passive and active exercises in a heated pool

The hot water aids relaxation, and is especially beneficial if there is severe spasticity.

Ice therapy and ultrasound

Ice therapy and ultrasound are used as and where suitable.

'Constant attack' is the motto for dealing with contractures. Treatment needs to be carried out several times a day using a variety of methods. For example, contracted biceps tendons have been successfully treated by giving daily passive movements, active exercises, ice therapy, ultra-sound and splinting; and hip and knee flexion contractures have been treated by giving passive movements, passive stretching on the plinth, ice therapy and exercises in a heated pool.

Surgical treatment

When no improvement has occurred for approximately 6 weeks in spite of intensive therapy, surgery may be considered.

Release of the iliopsoas by iliopsoas myotomy (Michaelis 1964), elongation of the tendo Achilles, and obturator neurectomy to release the adductor muscles are useful surgical procedures in cases of severe contractures which have not responded to conservative methods (Eltorai & Montroy 1990). If the patient has strong spasticity as well as contractures, other surgical procedures may be recommended (see p. 222).

HETEROTOPIC OSSIFICATION (HO) OR PARA-ARTICULAR CALCIFICATION

A special form of para-articular ossification, exclusively of non-infectious or traumatic aetiology, has been repeatedly observed in both complete and incomplete paraplegic and tetraplegic patients below the level of the lesion. There are numerous publications from many parts of the world on this subject, but the aetiology and pathology of the disease remain obscure.

The development of bone in the connective tissue always occurs below the level of the lesion and rarely after the first 6 months post-injury. The areas most commonly affected are the hips, knees and elbows, and the medial aspect of the femur. The joints themselves are not affected but the ossification can become massive enough to cause an extra-articular ankylosis. The therapist is often the first member of the team to notice the onset of the disease. When moving the limb, she becomes aware that the joint involved does not feel quite normal. Although there is no real resistance to movement, the joint does not 'feel' clear and free. It is as though the movement were taking place through sponge. At this very early stage, there will be no radiological evidence and there may not be any visible evidence, just the awareness of a vague abnormality on moving the limb. Swelling, and possibly some erythema, may occur within a few days.

Early X-ray evidence shows cloudy patches in the muscles involved but this may not show up for a further 2–3 weeks, and by this time there will be some joint stiffness. As the disease progresses, X-rays show calcerous deposits in the para-articular tissues and finally dense ossification of the ligaments, fasciae and muscles surrounding the joints. The degree of ossification which occurs before the disease burns itself out varies considerably. Some patients have very little residual loss of joint range, whilst others have severe loss of function and independence.

Banavic & Gonzalez (1997) suggest that bone scintigraphy in asymptomatic patients is a sensitive test for early diagnosis of HO. The study showed that epidronate (the most common drug used for HO) therapy, given in higher doses and started in asymptomatic patients, may prevent the development of HO.

Ultrasonography used by an experienced person can detect HO prior to seeing it on X-ray and it is being increasingly used to document clinically suspected HO. The sonographic appearance of early HO suggests that it might be due to a partial muscle tear with massive haemorrhage (Snoecx et al 1995). Passive movements on the

seven patients in the Snoecx et al (1995) study were started a week after injury. Silver (1995) suggests that contractures could have been already forming in the limbs, tears occurred when passive movements were commenced and HO was the result. If the direction of tear could be determined (longitudinal or transverse), it could be related to the movements performed and the possibility of a link investigated (Silver 1995).

Current physiotherapy

In the initial stage when the joint feels 'spongy' and the area may be red and swollen, passive movements to that joint are discontinued until the inflammation has subsided. This will take approximately a week; passive movements are then recommenced. The limb is moved slowly and carefully two or three times only, through as full a range as possible. No forced movements are given, but every effort is made to maintain the range. When the disease becomes less active, after approximately 4–8 weeks, the passive movements and general activity are increased and careful effort is made to increase the joint range. As it is possible that vigorous passive movements causing a small tear in a muscle may lead to HO, all passive movements must be given with extreme care.

Surgery

Gross para-articular ossification interferes with joint range and, as a result, with independence. If severe, it may even interfere with a comfortable sitting posture in the wheelchair.

To restore some independence, operations are performed to remove the bone, but surgery is only considered after the disease has completely burnt itself out, which is usually 18 months to 2 years after onset. Recurrence of ossification is not uncommon even after this time lapse.

OEDEMA
Feet and legs

Due to the poor vasomotor control and loss of muscle tone in the legs, some patients get oedema of the feet, ankles and lower legs when they first start sitting out of bed. This is, of course, severely aggravated if the patient has had a deep venous thrombosis.

Every effort must be made to correct this condition in the early stages so that it does not become chronic.

To stimulate the vasomotor system, the legs are elevated several times during the day, and if necessary the bed is elevated at night. Besides being elevated in the physiotherapy department, the patient should be responsible for putting his feet up on a chair at appropriate times during the day, e.g. at meal times, in the occupational therapy department and while watching television. The patient and therapist should work out a suitable programme.

Only if this procedure fails to reduce the swelling after 3–4 weeks are elastic stockings supplied. These are more frequently necessary for patients who have had a deep venous thrombosis. Full-length stockings are given. The patient may need to spend 24–48 hours in bed with the foot of the bed elevated to disperse the oedema before measurements for the stockings can be taken.

Hands

Patients with high lesions sometimes develop oedema in the hands. This is again due to impairment of the vasomotor control with consequent loss of vasoconstriction in the blood vessels and poor venous return. This always occurs below the level of the lesion. If the oedema is not dispersed, the collagen deposit is changed into fibrous tissue and contractures develop.

Elevation. To reduce the oedema, the hands are kept in elevation day and night except during occupational therapy and physiotherapy sessions.

Passive movements. Forced passive movements to oedematous joints can only cause trauma and encourage the formation of contractures. Therefore, movements are given to affected joints with extreme care and full range is obtained only when the swelling is reduced, which may take half an hour or several days. Treatment is given several times a day taking care to maintain full range of all the non-affected joints. After an initial period of elevation, boxing glove splints may be used if desired to keep the swelling down.

In tetraplegic patients, usually over the age of 30, oedema followed by contractures of the metacarpophalangeal and interphalangeal joints sometimes occurs in spite of regular and intensive treatment. In these cases, the joints often resemble rheumatoid arthritic joints. They are red and shiny as well as swollen. The aetiology of this complication is still obscure.

When the disease has ceased to be active, treatment can be given as described for contractures.

OSTEOPOROSIS

Research into the physiology of bone formation and absorption has shown that the mineral metabolism associated with atrophy of the muscular and skeletal systems changes as a result of prolonged bedrest. These changes are emphasized when the bedrest is combined with immobilization. Considering the inevitable immobility of the paralysed limbs, it is not surprising that osteoporosis is present to some degree, below the level of the lesion, in all tetraplegic and paraplegic patients. The degree of osteoporosis is considerably increased by chronic infection from any cause.

The natural history of the development of the atrophy of the skeleton below the level of the lesion is not well understood (Szollar et al 1997). The change in bone mass in patients with spinal cord lesions is different from that due to other causes, e.g. the menopause or age. Unlike vertebral collapse, in these other forms of osteoporosis there is mineral loss in the hips, no loss in the lumbar spine and, as far as can be detected by densitometry, the most dramatic loss in the femoral region (Szollar et al 1997). In young men, lumbar bone mass was found to be stable with a non-significant decline in tetraplegic persons 1–5 years post-injury.

With the advent of sensitive, non-invasive techniques to measure bone mineral density and the possibility of sensitive biochemical markers becoming available, future studies may be able to identify therapeutic strategies which will reduce the loss of bone density in these patients (Uebelhart et al 1995).

Spontaneous fractures

Osteoporotic bone is rarified and therefore easily fractured. Fractures can occur as a result of exceptionally minor injuries and are referred to as 'spontaneous' fractures. For example, a patient who has had his paraplegia for some time may fracture his femur whilst dressing or turning over in bed, or a child may receive a simple knock in school.

The therapist can easily fracture an osteoporotic limb through careless handling when giving strong and extensive passive movements, particularly if contractures are present.

Due to the lack of sensation, the patient may be unaware that a fracture has occurred until the area becomes swollen, or until he feels unwell or has a fever. The therapist and the nursing staff should inspect the legs for any swelling and report abnormal findings immediately.

The fractures are generally treated conservatively using well-padded splints. The splint is removed daily and the limb inspected for any areas of excessive pressure or skin damage. The padding is renewed before reapplying the splint. Where possible, passive movements are continued to maintain joint range.

PAIN

Pain causes emotional distress in addition to the distress caused by the spinal cord injury and is a significant problem for paraplegic and tetraplegic people (Anke et al 1995). Large variations are seen in the reported incidence and prevalence of pain, perhaps because there appears to be little consensus on the nature, terminology and definition of the various types of pain. A classification system has been suggested by Siddal et al (1997).

There are three types of pain with which the therapist should be familiar:

- pain due to periarticular and muscular contractures
- central cord pain
- referred pain.

Pain due to periarticular and muscular contractures

This pain is always found above the level of the lesion, most frequently in complete lesions of the cervical cord. Trauma to the cervical roots may cause some root irritation initially, but continuing pain appears to be due to contractures around the shoulder and shoulder girdle due to faulty positioning and lack of movement. The treatment given is general mobilization as for any contracted joint where sensation is unimpaired. It must be borne in mind that the patient's general condition and morale at this time are often poor and his pain tolerance low. Rough handling or indiscriminate stretching of a joint sets up involuntary protective spasm, the patient loses confidence and the desired result is considerably delayed.

Central cord pain

Central cord pain remains a problem for 5–10% of patients with spinal cord injury (Sweet et al 1995). It is described as 'burning', 'scalding' or 'shooting'/'stabbing', and patients with this type of pain have autonomic instability (Bowsher 1996). These sensations are 'felt' below the level of the lesion. The acute pain usually lasts a few seconds and is often followed by paroxysms of another type of pain which can be cramping in character. The number of attacks per day varies considerably from patient to patient and even from day to day in the same patient. There is no association between the severity of pain and level or completeness of injury (Anke et al 1995).

Management of this type of pain is difficult. Not many trials have been carried out, in spite of chronic central pain being a frequent complication following spinal cord injury (Drewes et al 1994). Anticonvulsant drug therapy (Balazy 1992), antidepressants and transcutaneous nerve stimulation (Hachen 1978) all have their advocates. Drewes et al (1994) in a double-blind crossover trial found no significant difference between drug and placebo groups. Clinicians agree that the present available pharmacological agents are most effective in patients with mild or moderate pain. Only mild analgesics are prescribed, as drugs are quickly habit-forming in these cases. Occasionally, due to the severity of the pain, destructive procedures may be undertaken, e.g. Dorsal Root Entry Zone (DREZ) lesions. Dorsal Column Stimulation (DST) and Deep Brain Stimulation (DBS) may be tried in order to change brain responses. Although each procedure has its advocates, no long-term benefits have as yet been documented.

Intensive physiotherapy may be useful, including some form of sport. The condition may show some spontaneous improvement as the patient learns to tolerate his pain by diversional activities.

Patients with complete lesions of the mid-thoracic and thoracolumbar cord sometimes develop a band of hyperpathia around the level of the lesion. The patient complains that there is a tight band around his chest, and occasionally it is so hypersensitive that he cannot bear anything to touch his skin.

Referred pain

Patients with cervical and high thoracic lesions can experience pain in the shoulder region when any abnormal visceral activity occurs. Impulses are carried from the paralysed to the non-paralysed area via the phrenic nerve. For example, a patient with a C4 lesion had a haematemesis due to a perforated ulcer. On looking back at the therapist's notes, it was seen that the patient had complained of nausea and pain across the upper part of the shoulders for at least 2 weeks previously.

Patients with cervical lesions can suddenly develop severe frontal headache. This may be due to overdistension of the bladder and should be investigated without delay.

PRESSURE SORES

The effects of pressure and its prevention are described in Chapter 6. Patients admitted early to a spinal unit have a significantly lower risk of developing pressure sores (Aung & El Masry 1997). In their study of 60 patients, Rodriguez & Garber (1994) found that the pressure sores developed within 2 years post-injury and were more frequent in those with lesions above T6. Of those who smoked, 36% got pressure sores, as compared with 26% of the non-smokers.

The treatment of established pressure sores

Conservative treatment

Relieve pressure. The first essential step in treating a pressure sore is to relieve the pressure on the sore totally and continuously. This means complete bedrest for patients who are already ambulant or wheelchair bound.

The patient must be turned every 3 hours, day and night, to prevent further sores from developing on unaffected areas, and positioned in such a way that no weight is thrown on the sore or sores. Rings around the heels to relieve localized pressure are contraindicated. The area of skin under the ring may receive sufficient pressure to cut off the blood supply to the area in the centre, which is the area most at risk.

A low air loss bed facilitates positioning a patient with multiple sores, or a sorbo pack bed or pillow packs spaced as for sorbo packs can be used on top of an ordinary mattress.

If pressure is not relieved over the sore, any other measures taken will prove unsuccessful.

General treatment. Blood transfusions may be required to keep the haemoglobin level in the upper limits of normal.

Local treatment. All slough and necrotic tissue is radically excised. This prevents the toxic effects which result from the absorption of dead tissue into the bloodstream. A wide range of lotions is used, including local antibiotics in solution, and the dressing is completely sealed off with wide porous elastoplast.

Surgical treatment

Various surgical procedures may be considered in selected cases.

Physiotherapy

Passive movements

Passive movements are given to the paralysed limbs to improve the circulation and to prevent contractures. Passive movements to the lower limbs are recommended after surgery when the surgeon considers it advisable. As a general rule, the patients can be divided into those with severe spasticity and those with flaccid lesions.

If the patient has severe spasticity or if any one movement causes violent spasm, all movements are avoided until the scar is healed. If the lesion is flaccid or the patient has minimum spasticity, it may be possible to commence moving the knees and feet after a week to 10 days.

Initially very gentle movements only are given. Whilst moving the joints involved, the therapist watches the scar to avoid excessive tension. The range of any movement which looks potentially dangerous is increased with extreme caution to avoid breakdown of the wound.

Grease massage

The pliability of the skin is an important factor when excision of the sore is considered. The more pliable the surrounding tissues, the easier is the approximation of the skin following the excision. When necessary, daily massage with lanolin is given to a wide area surrounding the sore. Deep finger kneading increases the circulation and improves the elasticity and mobility of the skin and subcutaneous tissue.

Exercise

The patient is encouraged to pull a chest expander or lift weights of suitable strength several times every hour to maintain strength in the arms and upper trunk.

Chest therapy

Pre- and postoperative therapy is given if a general anaesthetic is used for any surgical procedures.

Pressure consciousness

The patient must be educated, or re-educated, in 'pressure consciousness' and have his posture, cushion and wheelchair checked by the expert therapist in that field.

Transfers

In spite of any previous rehabilitation, once the patient is mobile all transfers are checked to see that due care is taken when lifting and moving the limbs.

SHOULDER–HAND SYNDROME (SHS)

The clinical features of the SHS are shoulder pain, wrist/hand pain, oedema, vasomotor changes, trophic changes and osteoporosis on X-ray. Aisen & Aisen (1994) found that almost one-third of the patients in their study had three or more of these symptoms. Almost all were satisfactorily resolved with conservative treatment after about 4 months.

The pathophysiology of this condition is unclear, although sympathetic hyperactivity appears to be important (Bennett 1991). The few studies reported are on SHS after stroke, where it is sometimes treated with corticosteroids and also by stellate block with good effect (Braus & Strobel 1991). Any shoulder problem causes delay in rehabilitation in spinal cord injured patients (Ohry et al 1978).

Treatment by physiotherapy is conservative, continuing movements without force and elevating the limb to reduce swelling.

SPASTICITY

During the period of spinal areflexia following complete transverse section of the cord, there is flaccid paralysis of all muscles below the level of the lesion. Subsequently, the isolated cord resumes some autonomous function and the motor paralysis becomes spastic.

The heightened reflex activity of the isolated cord is demonstrated by increased tone in the muscles and brisk tendon reflexes. The ensuing degree of spasticity varies. In some cases it may remain mild, while in others the afferent stimuli, uninhibited by higher centres, cause a mass response in the isolated cord, and a mass response of muscle action ensues. This can produce any combination of muscle spasm, e.g. total flexor or extensor patterns, or alternating flexor and extensor spasticity, or flexion of the knees with extension of the hips.

The increased muscular tension leads to an uneven distribution of pressure on joint cartilage. This may result in the destruction of cartilage, capsular contractures or partial dislocations of varying degrees. Spasticity is dealt with more extensively in Chapter 14.

Treatment of established spasticity

A combination of the following methods may be used:

- physiotherapy
- chemotherapy
- surgery.

Certain factors stimulate spasticity and these are excluded before deciding on a course of treatment:

- distension of internal organs below the level of the lesion, i.e. bladder and bowels
- septic conditions, such as urinary tract infections, or infected pressure sores
- contracted tendons and joints, which reduce the threshold of irritability of the stretch reflex
- local skin lesions, ingrowing toe nails, etc.

When considering treatment, the following facts are borne in mind:

- fatigue has a depressant effect on spasticity
- muscle accommodates to prolonged stretch
- posture influences reflexes
- spasticity is influenced by emotional factors.

Physiotherapy

Passive movements. These are always given to maintain mobility in all structures.

Prolonged passive stretching. The stretch may be given manually, or by utilizing one of the stretch positions as for contractures, or in the standing position.

Hydrotherapy. Passive movements and swimming exercises in a heated pool may provide temporary relief for some patients.

Reflex inhibiting postures. These may be useful to reduce spasticity or maintain relaxation during treatment. The position adopted when sleeping can be used to reduce spasticity. For example, sleeping prone for 3 or 4 hours reduces flexor spasticity in the lower limbs.

Standing and walking. Weight-bearing reduces spasticity. However, in some severely spastic cases, the standing position may be impossible without first reducing the spasticity by some other means, e.g. passive movements, a passive stretch or hydrotherapy.

Ice therapy. Ice towels may reduce spasticity when it is associated with contracture, but they have not proved valuable in treating the large muscle groups for spasticity alone.

Chemotherapy

Chemotherapy is used in the following ways.

Drug therapy. Antispasmodic drugs can be used with some effect on certain patients, although their effectiveness in reducing severe spasticity is extremely limited. They are usually prescribed with caution only after a period of physiotherapy has proved insufficient, as the side-effects, notably that of sedation, can affect the patient's rehabilitation.

Local temporary block and intrathecal injections. These are used for the relief of spasticity and are covered in Chapter 14.

Surgery

Surgical procedures on peripheral structures are preferred to those performed on the cord or roots. Methods used to reduce spasticity include diminishing the contraction potential of the muscle by elongating the tendon, or by severing the nerve supplying a large muscle group, and by tenotomy or capsulotomy (Eltorai & Montroy 1990).

In certain patients with complete or incomplete lesions, it appears that one muscle 'triggers' off the spastic pattern. In these cases, a surgical procedure may be performed to block conduction to the 'trigger' muscle. In most instances the result is an overall reduction in spasticity.

SPINAL DEFORMITY

Any patient confined to bed for some time is in danger of developing contractures and may also develop a scoliosis. Children and adolescents are in particular danger because of continuing growth and extreme joint mobility (Ch. 15).

When a patient spends a high proportion of time in an abnormal, incorrect posture for functional activities, convenience or comfort, whether in bed or in a wheelchair, deformities develop. Gross scoliosis or pelvic distortion will severely hamper the patient's rehabilitation and may prevent him from attaining complete independence or from functional weight-bearing.

In assessing the deformity, the exact nature of the problem needs to be identified, especially whether the posture is correctable or has become fixed.

Prevention and treatment

Every effort must be made to prevent such deformities by correct positioning in bed and when seated in the wheelchair, re-education of posture and muscle development. The correct choice of cushion, and the posture and fit of the patient in his wheelchair are dealt with in Chapter 6.

The following methods of treatment can be useful:

- strengthening the weaker or less used muscle groups, including the use of functional electrical stimulation and archery where appropriate
- stretching those muscles tending to shorten
- maintaining a passive stretch in the

overcorrected position for those muscles tending to shorten
- re-education of posture and regular reassessment of efficacy of cushion
- corrective sleeping postures
- bracing.

Corrective sleeping postures

Pillows can be used to support the spine in a corrected position at night. For example, a patient with a long 'C' curve to the left should have sufficient pillows under the thorax when lying on his left side to give maximum correction of the deformity.

Bracing

A spinal brace may be necessary to support the child or adolescent with a bad posture in sitting or standing. Occasionally an adult may also need a brace for this purpose.

Archery

Archery is an excellent exercise for the back and shoulder girdle muscles (see Fig. 17.1a). Correction of a scoliosis may be obtained at the full draw position. If the scoliosis is a simple one, the bow is held by the arm on the side of the concavity, as maximum strength is required by the arm pulling the bow string.

If the scoliosis is complex, an X-ray is taken at full draw using each arm in turn to see if correction can be obtained.

Surgery

Surgical procedures may be indicated in a few selected cases.

SYRINGOMYELIA

The major symptoms of this complication are pain, which may be localized centrally or which may radiate into the arm or trunk, sensory impairment and increasing weakness. It appears to be more common in tetraplegic than in paraplegic patients (Rossier et al 1985).

The results of conservative treatment have proved unsatisfactory. With the development of magnetic resonance imaging and the possibility of non-traumatic investigation, it is possible to detect syringomyelia earlier and to drain those producing significant symptoms or signs. This is a distressing condition where increasing weakness can rob the patient of his independence. Physiotherapy is directed towards re-education after surgery.

17

Sport in rehabilitation

THE THERAPEUTIC VALUE OF SPORT

Clinical sport has an important contribution to make in the rehabilitation of patients with spinal cord injury. It assists in restoring the patient's strength, balance, coordination and endurance. It stimulates activity of mind and encourages self-confidence and interaction with others. Some patients were enthusiastic sportsmen before becoming disabled and, once introduced to sport in a wheelchair, will continue when they leave hospital. Sports clubs provide a useful opportunity for mixing with the local community.

Swimming, archery and table tennis are particularly valuable during rehabilitation. Dartchery, snooker and basketball or volleyball are also useful (Guttmann 1976c).

SWIMMING

The pool

To enable patients to swim, the pool must be a reasonable length, if possible, a minimum of 8 m. If different depths are required, a sloped floor is preferable to steps. Skin damage can easily occur against the hard edges of steps as the paralysed legs trail in the water. As it is generally found that cold water increases spasticity, the water temperature is kept high: 32–36°C (90–96°F). At this temperature, spasticity is reduced in the majority of patients.

Hygiene

The pool should have some form of continuous flow system through a filter plant. The chlorine content is maintained and checked twice a day. Samples of the water are cultured regularly. The patient expresses his bladder prior to entering the pool and should have had a satisfactory bowel evacuation.

Entry into the water

Some type of hydraulic lift provides the safest method of entry for all tetraplegic patients and for those patients with lower lesions who are incapable of independent transfer. Active paraplegic patients enter over the side of the pool using a sorbo rubber pad placed over the edge to protect the skin from the hard surface.

Therapeutic uses

Increase of muscle strength

Swimming increases the strength of all innervated muscles. Motor power in patients with incomplete lesions can be increased by normal hydrotherapy techniques, using water to eliminate gravity or to assist or resist movement. In addition to swimming, exercises to increase muscle strength in patients with complete lesions can be given using the water to assist or resist movement as required.

Improved coordination

Coordination can be improved by all the strokes used in swimming, in particular the unilateral strokes.

Reduction of spasticity

This is achieved *passively* through the heated water, passive movements and passive stretching, and *actively* through swimming.

Swimming increases exercise tolerance, vital capacity and cardiovascular efficiency. Swimming prone increases the activity of the diaphragm and consequently lung volume in patients with cervical cord lesions because of the need to hold the breath in this position.

Reduction of contractures

Passive stretching of contractures is often facilitated by the heated water.

Psychological and social aspects

Mobility in the water is often the only experience of unaided body movement within the environment that most paralysed patients enjoy. Consequently, a new enthusiasm is often noted when pool activities are commenced. Swimming fosters the growth of independence and self-expression. It also provides a further opportunity to mix with the able-bodied, many patients enjoying swimming with family and friends.

Swimming instruction

The Halliwick method of teaching independence in the water is largely used in the UK as a recreational activity, but it also has great value in the therapeutic field (Martin 1981). The objective of this method is water safety leading to independent freedom of movement in water, which is achieved with no help other than a close instructor–swimmer relationship. The method suggests that the swimmer should first adjust to the water and then learn to change his position in the water so that he can always move himself into a position in which he is able to breathe.

Rolling

To roll in the water, the swimmer turns his head to one side, e.g. the left, and moves one arm, e.g. the right, across his body causing him to tip over until he is face down in the water. The same procedure is repeated to continue the roll to bring the swimmer face upwards again. The 360° roll needs to be practised until it can be done with ease.

Independence in the water is first achieved on the back, the prone position being more difficult to maintain without muscle power at the hip joints. Symmetrical strokes are taught initially, as asymmetrical activity causes the paralysed limbs to roll and the patient finds difficulty in maintaining a straight course.

Instruction for patients with thoracic or lumbar lesions

When supine in the water, the paralysed portion of the body lies at an angle of 45° from the site of the fracture. To compensate for the paralysed limbs, the head needs to be well extended.

Backstroke

The therapist supports the patient under the neck; the patient, maintaining his head in extension, moves his arms simultaneously away from the sides with the elbows flexed. He then extends the elbows and brings the arms back to *midline*, with the thumbs just breaking the surface of the water. Because the hips are lower in the water, the body will be pushed upwards if the arms are brought back to the *sides*. Similarly, when the patient relaxes the stroke, his body will sink again. In this way, a vertical as well as a horizontal component to the movement is produced with consequent wasted effort. Once the patient has become accustomed to his position in the water, the 'sculling' stroke is expanded, and the arms are brought out of the water close to the head, as in the Old English backstroke. To prevent his head submerging when the arms are in full elevation, the patient must relax his extended head for a second or two.

Breaststroke

The position of the body when the patient is prone in the water resembles an inverted U, with the head submerged and the buttocks floating to the surface. To counteract this tendency, the patient is initially taught to do the breaststroke with his head constantly out of the water, as strong extension of the head and upper trunk is needed to keep the buttocks submerged.

The therapist assists the patient with one hand under his chin and the other pressing down on his buttocks. As the patient becomes aware of his position in the water, the chin support is withdrawn. Later the pressure on the buttocks is gently released and the patient must work hard to maintain the necessary extension. When this is achieved, the patient begins to swim with his head under water for several strokes in the usual way. He must, however, *start* to extend his head much sooner than the able-bodied breaststroke swimmer. The head of the paraplegic swimmer will be forced under water just before his hands are level with his shoulders.

Unilateral strokes (crawl)

Without the necessary leg movement to prevent it, the lower half of the body will roll during a unilateral stroke. The roll can be prevented during back crawl by making small paddling movements with the non-stroke arm as the stroke arm pulls down.

Butterfly stroke

Patients with lesions at C6 and below who have been proficient in this stroke prior to their accident can relearn it.

Instruction for patients with cervical lesions

Patients with functional use of latissimus dorsi and triceps swim in the same way as patients with lower lesions. Patients with lesions at C6 can occasionally become independent swimmers, but the majority, although capable of swimming alone, need an attendant in case difficulties arise.

Rolling

This is discussed on page 226.

Backstroke

To gain extension at the elbow without triceps, the arm must be kept in lateral rotation and it can be lifted only a few degrees above shoulder level. As the arm returns to the water and pulls down, water pressure will keep the elbow straight.

Swimming prone

Without triceps, the true movements of the breaststroke are impossible. The patient with a lesion at C5–6 *pulls* his arms through the water towards his body using biceps, deltoid and the clavicular head of pectoralis major. While the patient is swimming face down, it is important that the therapist keeps one hand on the patient's shoulder where he has sensation. Initially, most patients will only be able to swim two or three strokes, but within six or seven sessions this can be increased up to an average of 8–10 m.

Leaving and returning to the side of the pool

To leave the side, the patient lies parallel with the side of the pool with the head extended and pushes off gently, with the arm just on the surface of the water. To return to the side, the patient swims in parallel with, and as close as possible to, the side of the pool, keeping the nearside arm under the surface of the water. He then rapidly flings the arm into the overflow trough and strongly flexes his neck. To maintain this position, paddling movements are performed with the free arm by pulling the water towards the body, as in the breaststroke movement.

Incomplete lesions

Patients with incomplete lesions with weak, scattered muscles and patchy sensation can gain strength and coordination from using all the available swimming strokes.

ARCHERY

From both the medical and recreational aspects, archery has proved to be an ideal sport for patients with spinal cord injury.

Therapeutic value

Increase of muscle strength

Archery develops and strengthens the essential muscles of the paraplegic patient, i.e. erector spinae, deltoid, pectorals, rhomboids, trapezius and latissimus dorsi (Fig. 17.1a).

Balance, control and coordination

When the bow arm is lifted and the centre of gravity consequently altered, skilled balance is required to maintain the erect posture. Initially patients with high thoracic lesions may need to bring the buttocks slightly forward in the chair and lean heavily against the backrest to achieve sufficient stability. As the balance improves, the upright posture is resumed.

Accurate marksmanship requires control, dexterity and judgement, and demands fine coordination of the eye, hand and arm.

Correction of scoliosis

Archery is used as a corrective exercise for many patients with scoliosis. The string is drawn by the arm on the side of the convexity, irrespective of the dominant eye, to strengthen the weaker muscles. For a simple scoliosis, the correction is usually obvious. With a multiple scoliosis, X-rays taken while sitting at rest and again at full draw are essential to confirm that the correct arm is being used to draw the string.

Social value

The disabled and the able-bodied can meet on equal terms. The wheelchair archer can join a club for the able-bodied which provides a further opportunity for integration with the local community.

Archery for patients with cervical cord lesions

Special equipment is necessary to enable the tetraplegic patient to shoot.

The release

To release the arrow without finger flexion or extension, a hook device is used. A small hook at the end of a metal splint is strapped to the palmar surface of the middle finger extending across

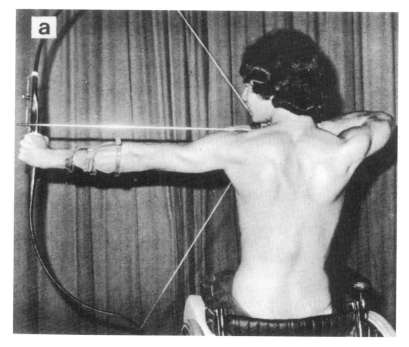

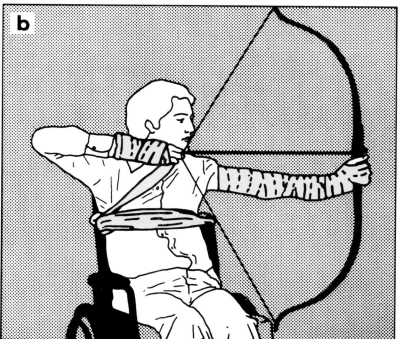

Figure 17.1   Archery. a: Patient with a complete lesion below T10. b: Patient with a complete lesion below C6.

the wrist of the drawing hand (Fig. 17.2). To release the string the archer slightly *pronates* his forearm. Pronation gives greater accuracy, as supination allows gravity to act on the unstable forearm. This causes the elbow to drop and results in inaccurate shooting. With the appropriate training, archers of ability who use the hook release can reach the longest international distance of 90 m.

The bow arm

The patient without triceps needs a splint to maintain the elbow in extension. If the wrist extensors are weak, a wrist splint is frequently necessary to prevent the wrist being forced into flexion by the tension of the bow. The bow needs bandaging into the hand. To gain the necessary stability, all patients with cervical cord lesions need to be tied into the chair. The tie is usually placed around the upper thorax and tied to the chair handle on the side of the drawing arm (Fig. 17.1b).

DARTCHERY

This game, played in pairs, was developed for paraplegic patients. Bow and arrows are used to shoot at a target face which is a replica of a dartboard. The target is set at a distance of 15 m from the players and the rules are basically the same as those governing dart play.

DARTS

The dart board must be at an appropriate height for wheelchair users. If the player cannot hold conventional darts, blow darts can be used. The rules are the same as for able-bodied players.

TABLE TENNIS
Therapeutic value

The therapeutic value of table tennis includes:

- improved coordination, especially that of eye and hand
- improved agility in the wheelchair.

The loss of sensation and lack of balance make the patient fearful of falling during his early days in a wheelchair. Consequently, the patient is often rigid, unwilling to move any part of his body except his head. In his desire to hit the ball, this fear is gradually forgotten and the patient comes to realize that he can move about within

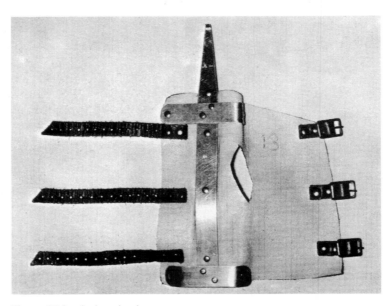

Figure 17.2   Archery hook.

the chair without either tipping it or falling out. The patient is taught to play with the chair stationary in the centre of the backline. The rules of play are the same as for the able-bodied, with the exception of the 'alternate shot rule' for doubles. This rule is amended so that either partner can return any shot except when receiving service. Patients with cervical cord lesions also enjoy table tennis. Those without finger movement need the bat bandaged or strapped into the hand. To play backhand shots, those without triceps use outward rotation of the shoulder. An adjustable table tennis bat has recently been developed for tetraplegic sportsmen where the angle of the head of the bat can be changed in relation to the grip. The bat is held firmly in the hand by an elasticated glove. This allows a greater range of shots (Taktak 1997).

BASKETBALL

Wheelchair basketball is a fast and exciting game which calls for team work and accurate control of the body, chair and ball. Mobility, strength, endurance and dexterity in wheelchair management are developed. It is a game for those patients with a good functional grip, as accurate and immediate control of the chair is essential. A less active form of this game, volleyball, can be played by patients in their first period of rehabilitation.

BOWLS

Bowls are played from the wheelchair with the same rules as for able-bodied players. This game can also be played on a carpet with 5 cm bowls for tetraplegic and 10 cm bowls for paraplegic players during their rehabilitation. It can also be played on a snooker table when the 3 cm bowls are bowled down a wooden slide.

FENCING

The weapon used for novices is the foil. No wheelchair skills are required as the chair remains static and tactics are all-important.

SNOOKER

This game provides excellent practice in coordination skills, particularly for patients with cervical cord lesions.

TENNIS

The rules are the same as for able-bodied tennis except that the ball is allowed to bounce twice before it must be hit.

WHEELCHAIR RUGBY

This game is for people with tetraplegia. It is similar to basketball, except that the goals are scored by having two wheels over the back line of the key area whilst being in possession of the ball.

Some of these games, if not all, are usually available in spinal units as the skills required to play contribute to the rehabilitation of patients with spinal cord injury.

RULES

All sports are conducted, as far as possible, under the rules of the game for the able-bodied; for example, archery under the rules of the Grand National Archery Association and swimming under those of the Amateur Swimming Association. Books of rules are available which cover all sports played by wheelchair competitors. The International Stoke Mandeville Sports Federation rule book for wheelchair sports now includes archery, athletics, basketball, cue sports, lawn bowling, fencing, shooting, swimming, table tennis, tennis, weight lifting, racquetball, wheelchair rugby and winter sports.

THE BENEFIT OF COMPETITIVE SPORT

In one sense, all sport is competitive. The sportsman always competes with his past performance. He also competes, consciously or unconsciously, with others taking part in the same swimming or archery session. A profitable physical and psychological stimulus is provided by competitive sport. These activities create a sense of comradeship and help to eliminate any self-consciousness suffered by patients in relation to their disability. They can give a sense of physical adequacy and increase self-esteem (Bedbrook 1981). Competitive sport is also of great value in integrating disabled people with the able-bodied community and the facilities of some sports centres are available for both groups.

Inter-spinal unit games offer a taste of competitive sport to patients still in hospital. They provide the opportunity to mix with people from other units, some of whom will be paralysed and some able-bodied, in a relaxed atmosphere where the social as well as the athletic skills of the recently paralysed patient will be required. Some patients become proficient and enter international sporting events.

Some wheelchair users are not interested in competitive sport but want to participate in sporting activities with family and friends (Kennedy & Smith 1990).

Due to the initiative, enterprise and enthusiasm of disabled individuals, the list of sports open to the paralysed person is continually being extended. Wheelchair users can now enjoy angling, cricket, sailing, scuba diving, snorkling, waterpolo, karting with hand controls and recently flying light aircraft with hand controls.

The majority of sports are unsuitable for open competition with able-bodied people. Exceptions are archery, angling, green bowling, snooker and table tennis. Basketball, fencing, field events, swimming, track racing and weight lifting are sports which can be competitive only amongst disabled people.

Competitive sport for patients with spinal cord injury is organized on a national and international level through the Stoke Mandeville Games for the Paralysed and Other Disabled.

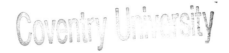

Appendices

Appendix 1
Standard neurological classification of spinal cord injury

STANDARD NEUROLOGICAL CLASSIFICATION OF SPINAL CORD INJURY

MOTOR

KEY MUSCLES

C2	
C3	
C4	
C5	Elbow flexors
C6	Wrist extensors
C7	Elbow extensors
C8	Finger flexors (distal phalanx of middle finger)
T1	Finger abductors (little finger)
T2	
T3	
T4	
T5	
T6	
T7	
T8	
T9	
T10	
T11	
T12	
L1	
L2	Hip flexors
L3	Knee extensors
L4	Ankle dorsiflexors
L5	Long toe extensors
S1	Ankle plantar flexors
S2	
S3	
S4-5	

0 = total paralysis
1 = palpable or visible contraction
2 = active movement, gravity eliminated
3 = active movement, against gravity
4 = active movement, against some resistance
5 = active movement, against full resistance
NT = not testable

Voluntary anal contraction (Yes/No)

TOTALS [ ] + [ ] = [ ] MOTOR SCORE
(MAXIMUM) (50) (50) (100)

SENSORY

KEY SENSORY POINTS

0 = absent
1 = impaired
2 = normal
NT = not testable

* Key Sensory Points

	LIGHT TOUCH		PIN PRICK	
	R	L	R	L
C2				
C3				
C4				
C5				
C6				
C7				
C8				
T1				
T2				
T3				
T4				
T5				
T6				
T7				
T8				
T9				
T10				
T11				
T12				
L1				
L2				
L3				
L4				
L5				
S1				
S2				
S3				
S4-5				

Any anal sensation (Yes/No)

TOTALS [ ] + [ ] [ ] + [ ] =
(MAXIMUM) (56) (56) (56) (56)

[ ] = PIN PRICK SCORE (max: 112)
[ ] = LIGHT TOUCH SCORE (max: 112)

Version 4p
GHC 1996

ZONE OF PARTIAL PRESERVATION
Partially innervated segments

	R	L
SENSORY		
MOTOR		

NEUROLOGICAL LEVELS
The most caudal segment with normal function

	R	L
SENSORY		
MOTOR		

COMPLETE OR INCOMPLETE
Incomplete = Any sensory or motor function in S4-55

ASIA IMPAIRMENT SCALE

This form may be copied freely but should not be altered without permission from the American Spinal Injury Association.

Maynard FM et al 1997 Figure 4 in *International Standards for Neurological and Functional Classification of Spinal Cord Injury*. Spinal Cord 35(5): 272 (with permission from American Spinal Injury Association)

Appendix 2
Functional independence measure

Functional Independence Measure (FIM)

LEVELS			No Helper
	7	Complete Independence (Timely, Safely)	No Helper
	6	Modified Independence (Device)	
	Modified Dependence		Helper
	5	Supervision	
	4	Minimal Assist (Subject = 75%+)	
	3	Moderate Assist (Subject = 50%+)	
	Complete Dependence		
	2	Maximal Assist (Subject = 25%+)	
	1	Total Assist (Subject = 0%+)	

	ADMIT	DISCH
Self Care		
A. Eating	☐	☐
B. Grooming	☐	☐
C. Bathing	☐	☐
D. Dressing-Upper Body	☐	☐
E. Dressing-Lower Body	☐	☐
F. Toileting	☐	☐
Sphincter Control		
G. Bladder Management	☐	☐
H. Bowel Management	☐	☐
Mobility		
Transfer:		
I. Bed, Chair, Wheelchair	☐	☐
J. Toilet	☐	☐
K. Tub, Shower	☐	☐
Locomotion	W ☐	W ☐
L. Walk/Wheelchair	C ☐	C ☐
M. Stairs	☐	☐
Communication	A ☐	A ☐
N. Comprehension	V	V
O. Expression	V ☐	V ☐
	N	N
Social Cognition		
P. Social Interaction	☐	☐
Q. Problem Solving	☐	☐
R. Memory	☐	☐
Total FIM	☐	☐

NOTE: Leave no blanks; enter 1 if patient not testable due to risk.

ASIA IMPAIRMENT SCALE

☐ **A = Complete:** No motor or sensory function is preserved in the sacral segments S4-S5.

☐ **B = Incomplete:** Sensory but not motor function is preserved below the neurological level and includes the sacral segments S4-S5.

☐ **C = Incomplete:** Motor function is preserved below the neurological level, and more than half of key muscles below the neurological level have a muscle grade less than 3.

☐ **D = Incomplete:** Motor function is preserved below the neurological level, and at least half of key muscles below the neurological level have a muscle grade of 3 or more.

☐ **E = Normal:** motor and sensory function is normal

CLINICAL SYNDROMES

☐ Central Cord
☐ Brown-Sequard
☐ Anterior Cord
☐ Conus Medullaris
☐ Cauda Equina

Maynard F M et al 1997 Figure 5 in *International Standards for Neurological and Functional Classification of Spinal Cord Injury* 35(5): 273 (with permission from American Spinal Injury Association)

Appendix 3
Major segmental innervation of the muscles of the upper limb

C2			
	+C3	Sternomastoid	

C3			
	+C4	Trapezius	
		+C5	Levator scapulae

C4	Diaphragm		

C5	Rhomboids		
	Deltoid		
	Teres minor		
	Supraspinatus		
	Infraspinatus		
	Subclavius		
	+C6	Biceps	

C6	Brachialis		
	Supinator		
	Brachioradialis		
	Subscapularis		
	Teres major		
	Coracobrachialis		
	+C7	Serratus anterior	
		Latissimus dorsi	
		Extensor carpi radialis longus	
		+C8	Pectoralis major

C7	Pronator teres		
	Pectoralis minor		
	Extensor digitorum		
	Extensor digiti minimi		
	Flexor carpi radialis		
	+C8	Triceps	
		Extensor carpi radialis brevis	
		Palmaris longus	

C8	Extensor carpi ulnaris	
	Flexor carpi ulnaris	
	Extensor indicis	
	Flexor digitorum profundus	
	Flexor digitorum sublimis	
	Abductor pollicis longus	
	Abductor pollicis brevis	
	Opponens pollicis	
	Flexor pollicis longus	
	Extensor pollicis longus	
	Extensor pollicis brevis	
	+T1	Adductor pollicis

T1	Flexor pollicis brevis
	Abductor digiti minimi
	Flexor digiti minimi
	Opponens digiti minimi
	Lumbricales
	Interossei

Appendix 4
Major segmental innervation of the muscles of the lower limb

L1	Psoas minor		
	+L2	Psoas major	
L2	Iliacus		
	+L3	Sartorius	
		+L4	Adductors
L3			
	+L4	Quadriceps	
L4	Obturator externus		
	+L5	Tensor fascia lata	
		Tibialis posterior	
		+S1	Tibialis anterior
			Extensor hallucis
			Extensor digitorum longus
			Peroneus tertius
			Popliteus
L5	Gluteus medius		
	Gluteus minimus		

+S1	Quadratus femoris		
	Semimembranosus		
	Semitendinosus		
	Biceps femoris		
	Peroneus longus		
	Peroneus brevis		
S1	Obturator internus		
	Gastrocnemius		
	+S2	Gluteus maximus	
S2	Flexor hallucis longus		
	Flexor digitorum longus		
	Soleus		
	+S3	Interossei	
S3	Abductor hallucis		
	Adductor hallucis		
	Lumbricales		
	Abductor digiti minimi		

Appendix 5
A guide to the functional control of joints of the upper and lower limbs

	C5	C6	C7	C8	T1
Shoulder	Minimal	Partial	COMPLETE		
Elbow	Minimal	Partial	COMPLETE		
Wrist		Minimal	Partial	COMPLETE	
Hand			Minimal	Partial	COMPLETE

	L2	L3	L4	L5	S1
Hip	Minimal	Partial	Partial	COMPLETE	
Knee		Minimal	Partial	COMPLETE	
Ankle			Partial	Partial	COMPLETE
Foot			Minimal	Partial	COMPLETE

Appendix 6
Functional independence

Segmental level	PERSONAL INDEPENDENCE	WHEELCHAIR MANAGEMENT	TRANSFERS	GAIT
C4	Type, turn pages, use telephone and computer with mouth-stick			
C5	Type Feed	Manipulate brake Push on the flat		
C6	Drink Wash, shave, brush hair Dress upper half Sit up/lie down in bed Write	Remove armrests/footplates Push on sloping ground Turn chair	Chair ↔ bed Chair ↔ car ? with sliding board	
C7	Turn in bed Dress lower half Skin care	Pick up objects from floor Wheel over uneven ground 'Bounce' over small elevations	Chair ↔ toilet Chair ↔ chair ? Chair ↔ bath	Stand in frame
C8	Bladder and bowel care	Negotiate kerbs	Chair ↔ bath	Stand in frame
T1–T5		Balance on rear wheels Pull wheelchair into car	Chair ↔ floor	Stand in frame Swing-to in bars
T6 –T9			Chair ↔ crutches	Swing-to on crutches or rollator ? Stairs
T10–L1				All three gaits on crutches Stairs Car ↔ crutches Floor ↔ crutches

Appendix 7
Segmental innervation of the skin

Upper limb

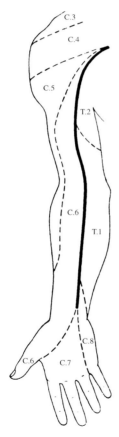

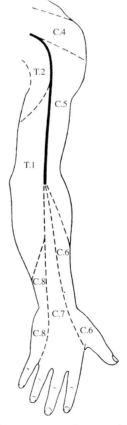

Arrangement of dermatomes on the anterior aspect of the upper limb. The solid black line represents the *ventral axial line*, and the overlap across it is *minimal*. Across the interrupted lines, overlap is considerable.

Arrangement of dermatomes on the posterior aspect of the upper limb. The solid black line represents the *dorsal axial line*, and the overlap across it is *minimal*. Across the interrupted lines, the overlap may be and often is considerable.

Figure A7.1 Reproduced from *Gray's Anatomy*, 35th edn with permission.

Lower limb

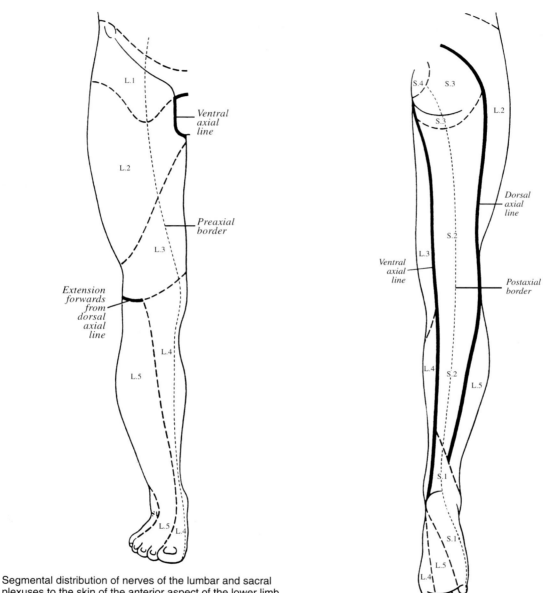

Segmental distribution of nerves of the lumbar and sacral plexuses to the skin of the anterior aspect of the lower limb.

Segmental distribution of nerves of the lumbar and sacral plexuses to the skin of the posterior aspect of the lower limb.

Figure A7.2   Reproduced from *Gray's Anatomy*, 35th edn with permission.

Appendix 8
Useful addresses and equipment suppliers

LIST OF USEFUL ADDRESSES

Access Travel (Lancs) Ltd Holidays for Disabled Persons
16 Haweswater Avenue
Astley
Lancs M29 7BL

Banstead Place Mobility Centre
Damson Way
Orchard Hill
Queen Mary's Avenue
Carshalton
Surrey SM5 4NR

British Paraplegic Sports Society Ltd and *The British Sports Association for the Disabled*
Stoke Mandeville Sports Stadium for the Paralysed and Other Disabled
Harvey Road
Aylesbury
Buckinghamshire

Carers National Association
Maidstone Community Support Centre
Marsham Street
Maidstone
Kent ME14 1HH

Centre for Accessible Environments
Nutmeg House
60 Gainsford Street
London SE1 2NY

Disabled Advice Service
305 Garratt Lane
London SW18

The Disabled Drivers' Association
4 Laburnum Avenue
Wickford
Essex

The Disablement Income Group
19 Wedmore Street
London N19

Disabled Living Foundation
380–384 Harrow Road
London W9 2HU

Disability Law Service
40 Bedford Row
London WC1

Equipment for the Disabled
Mary Marlborough Lodge
Nuffield Orthopaedic Centre
Oxford OX3 7LD

International Co-ordinating Committee of the World Sports Organisations for the Disabled and *International Stoke Mandeville Games Federation*
Hayward House
Ludwig Guttmann Sports Centre
Barnard Crescent
Aylesbury
Buckinghamshire HP21 9PP

Joint Committee on Mobility for the Disabled
Wanborough Manor
Wanborough
Guildford
Surrey

Keep Able
Fleming Close
Park Farm
Wellingborough
Northants NN8 6UF

3M Healthcare Ltd
3M House
Morley Street
Loughborough
Leics LE11 1ET

Motability
Goodman House
Station Approach
Harlow
Essex CM20 2ET

The Pain Relief Foundation
Walton Hospital
Rice Lane
Liverpool L9 1EA

Society for Tissue Viability
Wessex Rehabilitation Association
Odstock Hospital
Salisbury
Wiltshire SOSP2 8BJ

Spinal Injuries Association
Yeoman House
76 St James Lane
London N10 3DF

EQUIPMENT SUPPLIERS
Automatic transmissions

Reselco Engineering Ltd
72 Black Lion Lane
Hammersmith
London W6

Chair power products

Chair Power Products plc
Malcolm House
583 Moseley Road
Birmingham B12 9BL

Chariot

Lomax Thomson Ltd
Kingsway East
Dundee
Scotland DD4 8ED

Countryside buggy suppliers

Able Buggies Ltd
Lane End Farm
Bare Heath
Wareham
Dorset BH20 7NS

Egerton–Stoke Mandeville Tilting and Turning Bed

Egerton Hospital Equipment Ltd
Tower Hill
Horsham
Sussex

Environment control systems

The Gemini System
Scientific and Technical Developments
Melbourne Road
Wallington
Surrey SM6 8SD

Possum Ltd
Middleton Green Road
Langley
Slough
Berkshire SL3 6DF

Femupan suppliers

A. J. Products
6 Hollow Road
Elmden
Essex CB11 4NA

Gymnastic ball

Central Medical Equipment Ltd
7 Ascot Park Estate
Lenton Street
Sandiacre
Nottingham NG10 5DL

Incontinence products

Condom urinals

GU Manufacturing Co Ltd
28a Devonshire Street
London W1

Conveen penile sheaths

Colloplast Ltd
Peterborough Business Park
Peterborough PE2 0FX

Oswestry standing frames

Theo Davies
Berwyn Mill
Glyn Ceiriog
Llangollen
Wrexham
South Wales LL20 7HN

Power pack

Alfred Bekker
Longtoft
Driffield
North Humberside YO25 0TF

Rear and other access vehicles

Team Traction
130 Sturry Road
Canterbury
Kent CT1 1DP

Sorbo packs

Vitafoam Ltd
Don Mill
Middleton
Manchester M24 2DB

Wheelchairs

Gerald Simmonds Healthcare Ltd
Gerald Simmonds Wheelchairs
Stoke Mandeville
9 March Place
Gatehouse Way
Aylesbury
Buckinghamshire HP19 3UG

Mobility 2000
Telford Industrial Centre
Stafford Park 4
Telford
Shropshire TF3 3BA

Levo stand-up wheelchair

Valutec Ltd
Steigstrasse 2
Ch-8610 Uster 3/Zurich

Sports and other wheelchairs

Cyclone
Ellesmere Port
South Wirral L66 1BR

References

Ada L, Canning C 1990 Anticipating and avoiding muscle shortening. In: Ada L, Canning C (eds) Key issues in neurological physiotherapy: physiotherapy foundations for practice. Butterworth Heinemann, Oxford

Aisen P S, Aisen M L 1994 Shoulder-hand syndrome in cervical spinal cord injury. Paraplegia 32: 588–592

Anderson T J, Rivest J, Stell R, Steiger M J, Cohen H, Thompson P D, Marsden C D 1992 Botulinum toxin treatment of spasmodic torticollis. Journal of the Royal Society of Medicine 85: 524–529

Anke A G W, Stenchjem A E, Kvalvik Stanghelle J 1995 Pain and life quality within two years of spinal cord injury. Paraplegia 33: 555–559

Ashley E A, Laskin R D, Olenik L M, Burnham, Steadward R D, Cummimg D C, Wheeler G D 1993 Evidence of autonomic dysreflexia during functional electrical stimulation in individuals with spinal cord injuries. Paraplegia 31: 593–605

ASIA 1994 Reference manual. International standards for neurological and functional classification of spinal cord injury. American Spinal Injury Association

Aung T S, El Masry W S 1997 Audit of a British centre for spinal injury. Spinal Cord 35: 147–150

Bagley J C, Cochran T P, Sledge C B 1987 The impingement syndrome in paraplegia. Journal of Bone-Joint Surgery America 69: 676–678

Bajd T, Kralji A, Turk R, Benko H, Sega J 1989 Use of functional electrical stimulation in the treatment of patients with incomplete spinal cord injuries. Journal of Biomedical Engineering 11: 96–102

Balazy T E 1992 Clinical Management of pain in spinal cord injury. Clinical Journal of Pain 8: 102–110

Banavic K, Gonzalez F 1997 Evaluation and management of heterotopic ossification in persons with spinal cord injury. Spinal Cord 35: 158–162

Banja J D 1990 Rehabilitation and empowerment [commentary]. Archives of Physical Medicine and Rehabilitation 71: 614–615

Banta J V, Bell K J, Muik E A, Fezio J 1991 Parawalker energy cost of walking. Journal of Pediatric Surgery 1(suppl. 11): 7–19

Bar C A 1991 Evaluation of cushions using dynamic pressure measurement. Prosthetics and Orthotics International 15: 232–240

Barr F M D, Harper V J, Rushton D N, Taylor P N, Tromans

A, Phillips G F, Hagen S A, Wood D 1995 Screening and assessment for a lumbosacral anterior root stimulation implant programme. In: 5th Vienna International Workshop, August. Department of Biomedical Engineering and Physics, University of Vienna, p 95–98

Basmajian V J 1978 Muscles alive: their function revealed by electromyography, 4th edn. Williams and Wilkins, London, p 186

Bedbrook G 1981 The care and management of spinal cord injuries. Springer-Verlag, New York

Bedbrook G M 1985 A balanced viewpoint in the early management of patients with spinal cord injuries who have neurological damage. Paraplegia 23: 8–15

Bennett G J, 1991 The role of the sympathetic nervous system in painful peripheral neuropathy. Pain 45: 221–223

Bergborn-Engberg I, Haljamae H 1989 Assessment of patients' experience of discomforts during respirator therapy. Critical Care Medicine 17(10): 1068–1071

Bergström E M K 1994. Childhood spinal cord lesion: its effect on skeletal development, growth and lung function – a retrospective study. Master's thesis, Loughborough University of Technology

Bergström E M K, Frankel H L, Galer I A R, Haycock E L, Jones P R M, Rose L S 1985 Physical ability in relation to anthropometric measurements in persons with complete spinal cord lesions below the sixth cervical segment. International Rehabilitation Medicine 7(2): 51–55

Biss S, Fox B 1988 Functional electrical stimulation in incomplete tetraplegia. Physiotherapy Practice 4: 163–167

Bobath B 1985 Abnormal postural reflex activity caused by brain lesions. Heinemann Physiotherapy, London

Bobath B 1990 Adult hemiplegia: evaluation and treatment, 3rd edn. Heinemann Medical Books, Oxford

Bodenhamer E, Achterberg-Lawlis J, Kevorkian G et al 1983 Staff and patient perceptions of the psychosocial concerns of spinal cord injured persons. American Journal of Physical Medicine 62(4): 182–193

Bogie K M, Nuseibeh I, Bader D L, 1995 Progressive changes in tissue viability in the seated spinal cord injured subject. Paraplegia 33: 141–147

Boorman G L, Lee R G, Becker W J, Windhorst U R 1996 Impaired "natural reciprocal inhibition" in patients with spasticity due to incomplete cord injury. Electroencephalography and Clinical Neurophysiology 101: 84–92

Bowker P, Messenger N, Ogilvie C, Rowley D 1992 The energetics of paraplegic walking. Journal of Biomedical Engineering. 14: 344–350

Bowsher D 1996 Control pain of spinal origin. Spinal Cord 34: 707–710

Braus D F, Strobel J 1991 The shoulder-hand syndrome after stroke: a prospective study. Annual Neurology 30: 278–279

Bravo P, Labarta C, Alcaraz M A, Mendoza J, Verdu A 1996 An assessment of factors affecting neurological recovery after spinal cord injury with vertebral fracture. Paraplegia 34: 164–166

Brindley G S 1984 The fertility of men with spinal injuries. Paraplegia 22: 326–337

Brindley G S, 1994 The first 500 patients with sacral anterior root stimulator implants: general description. Paraplegia 32: 795–805

Brindley G S 1995 The first 500 anterior root stimulators: implant failures and their repair. Paraplegia 33: 5–9

Brindley G S, Rushton D N 1990 Long-term follow up of patients with sacral anterior root stimulator implants. Paraplegia 28: 469–475

Brooks V B 1986 The neural basis of motor control. Oxford University Press, Oxford

Brouwer B, Hopkins-Russel H 1997 Motor cortical mapping of proximal upper extremity muscles following spinal cord injury. Spinal Cord 35: 205–212

Brown P 1994 Pathophysiology of spasticity. Journal of Neurology, Neurosurgery and Psychiatry 57: 773–777

Burke D C 1972 Spinal cord trauma in children. Paraplegia 9: 1–14

Burke D C 1974 Traumatic spinal paralysis in children. Paraplegia 11: 268–276

Butler P B, Major R E 1971 The Para-Walker – a rational approach to the provision of reciprocal ambulation for paraplegic patients. Physiotherapy 73: 393–397

Cailliet R 1987 The shoulder in hemiplegia, 5th edn. F A Davis, Philadelphia

Calachis S C 1992 Autonomic hyperreflexia with spinal cord injury. American Paraplegia Society 15(3): 171–186

Capaul M, Zollinger H, Satz N, Diety V, Lehmann D, Schurch B 1994 Analyses of 94 consecutive spinal cord injury patients, using ASIA definition and modified Frankel score classification. Paraplegia 32: 583–58

Carr J H, Shepherd R B, Ada L 1995 Spasticity: research findings and implications for intervention. Physiotherapy 81: 421–429

Chawla J C, 1993 Rehabilitation of spinal cord injured patients on long term ventilation. Paraplegia 31: 88–92

Cheshire J E, Flack W J 1979 The use of operant physiotherapy techniques in respiratory rehabilitation of the tetraplegic. Paraplegia 16: 162

Cheshire D J E, Rowe G 1971 The prevention of deformity in the severely paralysed hand. Paraplegia 8: 48–56

Coghlan J K, Robinson C E, Newmarch B, Jackson G 1980 Lower extremity bracing in paraplegia – a follow up study. Paraplegia 188: 25–32

Collier P S, Wakeling L M 1982 Diaphragmatic pacing: a new procedure for high spinal cord lesions. Physiotherapy 68(2): 47

Cordo P J, Nashner L M 1982 Properties of postural adjustments associated with rapid arm movements. Journal of Neurophysiology 47: 287–302

Cosgrove A P, Corry I S, Graham H K 1984 Botulinum toxin in the management of the lower limb in cerebral palsy. Developmental Medicine & Child Neurology 36: 386–396

Craig A R, Hancock K M, Dickson H G 1994 A longitudinal investigation into anxiety and depression in the first 2 years following a spinal cord injury. Paraplegia 32: 675–679

Crawford H J, Jull G A 1993 The influence of thoracic posture and movement on range of arm elevation. Physiotherapy Theory and Practice 9: 143–148

Crozier K S, Graziani V, Ditunno J F, Herbison G J 1991 Spinal cord injury: Prognosis for ambulation based on sensory examination in patients who are initially motor complete. Archives of Physical Medicine 72: 119–121

Curtin M 1994 Development of a tetraplegic hand assessment and splinting protocol. Paraplegia 32: 159–169

Curtis K A, Roach K E, Brooks Applegate E, Amar T, Benbow C S, Genecco T D, Guelano J 1995 Development of the Wheelchair Users' Shoulder Pain Index (WUSPI). Paraplegia 33: 290–293, 595–601

Cushman L A, Dijkers M 1991 Depressed mood during rehabilitation of persons with spinal cord injury. Journal of Rehabilitation 57(2): 35–38

Cushman L A, Marcel P, Dijkers P 1990 Depressed mood in spinal cord injury patients: staff perceptions and patient realities. Archives of Physical Medicine and Rehabilitation 71: 191–196

Danon J, Dauz I S S, Goldberg N B, Sharpe J T 1979 Function of the isolated paced diaphragm and the cervical accessory muscles in CI quadriplegia. American Review of Respiratory Diseases 119: 909

Das T K, Park D M 1989 Botulinum toxin in treating spasticity. British Journal of Clinical Practice 43: 401–403

Dattola R, Girlanda P, Vita G, Santoro M, Tascano A, Venuto C, Baradello A, Messina C 1993 Muscle rearrangement in patients with hemiparesis after stroke: an electrophysiological and morphological study. European Neurology 33: 109–114

Daverat P, Petit H, Kamoun G, Dartigues J F, Barat M 1995 The long term outcome in 149 patients with spinal cord injury. Paraplegia 33: 665–668

Davidoff R A 1992 Skeletal muscle tone and the misunderstood stretch reflex. Neurology 42: 951–963

Davies P M 1990 Right in the middle. Springer-Verlag, Berlin

Davies P M 1994 Starting Again. Springer-Verlag, Berlin

Davies S, Illis L S, Raisman G 1995 Regeneration in the central nervous system and related factors. Summary of the Bermuda Paraplegia Conference, April 1994. International Spinal Research Trust

De Troyer A, Estenne M 1991 The expiratory muscles in tetraplegia. Paraplegia 29: 359–363

De Troyer A, Kelly S, Zin Wa 1983 Mechanical action of the intercostal muscles on the ribs. Science 220: 87–88

De Vivo M J, Rutt R D, Black K J, Go B K, Stover S L 1992 Trends in spinal cord injury demographics and treatment outcomes between 1973 and 1986. Archives of Physical Medicine and Rehabilitation 73: 424–430

Dietz V 1992 Human neuronal control of automatic functional movements: interaction between central programs and afferent input. Physiological Reviews 72(1): 33–69

Dietz V, Colombo G, Jensen L, Baumgartner L 1995 Locomotor capacity of spinal cord in paraplegic patients. Annual Neurology 37: 574–578

Dimitrijevic M R, Faganel J, Lehmkuhl D, Sherwood A 1983 Motor control in man after partial or complete spinal cord injury. In: Desmedt J E (ed) Motor control mechanisms in health and disease. Raven Press, New York

Ditunno J F, Young W, Donovan W H, Creasey G 1994 The international standards booklet for neurological and functional classification of spinal cord injuries. Paraplegia 32: 70–80

Dobkin B H 1994 New frontiers in SCI rehabilitation. Journal of Neuro-rehabilitation 8: 33–39

Dollfus P, Ball J M, Zimmerman M D R, Claudron J 1983 A driving adaptation for tetraplegic persons and a travelling adaptation device for paraplegic persons. Paraplegia 21: 127–130

Douglas R, Larsonn P F, D'Ambrosia R, McCall R E 1983 The L S U reciprocating gait orthosis. Orthopaedics 6: 834–839

Dover H, Pickard W, Swain I, Grundy D 1992 The effectiveness of a pressure clinic in preventing pressure sores. Paraplegia 30: 267–272

Drewes A M, Andreason A, Poulsen L H 1994 Valproate for treatment of chronic central pain after spinal cord injury. A double-blind cross-over study. Paraplegia 32: 565–569

Duffus A, Wood J 1983 Standing and walking for the paraplegic. Physiotherapy 79(2): 45–46

Edwards S 1996 Neurological physiotherapy: a problem-solving approach. Churchill Livingstone, Edinburgh

Edwards S, Charlton P 1996 Splinting and the use of orthoses in the management of patients with neurological disorders. In: Edwards S (ed) Neurological physiotherapy: a problem-solving approach. Churchill Livingstone, Edinburgh

El Masry W S 1993 Physiological instability of the spinal cord following injury. Paraplegia 31: 273–275

El Masry W S, Katoh S, Khan A 1993 Reflections on the neurological significance of bony canal encroachment following traumatic injury of the spine in patients with Frankel C D E presentation. Journal of Neurotrauma 10 (suppl. 1): 70

El Masry W S, Silver J R 1981 Prophylactic anticoagulant therapy in patients with spinal cord injury. Paraplegia 19: 334–342

El Masry W S, Tsubo M, Katoh M, El Miligui Y H S, Khan A 1996 Validation of the American Spinal Injury Association (ASIA) Motor Score and the National Acute Spinal Cord Injury Study (NASCIS) Motor Score. Spine 21(5): 614–619

Ellis R 1995 The patient's evaluation of reciprocating gait orthoses. Secretariat of 8th World Congress of International Society of Prosthetics and Orthotics, Melbourne, Australia

Eltorai I, Montroy R 1990 Muscle release in the management of spasticity in spinal cord injury. Paraplegia 28(7): 433–440

Ersmarke H, Dalan N, Kalan R 1990 Cervical spine injuries: a follow-up of 332 patients. Paraplegia 28: 25–40

Esclarin A, Bravo P, Arroyo O, Mazaira J, Garrido H, Alcaraz M A 1994 Tracheostomy ventilation versus diaphragmatic pacemaker ventilation in high spinal cord injury. Paraplegia 32: 687–693

Figoni S F 1984 Cardiovascular and haemodynamic response to tilting and to standing in tetraplegic patients. Paraplegia 22: 99–109

Foo D, Subrahmanyan T S, Rossier A B 1981 Post-traumatic acute anterior spinal cord syndrome. Paraplegia 19: 201–205

Frank R G, Elliott T R 1989 Spinal cord injury and health locus of control beliefs. Paraplegia 27: 250–256

Frankel H L 1968 Associated chest injuries. Paraplegia 5: 221–225

Frankel H L 1974 Intermittent catheterization. Urologic Clinics of North America 1(1): 115–124

Frankel H L, El Masry W S, Ravichandran G 1987 Non-operative treatment: rehabilitation and outcome. In: Advances in Neurotraumatology, vol 2. Springer Verlag, Vienna

Frankel H L, Hancock D O, Hyslop G, Melzak J, Michaelis L S, Vernon J D S, Walsh J J 1970 The value of postural reduction in the initial management of closed injuries of the spine with paraplegia and tetraplegia. Paraplegia 7: 179–192

Fung J, Stewart J E, Barbeau H 1990 The combined effects of clonidine and cyproheptadine with interactive training on modulation of locomotion in spinal cord subjects. Journal of Neurological Sciences 100: 85–93

Furher M J, Rintola D H, Hart K A et al 1992 Relationship of life satisfaction to impairment, disability and handicap among persons with spinal cord injuries living in the community. Archives of Physical Medicine and Rehabilitation 73: 552–557

Gage J R 1991 Gait analysis in cerebral palsy. Mac Keith Press, London, pp 92, 93, 95

Gage J R 1992 An overview of normal walking. In: Perry J (ed) Gait analysis: normal and pathological function. Slack Inc., New Jersey

Gerhart K A, Bergström E, Charlifue S W, Menter R R, Whiteneck G G 1993 Long-term spinal cord injury: functional changes over time. Archives of Physical Medicine and Rehabilitation 74: 1030–1034

Gianino J 1993 Intrathecal baclofen for spinal spasticity: implications for nursing practice. Journal of Neuroscience Nursing 25(4): 254–264

Given J D, Dewald J P A, Rymer W Z 1995 Joint dependent passive stiffness in paretic and contralateral limbs of spastic patients with hemiparetic stroke. Journal of Neurology, Neurosurgery and Psychiatry 59: 271–279

Glass C A 1993 The impact of home based ventilator dependence on family life. Paraplegia 31: 93–101

Glenn W L, Hogan J F, Loke J S O, Ciesielski T E, Phelps M L, Rowedder R 1984 Ventilatory support by pacing of the conditioned diaphragm in quadriplegia. The New England Journal of Medicine 310(18): 1150–1155

Glenn W L, Phelps M L, Elefteriades J A, Dentz B, Hogan J F 1986 Twenty years of experience in nerve stimulation to pace the diaphragm. Pace 9(1): 780–784

Goldman J M, Rose L S, Williams S J, Silver J R, Dension D M 1986 The Effect of abdominal binders on breathing in tetraplegic patients. Thorax 41(12): 940–945

Goldspink G, Williams P 1990 Muscle and connective tissue changes associated with use and disuse. In: Ada L, Canning C (eds) Key issues in neurological physiotherapy: physiotherapy foundations for practice. Butterworth Heinemann, Oxford

Granat M H, Ferguson A C B, Andrews B J, Delargy M 1993 The role of functional electrical stimulation in the rehabilitation of patients with incomplete spinal cord injury-observed benefits during gait studies. Paraplegia 31: 207–215

Gray's Anatomy 1995 Gray's Anatomy, 38th edn. Churchill Livingstone, Edinburgh

Green B C, Pratt C C, Grisby T E 1984 Self-concept among persons with long-term spinal cord injury. Archives of Physical Medicine and Rehabilitation 65: 751–754

Green E M, Nelham R L, 1991 Development of sitting ability, assessment of children with a motor handicap and prescription of appropriate seating systems. Prosthetica and Orthotics International 15: 203–216

Gupta A, McClelland M R, Evans A, El Masry W S 1989 Mini-tracheostomy in the early respiratory management of patients with spinal injury. Paraplegia 27: 269–277

Guttmann L 1945 New hope for spinal cord sufferers. New York Medical Times 73: 318

Guttmann L 1946a Rehabilitation after injury to spinal cord and cauda equina. British Journal of Physical Medicine 9: 130–160

Guttmann L 1946b Postural reduction. Nursing Times 42: 798

Guttmann L 1970 Spinal shock and reflex behaviour in man. Paraplegia 8: 100–111

Guttmann L, Sir 1976 Spinal cord injuries. Comprehensive management and research: (a) Hypertrophy of muscle, p 577; (b) Postural sensibility, p 582; (c) Sport, p 617–627; (d) Guttmann's sign, p 261

Guttmann E, Guttmann L 1942 The effect of electrotherapy on denervated muscles in rabbits: muscle bulk increased. Lancet 1: 169

Guttmann E, Guttmann L 1944 The effect of galvanic exercise on denervated and re-innervated muscles. Journal of Neurology and Neurosurgery 7: 7

Guttmann L, Sir, Silver J R 1965 Electromyographic studies on reflex activity of the intercostal and abdominal muscles in the cervical cord lesion. Paraplegia 3: 1–22

Hachen H J 1978 Psychological, neurophysiological and therapeutic aspects of chronic pain. Preliminary results with transcutaneous electrical stimulation. Paraplegia 15: 353–367

Haffner D L, Hoffer M M 1993 Etiology of children's spinal injuries at Rancho Los Amigos. Spine 18: 679–684

Hallett M, Cohen L G, Pascual-Leone A, Brasil-Nelo J, Wassermann E M, Commarota A N 1993 Plasticity of human motor cortex spasticity: mechanisms and management. Springer-Verlag, Berlin

Haln H R 1970 Lower extremity bracing in paraplegia with usage follow up. Paraplegia 8(3): 147–153

Hammell K W 1995 Spinal cord injury rehabilitation. Therapy in practice series. Chapman and Hall, London

Harris-Warwick R M, Sparks D L 1995 Neural control: editorial overview. Current Opinion in Neurology 5: 721–726

Harvey L A, Ellis E R 1993 The effect of continuous positive airway pressures on lung volumes in tetraplegic patients. Paraplegia 34: 54–58

Hasler D 1981 Developing a sense of symmetry. Therapy Weekly Aug 27: 3

Haymaker W 1969 Bing's local diagnosis in neurological diseases, 15th edn. Mosby, St Louis

Heckman C J 1994 Alterations in synaptic input to motorneurons during partial spinal cord injury. Medicine and Science in Sports and Exercise 26: 1480–1490

Henderson J L, Price S H, Brandstater M E, Mandac B R 1994 Efficacy of three measures to relieve pressure in seated persons with spinal cord injury. Archives of Physical Medicine and Rehabilitation 75: 535–539

Herbert R 1988 The passive mechanical properties of muscle and their adaptations to altered patterns of use. Australian Journal of Physiotherapy 34: 141–149

Hermens H J et al 1994 Advances in hybrid systems. A paper presented at the 10th Congress of the International Society of Electrophysiology and Kinesiology, Charleston, USA June 1994

Hill V B, Davies W E 1988 A swing to intermittent clean self-catheterisation as a preferred mode of management of the neuropathic bladder for the dextrous spinal cord person. Paraplegia 26: 405–412

Hirsch I H, Sager S W J, Seder J, King L, Staas W E 1990 Electro-ejaculatory stimulation of quadriplegic man. Archives of Physical Medicine and Rehabilitation 71: 54–57

Hong C, Sna Luis E B, Chung S 1990 Follow up study on the use of leg braces issued to spinal cord injury patients. Paraplegia 28: 172–177

Horak F B, Esselman P, Anderson M E, Lynch M K 1984 The effects of movement velocity, mass displaced, and task certainty on associated postural adjustments made by normal and hemiplegic individuals. Journal of Neurology, Neurosurgery and Psychiatry 47: 1020–1028

Horn S 1989 Coping with Bereavement. Thorsons, Wellingborough, p 104

Houston J M 1984 Comprehensive education for those concerned with spinal cord injury patients. Paraplegia 22(4): 244–248

Hughes J T 1984 Regeneration in the human spinal cord: a review of the response to injury of the various constituents of the human spinal cord. Paraplegia 22: 131–137

Hunter Peckham P 1987 FES: current status and future prospects of applications to the neuromuscular system in spinal cord injury. Paraplegia 25: 279–288

Jackson S E 1983 IPPB. In: Downie P A (ed) Cash's textbook of chest, heart and vascular disorders for physiotherapists, 3rd edn. Faber and Faber, London

Jacob K S, Zachariah K, Bhathachargi S 1995 Depression in individuals with spinal cord injury : methodological issues. Paraplegia 33: 377–380

Jaeger R J, Yarkany G M, Roth E J, Lovell L 1990 Estimating the population of a simple electrical stimulation system for standing. Paraplegia: 505–511

Jansen T W J, van Oers C A J M, Veegen H E J, Hollander A P, van der Woude L H V, Rozendal R H 1994 Relationship between physical strain during standardised ADL tasks and physical capacity in men with spinal cord injury. Paraplegia 32: 844–859

Johnson J E, Dabbs J M, Leventhal H 1970 Psychosocial factors in the welfare of surgical patients. Nursing Research 19: 18–19

Johnston M, Gilbert P, Partridge C, Collins J 1992 Changing perceived control in patients with physical disabilities: an intervention study with patients receiving rehabilitation. British Journal of Psychology 31: 89–94

Judd F K 1986 Depression following spinal cord injury: a prospective inpatient study. British Journal of Psychiatry 156: 668–671

Judd F K, Burrows G D 1986 Liaison psychiatry in a spinal unit (Australia). Paraplegia 24: 6–19

Judd F K, Franz C P, Brown D J 1988 The psychosocial approach to rehabilitation of the spinal cord injured patient. Paraplegia 26: 419–424

Katz R T, Rymer W Z 1989 Spastic hypertonia: mechanisms and measurement. Archives of Physical Medicine and Rehabilitation 70: 144–155

Keith M W, Hunter Peckham P, Thrope G B, Stroh K C, Smith B, Buckett J R, Kilgore K L 1989 Implantable functional neuromuscular stimulation in the tetraplegic hand. Journal of Hand Surgery (American volume)14A: 524–530

Kennedy D W, Smith R W 1990 A comparison of past and future leisure activity participation between spinal cord injured and non-disabled persons. Paraplegia 28: 130–136

Kilgore K L, Hunter Peckham P, Keith M W, Thorpe G B, Wuolie K S, Bryden A S, Hart R L 1997 An implanted upper extremity neuroprosthesis: follow-up of 5 patients. Journal of Bone and Joint Surgery 79-A(4): 533–541

Knott M, Voss D E 1968 Proprioceptive neuromuscular facilitation. Baillière Tindall and Cassel, London

Lance J W 1980 Symposium synopsis. In: Feldman R G, Young R R, Koella W P (eds) Spasticity: disordered motor control. Year Book Medical Publishers, Chicago

Lancourt J E, Dickson J H, Carter R E 1981 Paralytic spinal deformity following traumatic spinal cord injury in children and adolescents. The Journal of Bone and Joint Surgery 63A (1): 47–53

Ledsome J R, Sharp J M 1981 Pulmonary function in an acute cervical cord injury. American Review of Respiratory Diseases 124: 41

Levy W J, Amassian V E, Traad M, Cadwell J 1990 Focal magnetic coil stimulation reveals motor cortical systems reorganised after traumatic quadriplegia. Brain Research 501: 130–134

Lewis Y 1989 Use of the gymnastic ball in the treatment of adult hemiplegia. Physiotherapy 75(7): 421–424

Losseff N, Thompson A J 1995 The medical management of increased tone. Physiotherapy 81: 480–484

Lotta S, Fiocchi A, Giovannini R, Silvestrin R, Tesio L, Raschi A, Macchia L et al 1994 Restoration of gait with orthoses in thoracic paraplegia: a multicentre investigation. Paraplegia 31: 608–615

Lynch M, Grisogono V 1991 Strokes and head injuries. John Murray, London

McGarry J, Woolsey R, Thompson C W 1982 Autonomic hyperreflexia following passive stretching to the hip joint. Physical Therapy 62(1): 30–31

McGowan M B, Roth S 1987 Family functioning and family independence in spinal cord injury adjustment. Paraplegia 25: 357–365

MacLeod A D 1988 Self-neglect of spinal injured patients. Paraplegia 26: 340–349

MacLeod G M, MacLeod L 1996 Evaluation of client and staff satisfaction with a goal planning project implemented with people with spinal cord injury. Spinal Cord 34: 525–530

Martin J 1981 The Halliwick method. Physiotherapy 67(10): 288–291

Maroon J C, Abla A A, Wilberger J I, Bailes J E, Sternau L L 1991 Central cord syndrome. Clinical Neurosurgery 37: 612–621

Mathson-Prince J 1997 A rational approach to long term care: comparing the independent living model with agency-based care for persons with high spinal cord injuries. Spinal Cord 35: 326–331

Mayfield J K, Erkkila J C, Winter R B 1981 Spine deformity subsequent to acquired childhood spinal cord injury. The Journal of Bone and Joint surgery 63a.9: 1401–1411

Maynard F M, Karunas R S, Warung W P 1990 Epidemiology of spasticity following traumatic spinal cord injury. Archives of Physical Medicine and Rehabilitation 71: 566–569

Mazur J M, Shurtleff D, Menelaus M, Colliver J 1989 Orthopaedic management of high-level spina bifida. Journal of Bone and Joint Surgery 71A: 56–61

Melia J L 1997 Development of orthoses for people with paraplegia. Physiotherapy 83: 23–25

Michaelis L S 1964 Myotomy of iliopsoas and obliquis externus abdominis for severe spastic flexion contracture at the hip. Paraplegia 2: 287–294

Moore P, Stallard J 1991 A clinical review of adult paraplegia patients with complete lesions using the ORLAU Para Walker. Paraplegia 29: 191–196

Morgan M D L, De Troyer A 1984 The individuality of chest wall motion in tetraplegia. Thorax 39: 237

Morgan M D L, Gourlay A R, Denison D M 1984 An optical method of studying shape and movement of the chest wall in recumbent patients. Thorax 101: 235

Morse S D 1982 Acute central cervical cord syndrome. Annals of Emergency Medicine 11: 436–439

Motlock W M 1992 Principles of orthotic management for child and adult paraplegia and clinical experience with the isocentric RGO. In: Proceedings of the 7th World Congress of the International Society of Prosthetics and Orthotics, Chicago, p 28

Muir G D, Steeves J D 1997 Sensorimotor stimulation to improve locomotor recovery after spinal cord injury. TINS 20: 72–77

Nakajima M, Hirayama K 1995 Midcervical central cord syndrome: numb and clumsy hands due to midline disc protrusion at the C3–4 intervertebral level. Journal of Neurology, Neurosurgery and Psychiatry 58: 607–613

Nene A V, Hermens H T, Zilvold G 1996 Paraplegic locomotion: a review. Spinal Cord 34: 507–524

Nene A V, Patrick J H 1990 Energy cost of paraplegic locomotion using the parawalker electrical stimulation 'hybrid' orthosis. Archives of Physical Medicine and Rehabilitation 71: 116–120

Noble P C 1981 The prevention of pressure sores in persons with spinal cord injury. Monograph 11 International Exchange of Information in Rehabilitation, World Rehabilitation Fund, Inc., New York

Nordholm L, Westbrook M 1986 Effects of depression, self blame and dependency on health professionals' evaluation of paraplegic patients. Australian Occupational Therapy Journal 33(2): 59–70

Ohry A, Brooks M E, Steinbach T V, Rogin R 1978 Shoulder complications as a cause of delay in rehabilitation of spinal cord injured patients. Paraplegia 16: 310–316

Oliver M, Zarb G, Silver J, Moore M, Salisbury V 1991 Walking into darkness. The experience of spinal cord injury. MacMillan, Basingstoke

Osenbach R K, Menezes A H, 1989 Spinal cord without radiographic abnormality in children. Pediatric Neuroscience 15: 168–175

Ozer M N 1988 The management of persons with spinal cord injuries. Demos, New York, p 107–113

Pachalski A, Pachalski M M 1984 Programme of active education in the psycho-social integration of paraplegics. Paraplegia 22(4): 238–243

Pang D, Pollack I F 1989 Spinal cord injury without radiographic abnormality in children – the SCIWORA syndrome. Journal of Trauma 29: 654–664

Partridge C, Johnston M 1989 Perceived control of recovery from physical disability: measurement and prediction. British Journal of Clinical Psychology 28: 53–59

Peacock W J, Shrosbree R D, Key A G 1977 A review of 450 stab wounds of the spinal cord. South African Medical Journal 51: 961–964

Peloquin S M 1990 The patient-therapist relationship in occupational therapy: understanding visions and images. American Journal of Occupational Therapy. 44: 13–21

Pelser H, van Gijn J 1993 Spinal infarction. A follow-up study. Stroke 24(6): 896–898

Penrod L E, Hegde S K, Ditunno J F 1990 Age effect on prognosis for functional recovery in acute, traumatic central cord syndrome. Archives of Physical Medicine and Rehabilitation 71: 963–968

Pentland W E, Twomey P L D 1994 Upper limb function in persons with long term paraplegia and implications for independence: parts 1 and 2. Paraplegia 32: 211–224

Perry J 1992 Pathological gait. In: Perry J (ed) Gait analysis: normal and pathological function. Slack Inc., New Jersey

Petrofsky J S, Phillips C A, Larson P, Douglas R 1985 Computer synthesised walking: an application of orthosis and functional electrical stimulation (FES). Journal of Neurological and Orthopaedic Medicine and Surgery 63: 219–230

Phillips C A 1989 Electrical muscle stimulation in combination with a reciprocating gait orthosis for ambulation by paras. Journal of Biomedical Engineering 11: 338–344

Pool G M, Weerden G J V 1973 Experiences with frog breathing tetraplegic polio victims as telephone operators. Paraplegia 11: 253

Porter B 1997 Review of intrathecal baclofen in the management of spasticity. British Journal of Nursing 6: 253–262

Quencer R M, Bunge R P, Egnor M, Green B A, Puckett W, Naidich T P, Post M J D, Norenberg M 1992 Acute traumatic central cord syndrome: MRI-pathological correlations. Neuroradiology 34: 85–94

Rasch P J, Burke R K 1971 Kinesiology and applied anatomy. Febiger, Philadelphia

Ray C 1984 Social, sexual and personal implications of paraplegia. Paraplegia 22: 75–86

Reswick J B, Rogers J E 1976 Maximum suggested pressure/time application over bony prominences. In: Barbenel, Forbes and Lowe (eds) Pressure sores. Macmillan, London

Rodriguez G P, Garber S L 1994 Prospective study of pressure ulcer risk in spinal cord injury patients. Paraplegia 32: 150–158

Rose G K, Butler P, Stallard J 1982 Gait: principles, biomechanics and assessment. Orlau, Oswestry

Rose L, Geary M, Jackson J, Morgan M 1987 The effect of lung volume expansion in tetraplegia. Physiotherapy Practice 3: 163–167

Rossier A B, Foo D, Shillito J, Dyro F M 1985 Post traumatic cervical syringomyelia. Brain 108: 439–461

Roth E J, Lawler M H, Yarkony G M 1990 Traumatic central cord syndrome: clinical features and functional outcomes. Archives of Physical Medicine and Rehabilitation 71: 18–23

Rothery F A 1989 Preliminary evaluation of a pressure clinic in a new spinal injuries unit. Paraplegia 27: 36–40

Rothwell J 1994 Control of human voluntary movement, 2nd edn. Chapman and Hall, London

Rotter J B 1966 Generalised expectations for internal control of reinforcement. Psychological Monographs 80(1): 609

Rushton D N 1996 Surface versus implanted electrodes in the daily application of FES. In: Pedotti A, Ferrarin M (eds) Restoration of walking for paraplegics: recent advances and trends. 10S Press, Oxford

Rushton D N, de N Donaldson, Barr F M D, Harper V J, Perkins T A, Taylor P N, Tromans A M 1995 Lumbar root stimulation for restoring leg function: results in Paraplegia 5th Vienna International Workshop on FES, August. Department of Biomedical Engineering and Physics, University of Vienna, p 39–42

Scher A T 1995 Body surfing injuries of the spinal cord. South African Medical Journal 82: 1022–1024

Schmidt R A 1991 Motor learning principles for physical therapy. In: Lister M (ed) Contemporary management of motor control problems. Foundations for Physical Therapy, Alexandria, VA

Schneider R C, Cherry G L, Pantek H E 1954 The syndrome of acute central cervical spinal cord injury. Journal of Neurosurgery 11: 546–577

Schuren J 1994 Working with soft cast. 3M Minnesota Mining and Manufacturing, Germany

Scott B A 1971 Engineering principles and fabrication techniques for the Scott–Craig long leg brace for paraplegics. Orthotics and Prosthetics 25: 14 –19

Scrutton D R 1971 A reciprocating brace with polyplanar hip hinges used on spina bifida children. Physiotherapy 57: 61–66

Scrutton J, Edwards S, Sheean G, Thompson A 1996 A little bit of toxin does you good? Phys. Res. Int. 3: 141–147

Shadish W R, Hickman D, Arvick M C 1981 Psychological problems of spinal cord injury patients, Emotional distress as a function of time and locus of control. Journal of Clinical and Consulting Psychology 49: 297

Shaw E 1995 Central cord syndrome presenting as unilateral weakness. American Journal of Medicine 13: 41–42

Short D I, Silver J R, Lehr R P 1991 Electromagnetic study of sternomastoid and scalene muscles in tetraplegic subjects. International Disability Studies 13: 46–49

Shumway-Cook A, Wollacott 1995 Motor control: theory and practical applications. Williams and Wilkins, London

Siddall P J, Taylor D A, Cousins M J, 1997 Classification of pain following spinal cord injury. Spinal Cord 35: 69–75

Silva A, Luginbuhl M 1981 Balancing act treatment. Therapy Weekly, Aug 27: 3

Silver J R 1975 The prophylactic use of anticoagulant therapy in the prevention of pulmonary emboli in one hundred consecutive spinal patients. Paraplegia 12: 188–196

Silver J R 1996 Association between muscle trauma and heterotopic ossification in spinal cord injured patients. Spinal Cord 34: 499–500

Silver J R, Moulton A 1970 The physiological sequelae of paralysis of the intercostal and abdominal muscles in tetraplegic patients. Paraplegia 7: 131–141

Sinderby C, Ingvarsson P, Sullivan L 1992 The role of the diaphragm in trunk extension in tetraplegia. Paraplegia 30: 389–395

Snoecx M, De Muynck M, Van Laere M 1995 Association between muscle trauma and heterotopic ossification in spinal cord injured patients: reflections on their causal relationship and the diagnostic value of ultrasonography. Paraplegia 33: 464–468

Snow B J, Tsui J K C, Varelas M, Hashimoto S A, Calne D B 1990 Treatment of spasticity with botulinum toxin: A double-blind study. Annals of Neurology 28: 512–515

Soryal I, Sinclair E, Hornby J, Pentland B 1992 Impaired joint mobility in Guillain–Barre syndrome : a primary or secondary phenomenon? Journal of Neurology, Neurosurgery and Psychiatry 55: 1014–1017

Stallard J 1986 Reciprocal walking orthoses for paraplegic patients. British Journal of Therapy and Rehabilitation 3(8): 420–425

Stallard J 1993 The case for lateral stiffness in walking orthoses for paraplegic patients. Prosthetics Institute Mechanical Engineers 207: 2–7

Stallard J, Major R E 1995 The influence of orthosis stiffness on paraplegic ambulation. Prosthetics and Orthotics International 19: 108–114

Stallard J S, Major R E, Patrick J H 1989 A review of fundamental design problems of providing ambulation for

paraplegic patients. Paraplegia 27: 70–75

Steele J, Blackwell B, Gutman M C, Jackson T C 1987 The activated patient dogma, dream or desideratum? Beyond advocacy: a review of the active patient concept. Patient Education and Counselling 10: 3–23

Stein R B, Belanger M, Wheeler G, Wieler M, Popovic D B, Prochazka A, Davis L A 1993 Electrical systems for improving locomotion after incomplete spinal cord injury: an assessment. Archives of Physical Medicine and Rehabilitation 74: 954–959

Stein R B, Brucker B S, Ayyar D R 1990 Motor units in incomplete spinal cord injury: electrical activity, contractile properties and the effects of biofeedback. Journal of Neurology, Neurosurgery and Psychiatry 53: 880–885

Stevenson V L, Playford E D, Langdon D W, Thompson A J 1996 Rehabilitation of incomplete spinal cord pathology: factors affecting prognosis and outcome. Journal of Neurology 243: 644–647

Stiller K, Simionato R, Rice K, Hall B 1992 The effect of intermittent positive pressure breathing on lung volume in acute quadriparesis. Paraplegia 30: 121–126

Stocking B 1996 King's Fund News 19(3): 3

Stover S L, De Lisa J A, Whiteneck G G, 1995 Spinal cord injury: clinical outcomes from model systems. Asper Publishers, Inc., Gaitlersburg, MD

Sullivan J 1989 Incomplete spinal cord injuries – nursing diagnoses. Dimensions of Critical Care Nursing 8: 338–346

Sutherland D H 1992 Gait analysis in neuromuscular diseases. In: Perry J (ed) Gait analysis: normal and pathological function. Slack Inc., New Jersey

Sutherland D H, Cooper L, Daniel D 1980 The role of the ankle plantar flexors in normal walking. Journal of Bone and Joint Surgery 62A: 354–363

Sweet W H, Poletti C E, Gybels J M 1995 Operations in the brainstem and spinal canal with an appendix on the relationship of open to percutaneous cordotomy. In: Wall P D, Melzack R (eds) Textbook of pain. 3rd edn. Churchill Livingstone, Edinburgh

Sykes L, Edwards J, Powell E S, Raymond E, Ross S 1995 The reciprocating gait orthosis: long term usage patterns. Archives of Physical Medicine and Rehabilitation 76: 779–783

Szollar S M, Martin E M E, Parthemore J G, Sartoris D J, Deflos L J 1997 Demineralisation in tetraplegic and paraplegic man over time. Spinal Cord 4: 223–228

Taktak D M 1997 An adjustable table tennis bat and grip system for tetraplegics. Spinal Cord 35: 61–63

Tetsuo O, Kagulo A, Masaaki N, Shigenu S, Kaguhisa D, Masaru S, Naoichi C 1996 Functional assessment of patients with spinal cord injuries measured by the motor score and the F I M. Spinal Cord 34: 531–535

Topka H, Cohen L G, Cole R A, Hallet M 1991 Reorganisation of corticospinal pathways following spinal cord injury. Neurology 41: 1276–1283

Trieschmann G 1988 Spinal cord injury, psychological, social and vocational rehabilitation, 2nd edn. Demos, New York

Tucker 1984 Patient-staff interaction with the spinal cord patient. In: Kruger D W (ed) Rehabilitation psychology. Aspin, Rockville MD, p 262

Turton A, Fraser C, Flament D, Werner W, Bennett K M B, Lemon R N 1993 Organisation of cortico-motorneural projections from the primary motor cortex: evidence for task-related function in monkey and in man. In:

Thilmamm A F, Burke D J, Rymer W Z (eds) Spasticity: mechanisms and management. Springer-Verlag, London

Uebelhart D, Demiaux-Domenech B, Roth M, Chantraine A 1995 Bone metabolism in spinal cord injured individuals, and in others who have prolonged immobilisation. A review. Paraplegia 33: 669–673

Uzerman M J, Stoffers T, Groen F, Klatte M, Snoek G, Vorsteveld H, Nathan R, Hermans H 1996 The NESS Handmaster orthosis: restoration of hand function in C5 and stroke patients by means of electrical stimulation. Journal of Rehabilitation Sciences 9(3): 208

Wallston K A, Wallston B S 1978 Locus of control and health, a review of the literature. Health Education Monographs (Spring): 107–117

Wallston K A, Wallston B S, Smith S, Dobbins C J 1987 Perceived control and health. Current Psychological Research and Reviews 6(1): 5–15

Waters R L, Sie I, Adkins R H, YaKura J S 1995 Motor recovery following spinal cord injury caused by stab wounds: a multicenter study. Paraplegia 33: 98–101

Webber B A, Proyer J A 1995 Physiotherapy for respiratory and cardiac problems. Churchill Livingstone, Edinburgh

Weiner, Laurie J A 1969 Human Biology: A guide to field methods. International biological programme handbook, no. 9. Blackwell Scientific Publications, Oxford

Whiteneck G G, Charlifue S W, Frankel H L, Fraser M H, Gardner B P, Gerhart K A, Krishnan K R et al 1992a Mortality, morbidity, and psychosocial outcomes of persons spinal cord injured more than 20 years ago. Paraplegia 30: 617–630

Whiteneck G G, Charlifue S W, Gerhart K A, Lammertse D P, Manley S, Menter R R, Seedroff K R 1992b Ageing with spinal cord injury. Demos Publications, New York

Whittle M W, Cochrane G M 1989 A comparative evaluation of the hip guidance orthosis (HGO) and the reciprocating gait orthosis (RGO). Health Equipment Information National Health Service Procurement Directorate, London

Whittle M W, Cochrane G M, Chase A P, Copping A V, Jefferson R G, Staples D J, Fenn P T, Thomas D C 1991 A comparative trial of two walking systems for paralysed people. Paraplegia 29: 97–102

Winchester P K 1993 A comparison of paraplegic gait performance using two types of reciprocating gait orthoses. Prosthetics and Orthotics International 17: 101–106

Wing P C, Tedwell S J 1983 The weight bearing shoulder. Paraplegia 21: 107–113

Woodbury B, Radd C 1987 Psychosocial issues and approaches in spinal cord injury: concepts and management. In: Buchanan L E, Nawoczenski D A (eds) Concepts and management approaches. Williams & Williams, Baltimore, MD, p 191

Yang L, Granot M H, Paul J P, Condie D N, Rowley D I 1996 Further development of hybrid FES orthosis. Spinal Cord 34: 611–614

Yarkony G M, Roth E J, Heinemann A W 1988 Rehabilitation outcomes in C6 tetraplegia. Paraplegia 26: 177–185

Yarkony G, Sahgal V 1987 Contractures: a major complication of craniocerebral trauma. Clinical Orthopaedic Related Research 219: 93–96

Young W 1994 Neurorehabilitation of spinal cord injury. Journal of Neuro-rehabilitation 8: 3–9

Further reading

Adkins H V (ed) 1985 Spinal cord injury. Churchill Livingstone, New York

Bedbrook G, Sir (ed) 1981 The care and management of spinal cord injuries. Springer-Verlag, Heidelberg

Bedbrook G, Sir 1985 Lifetime care of the paraplegic. Churchill Livingstone, Edinburgh

Brain Lord 1985 Clinical neurology, 6th edn. (revised by Roger Bannister). Oxford University Press, Oxford

Cole J H, Furness A L, Twomey L T 1988 Muscles in action: an approach to manual muscle testing. Churchill Livingstone, Melbourne

Fallon B 1979 Able to work. Spinal Injuries Association, London

Fallon B 1982 The sexual lives of disabled people. West Sussex Disabilities Study Unit, Arundel

Ford R J, Duckworth B 1987 Physical management for the quadriplegic patient. F A Davis, USA

Gatehouse M 1995 Moving forward. The guide to living with spinal cord injury. Spinal Injuries Association, London

Guttmann L, Sir 1976 Textbook of sport for the disabled. H M & M Publishers, Aylesbury, Buckinghamshire

Hancock C 1996 Hoists, lifts and transfers. The Disability Trust, Mary Marlborough Centre, Oxford

Lanig I S, Chase T M, Butt L M, Hulse K L, Johnson K M M 1996 A practical guide to health promotion after spinal cord injury. Aspen Publications

Mandelstam D (ed) 1986 Incontinence and its management, 2nd edn. Croome Helm, Beckenham

Mandelstam D 1989 Understanding incontinence: a guide to the nature and management of a very common complaint. Chapman and Hall, London

Rasch P J, Burke R K 1971 Kinesiology and applied anatomy. Lee & Febiger, Philadelphia

Rogers M A 1978 Paraplegia: a handbook of practical care and advice. Faber & Faber, London

Spinal Injuries Association 1980 Nursing management in the general hospital: the first 48 hours following injury. Spinal Injuries Association, London

Spinal Injuries Association 1984 Spinal cord injuries: guidance for general practitioners and district nurses. Spinal Injuries Association, London

Stover S L, De Lisa J A, Whiteneck G G 1995 Spinal cord injury: clinical outcomes from the model systems. Aspen Publications, Gaithersburg, MD

Index